Order Additional FACTS Publications

- ☐ **American Drug Index** (Annual hardbound) $37.95
- ☐ **Approved Bioequivalency Codes** (Loose-leaf with monthly updates) $64.95
- ☐ **Drug Facts and Comparisons** (Loose-leaf with monthly updates) $165.00
- ☐ **Drug Facts and Comparisons** (Annual hardbound) $95.50
- ☐ **Drug Interaction Facts** (Loose-leaf with quarterly updates) $82.50
- ☐ **Drug Interaction Facts** (Hardbound) $44.95
- ☐ **Drug Newsletter** (12 issues) $54.00   ☐ Binder $6 additional
- ☐ **Lawrence Review of Natural Products Newsletter** (12 issues) $35.95
- ☐ **Ophthalmic Drug Facts** (Annual hardbound) $36.95
- ☐ **Patient Drug Facts** (Loose-leaf with quarterly updates) $65.95
- ☐ **Pharmacy Law Digest** (Loose-leaf with one update) $65.50

Method of Payment

- ☐ Payment enclosed.* Make check payable to Facts and Comparisons.
- ☐ Bill me (plus handling).
- ☐ Charge to my credit card number:
  - ☐ MasterCard   ☐ VISA   ☐ Am Exp

Card # _____

Exp. date _____

Signature _____

Send to:

Name _____

Institution _____

Address _____

City, State, Zip _____

Phone _____

Profession _____

* Include sales tax where applicable. Prices quoted in US funds and subject to change.   OD 93

Send A FACTS Publication For The Perfect Gift

- ☐ **American Drug Index** (Annual hardbound) $37.95
- ☐ **Approved Bioequivalency Codes** (Loose-leaf with monthly updates) $64.95
- ☐ **Drug Facts and Comparisons** (Loose-leaf with monthly updates) $165.00
- ☐ **Drug Facts and Comparisons** (Annual hardbound) $95.50
- ☐ **Drug Interaction Facts** (Loose-leaf with quarterly updates) $82.50
- ☐ **Drug Interaction Facts** (Hardbound) $44.95
- ☐ **Drug Newsletter** (12 issues) $54.00   ☐ Binder $6 additional
- ☐ **Lawrence Review of Natural Products Newsletter** (12 issues) $35.95
- ☐ **Ophthalmic Drug Facts** (Annual hardbound) $36.95
- ☐ **Patient Drug Facts** (Loose-leaf with quarterly updates) $65.95
- ☐ **Pharmacy Law Digest** (Loose-leaf with one update) $65.50

Method of Payment

- ☐ Payment enclosed.* Make check payable to Facts and Comparisons.
- ☐ Bill me (plus handling).
- ☐ Charge to my credit card number:
  - ☐ MasterCard   ☐ VISA   ☐ Am Exp

Card # _____

Exp. date _____

Signature _____

Send to:

Name _____

Institution _____

Address _____

City, State, Zip _____

Phone _____

Profession _____

* Include sales tax where applicable. Prices quoted in US funds and subject to change.   OD 93

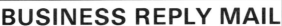

BUSINESS REPLY MAIL

FIRST CLASS MAIL   PERMIT NO. 3515   ST. LOUIS, MO

POSTAGE WILL BE PAID BY ADDRESSEE

Facts and Comparisons
111 West Port Plaza, Suite 423
St. Louis, MO 63146-9811

BUSINESS REPLY MAIL

FIRST CLASS MAIL   PERMIT NO. 3515   ST. LOUIS, MO

POSTAGE WILL BE PAID BY ADDRESSEE

Facts and Comparisons
111 West Port Plaza, Suite 423
St. Louis, MO 63146-9811

Ophthalmic Drug Facts

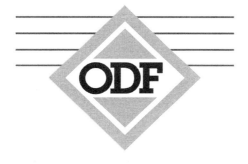

1993

Facts and Comparisons

A **Wolters Kluwer** Company

St. Louis

Ophthalmic Drug Facts

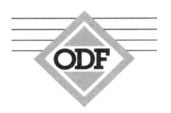

Ophthalmic Drug Facts®

Adapted from *Drug Facts and Comparisons®* loose-leaf drug information service.

ISBN 0-932686-69-9
ISSN 1043-1780

Printed in the United States of America

Published by
Facts and Comparisons
A **Wolters Kluwer** Company
111 West Port Plaza, Suite 423
St. Louis, Missouri 63146-3098
314/878-2515
800/223-0554 Customer Service

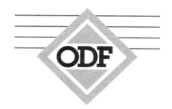

Facts and Comparisons Editorial Advisory Panel:

Dennis J. Cada, PharmD
Executive Editor, The Formulary
Director of Pharmacy
South Coast Medical Center

Timothy R. Covington, PharmD, MS
Professor and Chairman
Department of Pharmacy Practice
Samford University

Daniel A. Hussar, PhD
Remington Professor of Pharmacy
Philadelphia College of Pharmacy and Science

Louis Lasagna, MD
Dean, Sackler School of
    Graduate Biomedical Sciences
Academic Dean, School of Medicine Tufts University

James R. Selevan, BSEE, MD
Executive Director, The Formulary
Chairman, Pharmacy and Therapeutics Committee
South Coast Medical Center

Richard W. Sloan, RPh, MD
Chairman and Residency Program Director
Department of Family Medicine
York Hospital, Pennsylvania

David S. Tatro, PharmD
Associate Director of Pharmacy
Director of Drug Information
Stanford University Hospital
Assistant Clinical Professor
University of California, San Francisco

Thomas L. Whitsett, MD
Professor of Medicine and Pharmacology
Director of Clinical Pharmacology Program
University of Oklahoma Health Sciences Center

Facts and Comparisons Staff:

C. Sue Sewester
president

Bernie R. Olin, PharmD
editor-in-chief

Mary K. Hulbert, BA
coordinating editor

Steven K. Hebel, BS Pharm
associate editor

Charles E. Dombek, BS Pharm, MIM
assistant editor

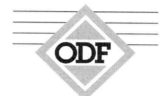

Table of Contents

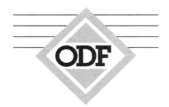

Editor's Preface

The mission of *Ophthalmic Drug Facts* is to provide reliable and objective ophthalmic drug information and facilitate therapeutic decision making. This book is intended to promote efficient, quality eye health care. Although general information is available for ophthalmic drugs, there are very few sources that provide comparative drug and drug product information in a concise format; none is as comprehensive.

Ophthalmic Drug Facts was conceived and developed through a team approach and will be of value to both the student and eyecare practitioner. Ophthalmologists, optometrists and opticians should find this text particularly valuable in their daily practices.

Ophthalmic Drug Facts provides a broad range of information including pharmacologic and pharmacokinetic information on drug entities, commercial product information, specific formulation availability and a cost index. The text is arranged in a pharmacotherapeutic format, with emphasis on drug action and current product availability rather than on pathophysiology of disease states.

Ophthalmic Drug Facts is a comprehensive ophthalmic drug information resource. We include detailed information on specific entities as well as many drug combinations. There is also a comprehensive section of contact lens products. Selected bibliographies are provided for all chapters. In addition, *Ophthalmic Drug Facts* includes valuable information on:

- ♦ Systemic drugs affecting the eye
- ♦ Unlabeled uses for FDA-approved drugs
- ♦ Orphan ophthalmic agents and investigational drugs
- ♦ Excipient glossary
- ♦ Ophthalmic product manufacturer index

The fourth edition of *Ophthalmic Drug Facts* has been significantly revised, reflecting the myriad number of changes taking place in the market since the previous edition. Certain chapters have been rearranged in order to reflect a more logical sequence from diagnostic to therapeutic agents.

New drug entities include: Fluoromethalone acetate (*Flarex,* by Alcon), ketorolac (*Acular,* by Allergan), hydroxyamphetamine/tropicamide (*Paremyd,* by Allergan), hydroxyamphetamine (*Paredrine,* by Pharmics) and carteolol (*Ocupress,* by Otsuka).

A new table has been adapted and incorporated into the Beta-Adrenergic Blocker monograph in order to facilitate cost comparisons of those products. A new chapter, Nonsurgical Adjuncts, has been added. The orphan drug and investigational drug sections have been greatly expanded. In addition, hundreds of product changes have been incorporated.

We hope the reader finds this a valuable guide in ophthalmic drug product selection and use. As any practitioner is aware, ophthalmic practice is constantly adapting to incorporate the latest information. We intend to continue the effort with future editions; therefore, your comments, criticisms and suggestions are always welcome.

> Jimmy D. Bartlett, OD, DOS
> N. Rex Ghormley, OD, FAAO
> Siret D. Jaanus, PhD
> J. James Rowsey, MD
> Thom J. Zimmerman, MD, PhD

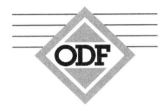

Introduction

Ophthalmic Drug Facts is a comprehensive ophthalmic drug information compendium. Organized by therapeutic drug class, the unique format is designed to facilitate comparisons between drugs. A table of contents, a comprehensive alphabetical index and extensive cross-referencing enable the reader to quickly locate needed information. The following pages explain the organization and contents of *Ophthalmic Drug Facts* in detail. All readers are urged to review this information to assure efficient and effective use of *Ophthalmic Drug Facts*.

◆ Editorial Policy

The principle editorial guidelines are: Accurate, unbiased information; concise, standardized presentation; comparative, objective format; timely delivery. Review of FDA-approved product labeling, hundreds of journal articles and textbooks and policies and recommendations from many authoritative and official groups form the base of evaluation of information for *Ophthalmic Drug Facts*. FDA-approved indications and dosage recommendations are included. In addition, other established or potential uses are discussed and are designated as *"Unlabeled Uses."*

Most of the products listed are protected by letters of patent and their names are trademarked and registered by the firm whose name appears with the product. Identification of the product distributor is given in parentheses next to the brand name. The distributor may or may not be the actual manufacturer or fabricator of the final dosage form. Listing of specific products is an indication only of availability on the market and does not constitute an endorsement or recommendation.

Products which contain identical amounts of active ingredients are listed together for comparison as an aid in product selection. Drug product interchange is regulated by state laws; listing of products together does not imply that they are therapeutically equivalent or legally interchangeable. Caution is particularly advised when comparing sustained release, timed release or repeat action dosage forms.

◆ Editorial Panel

The Editorial Panel for *Ophthalmic Drug Facts* is an interdisciplinary group of established, respected and renowned clinicians and researchers. The panel includes recognized experts in the fields of ocular pharmacology, therapeutics and drug information. These experts contribute the introductory material, review monographs and provide direction for *Ophthalmic Drug Facts*.

The *Drug Facts and Comparisons* Editorial Advisory Panel consists of a very distinguished group of physicians, pharmacologists and pharmacists. This panel reviews monographs and provides editorial direction for the entire Facts and Comparisons data base.

◆ Organization

Information in *Ophthalmic Drug Facts* is organized by therapeutic use. Eleven chapters are divided into groups and subgroups to facilitate comparisons of drugs and drug products with similar uses. The remaining chapters provide information on ophthalmic dose forms and routes of administration, systemic drugs affecting the eye, drugs with unlabeled ophthalmic uses and investigational and orphan drugs.

Products most similar in content or use are listed together. This format of presenting the facts makes it easy to make comparisons of identical, similar or related products. Because drugs are listed by use, some drugs may be listed in more than one section of the book.

◆ Index

The alphabetical index includes page references for drugs by their generic name, brand name *(italics)*, and therapeutic group names. Additionally, many synonyms, pharmacological actions and therapeutic uses for agents are included.

◆ Chapter Introductions

The introduction to the chapter provides information about the drugs in each therapeutic class. It also discusses general treatment guidelines. A selected bibliography is located at the end of each chapter introduction to provide additional sources of information.

◆ Drug Monographs

Prescribing information is presented in comprehensive drug monographs. General information on a group of closely related drugs may be presented in a group monograph. Specific information relating to a particular drug is presented in an individual monograph under the generic name of the drug. All monographs are divided into sections identified with bold titles for ease in locating the desired information.

Actions: This section gives a brief summary of the known pharmacologic and pharmacokinetic properties.

Indications: All FDA approved indications or uses are listed. When available, drug monographs also include "Unlabeled Uses." These include investigational uses for drugs and uses not yet approved by the FDA.

Contraindications: This section specifies those conditions in which the drug should NOT be used.

Warnings and Precautions: These sections list conditions in which use of the drug may be hazardous, precautions to observe and parameters to monitor during therapy.

Drug Interactions: A brief summary of documented, clinically significant drug-drug, drug-food and drug-lab test interactions is provided.

Adverse Reactions: Reported adverse reactions are presented. Incidence data on adverse effects are included when available.

Overdosage: The clinical manifestations of toxicity and treatment of overdosage are given for most agents.

Patient Information: This section provides the essential information to be communicated to the patient by the health professional to allow the patient to safely and effectively administer the medication.

Administration and Dosage: Dosage ranges and methods of administration are presented.

◆ Charts and Tables

Charts and tables are included in many monographs to make drug-to-drug comparisons easier. Examples of tables include: Pharmacokinetics (onset, peak and duration of action), routes of administration, dosage ranges and adverse reactions.

◆ Special Features

Contact Lens Care Products: Chapter 12 provides guidelines and product information for hard, soft and rigid gas permeable contact lens care.

Systemic Drugs Affecting the Eye: Chapter 13 discusses the effects systemic drugs have on ocular structures and functions.

Drugs with Unlabeled Ophthalmic Uses: Chapter 14 discusses FDA approved drugs which are being used for unlabeled ophthalmic purposes.

Orphan Drugs: Chapter 15 briefly describes Orphan Drug legislation and includes a table which provides generic name, trade name, indication and manufacturer information on Orphan Drugs for ophthalmic conditions.

Investigational New Drugs: Chapter 15 outlines the FDA drug approval process and includes a table which provides generic name, trade name (if available), therapeutic class and/or use and manufacturer information for ophthalmic drugs on the horizon. Selected bibliographies are available at the end of the chapter.

Excipient Glossary: This glossary, which is located in the appendix, lists pharmaceutical excipients found in ophthalmic products. The functions and strengths of these adjuncts are briefly described.

Manufacturer Index: This index, which is located in the appendix, provides the addresses and phone numbers of the manufacturers and distributors of ophthalmic products listed in *Ophthalmic Drug Facts*.

◆ Product Listings

Individual products are listed following each monograph. The format and components of the product listings are discussed below and illustrated on the opposite page.

◇1 **Chapter title** is located at the top of the right-hand page.

◇2 **Generic titles** appear at the beginning of general drug monographs and individual drug monographs.

◇3 **Cross references** to the appropriate drug monograph appear for complete prescribing information.

◇4 **The Cost Index,** located on the right side of the product listings, is designed to quickly determine the *relative cost* of similar or identical products. It is not a dollar-and-cents figure, but a ratio of the average wholesale prices for equivalent quantities of a drug. The Cost Index is calculated on average wholesale prices for standard package sizes and does not reflect any special purchasing considerations such as special discounts, quantity discounts or contract prices. The basis for the Cost Index calculation is given at the bottom of each table of product listings.

As an example of the Cost Index, if product A has a Cost Index of 45, and product B has a Cost Index of 15, product A is 3 times as expensive as product B (based on average wholesale cost).

The Cost Index is only an indication of *relative wholesale costs.* It is NOT a rating or recommendation. It is presented for informational purposes only, without consideration of potential differences in the quality of similar products.

◇5 **Distribution status** of products is indicated as *Rx* or *otc*.

◇6 **Products are grouped** by dosage form or strength.

◇7 **Identical brand name products** are listed in alphabetical order. Combination products are listed in tables to facilitate comparisons. Products most similar in formulation are listed next to each other.

◇8 **Package sizes** are given for all dosage forms and strengths of each product.

◇9 **Products available by their generic name** from multiple sources are indicated as available from (Various) distributors. Selected multiple source distributors and manufacturers are provided. The list of distributors and manufacturers is intended to provide an example, and is not an attempt to be comprehensive.

◇10 **Distributor's name** is given in parentheses next to the product name.

ATROPINE SULFATE

For complete prescribing information see General Monograph p. 46.

Indications:

A potent parasympatholytic agent for use in producing cycloplegia and mydriasis. Useful for cycloplegic refraction or for pupil dilation in acute inflammatory conditions of the iris and uveal tract.

Administration and Dosage:

Solution:

Adults:

For uveitis – Instill 1 or 2 drops into the eye(s) up to 4 times daily.

For refraction – Instill 1 or 2 drops of the 1% solution into the eye(s) 1 hour before refracting.

Children:

For uveitis – Instill 1 or 2 drops of 0.5% solution into the eye(s) up to 3 times daily.

For refraction – Instill 1 or 2 drops of 0.5% solution into the eye(s) twice daily for 1 to 3 days before examination.

Ointment: A small amount in the conjunctival sac up to 3 times daily.

Compress the lacrimal sac by digital pressure for 1 to 3 minutes after instillation.

Individuals with heavily pigmented irides may require larger doses.

Storage: Store at 46° to 86°F (8° to 30°C).

			C.I.*
Rx **Atropisol** (Iolab)	**Solution:** 0.5%	In 1 ml Dropperettes.[1]	54
Rx **Isopto Atropine** (Alcon)		In 5 ml Drop-Tainers.[2]	53
Rx **Atropine Sulfate** (Various, eg, Alcon, Allergan, Bausch and Lomb, Fougera, Moore, Rugby, Schein, Steris)	**Solution:** 1%	In 2, 5 and 15 ml and UD 1 ml.	6+
Rx **Atropine Care** (Akorn)		In 2, 5 and 15 ml.[3]	25
Rx **Atropine-1** (Optopics)		In 2, 5 and 15 ml.	17
Rx **Atropisol** (Iolab)		In 5[4] and 15[4] ml and 1 ml Dropperettes.[1]	36
Rx **Isopto Atropine** (Alcon)		In 5 and 15 ml Drop-Tainers.[2]	60
Rx **Atropine Sulfate** (Alcon)	**Solution:** 2%	In 2 ml.	53
Rx **Atropisol** (Iolab)		In 1 ml Dropperettes.[1]	54
Rx **Isopto Atropine** (Alcon)	**Solution:** 3%	In 5 ml Drop-Tainers.[2]	67
Rx **Atropine Sulfate S.O.P.** (Allergan)	**Ointment:** 0.5%	In 3.5 g.	64

* Cost Index based on cost per g or ml.
[1] With benzalkonium chloride.
[2] With 0.01% benzalkonium chloride and 0.5% hydroxypropyl methylcellulose.
[3] With 0.01% benzalkonium chloride and hydroxypropyl methylcellulose.
[4] With benzalkonium chloride and EDTA.

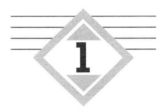

Dosage Forms and Routes of Administration

For ophthalmic drugs to be effective, they must reach ocular tissues in relatively high concentrations. Depending on the specific diagnostic or therapeutic objective, ophthalmic drugs may be delivered to the eye through various routes of administration, including:

- Topical
- Oral
- Parenteral
- Periocular
- Intracameral
- Intravitreal

TOPICAL ADMINISTRATION

Topical application is the most common route of administration for ophthalmic drugs. Advantages of topical administration include convenience, simplicity, its noninvasive nature and the ability of the patient to self-administer the medication. Because of blood and aqueous losses of drug, topical medications do not typically penetrate in useful concentrations to the posterior ocular tissues and therefore are of no therapeutic benefit for diseases of the retina, optic nerve and other posterior segment structures.

Inactive Ingredients

The following inactive agents may be present in ophthalmic products:

Preservatives destroy or inhibit multiplication of microorganisms introduced into the product by accident.

benzalkonium chloride
benzethonium chloride
cetylpyridinium chloride
chlorobutanol
EDTA

mercurial preservatives
  (phenylmercuric nitrate,
  phenylmercuric acetate,
  thimerosal)
methyl and propylparabens

phenylethyl alcohol
sodium benzoate
sodium propionate
sorbic acid

Viscosity-Increasing Agents slow drainage of the product from the eye, thus increasing retention time of the active drug. Increased bioavailability may result.

acetylated polyvinyl alcohol	hydroxyethyl cellulose	polyvinyl alcohol 2%
carboxymethylcellulose sodium	hydroxypropyl methylcellulose	polyvinylpyrrolidone (povidone)
dextran 70	methylcellulose	propylene glycol
gelatin	polyethylene glycol 300	
glycerin	polysorbate 80	

Antioxidants prevent or delay deterioration of products by oxygen in the air.

EDTA	sodium metabisulfite	thiourea
sodium bisulfite	sodium thiosulfate	

Wetting Agents reduce surface tension, allowing the drug solution to spread over the eye.

polysorbate 20	poloxamer 282	tyloxapol (Triton WR-1339)
polysorbate 80	(Pluronic L-92)	

Buffers help maintain ophthalmic products in the range of pH 6 to 8.

acetic acid	potassium carbonate	sodium biphosphate
boric acid	potassium citrate	sodium borate
hydrochloric acid	potassium phosphates	sodium carbonate
phosphoric acid	potassium tetraborate	sodium citrate
potassium bicarbonate	sodium acetate	sodium hydroxide
potassium borate	sodium bicarbonate	sodium phosphate

Tonicity Agents help the ophthalmic product solutions to be isotonic with natural tears. Products in the sodium chloride equivalence range of 0.9% ± 0.2% are considered isotonic and will help prevent ocular pain and tissue damage. A range of 0.6% to 1.8% can usually be tolerated without damage.

buffers	glycerin	propylene glycol
dextran 40 and 70	potassium chloride	sodium chloride
dextrose		

Packaging Standards

To help reduce confusion in labeling and identification of various topical ocular medications, drug packaging standards have been proposed. When fully implemented by the ophthalmic drug industry, the standard colors for drug labels and bottle caps will include the following:

RECOMMENDED STANDARD COLORS FOR OPHTHALMIC DRUG LABELING	
Therapeutic Class	**Proposed Color**
Beta blockers	Yellow, blue or both
Mydriatics and cycloplegics	Red
Miotics	Green
Nonsteroidal anti-inflammatory agents	Gray
Anti-infectives	Brown, tan

Medications

Solutions and Suspensions: Most topical ocular preparations are commercially available as solutions or suspensions that are applied directly to the eye from the bottle, which serves as the eye dropper. The patient should avoid touching the dropper tip to the eye because this can lead to contamination of the medication and may also cause ocular injury. Suspensions (notably, many ocular steroids) should be resuspended by shaking to provide an accurate dosage of drug.

RECOMMENDED PROCEDURES FOR ADMINISTRATION OF SOLUTIONS AND SUSPENSIONS

1. Wash hands thoroughly before administration.
2. Tilt head backward or lie down and gaze upward.
3. Gently grasp lower eyelid below eyelashes and pull the eyelid away from the eye to form a pouch.
4. Place dropper directly over eye. Avoid contact of the dropper with the eye, finger or any surface.
5. Look upward just before applying a drop.
6. After instilling the drop, look downward for several seconds.
7. Release the lid slowly.
8. With eyes closed, apply gentle pressure with fingers to the inside corner of eye for 3 to 5 minutes (see figure 1). This retards drainage of solution from the intended area.
9. Do not rub the eye. Minimize blinking.
10. Do not rinse the dropper.
11. Do not use eye drops that have changed color.
12. If more than one type of ophthalmic drop is being employed, wait at least 5 minutes before administering the second agent.
13. When the instillation of eye drops is difficult (eg, pediatric patients, adults with particularly strong blink reflex), the closed-eye method may be used. This involves lying down, placing the prescribed number of drops on the eyelid in the inner corner of the eye, then opening the eye so that drops will fall into the eye by gravity.

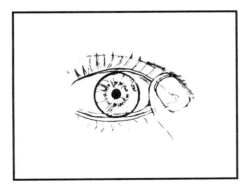

Figure 1.

Ointments: The primary purpose for an ophthalmic ointment vehicle is to prolong drug contact time with the external ocular surface. This is particularly useful for treating children, who may "cry out" topically applied solutions, and for medicating ocular injuries, such as corneal abrasions, when the eye is to be patched. Administer solutions before ointments. Ointments retard entry of subsequent drops.

RECOMMENDED PROCEDURES FOR ADMINISTRATION OF OINTMENTS
1. Wash hands thoroughly before administration.
2. Holding the ointment tube in the hand for a few minutes will warm the ointment and facilitate flow.
3. When opening the ointment tube for the first time, squeeze out and discard the first 0.25 inch of ointment as it may be too dry.
4. Tilt head backward or lie down and gaze upward.
5. Gently pull down the lower lid to form a pouch.
6. Place 0.25 to 0.5 inch of ointment with a sweeping motion inside the lower lid by squeezing the tube gently.
7. Close the eye for 1 to 2 minutes and roll the eyeball in all directions.
8. Temporary blurring of vision may occur. Avoid activities requiring good visual acuity until blurring clears.
9. Remove excessive ointment around the eye or ointment tube tip with a tissue.
10. If using more than one kind of ointment, wait about 10 minutes before applying the second drug.

Gels: Ophthalmic gels are similar in viscosity and clinical usage to ophthalmic ointments. Pilocarpine *(Pilopine HS)* is currently the only ophthalmic preparation available in gel form, and it is intended to serve as a "sustained-release" pilocarpine, requiring only once-daily administration (at bedtime).

Sprays: Although not commercially available, some practitioners use mydriatics or cycloplegics, alone or in combination, administered as a spray to the eye to dilate the pupil or for cycloplegic examination. This is most often used for pediatric patients, and the solution is administered using a sterile perfume atomizer.

Lid Scrubs: Commercially available eyelid cleansers or antibiotic solutions or ointments can be applied directly to the lid margin for the treatment of blepharitis. This is best accomplished by applying the medication to the end of a sterile cotton-tipped applicator and then scrubbing the eyelid margin several times daily. The gauze pads supplied with commercially available eyelid cleansers are also convenient for applying eyelid scrubs.

Devices

Contact Lenses: Soft contact lenses can absorb water-soluble drugs and release them to the eye over prolonged periods of time. This has the clinical advantage of promoting sustained-release of solutions or suspensions that would otherwise be removed quickly from the external ocular tissues. Soft contact lenses as drug delivery devices are most often used in the management of dry eye disorders, but the technique is occasionally used for the treatment of ocular infections, including corneal ulcers.

Corneal Shields: A non-cross-linked, homogenized, porcine scleral collagen shield is available *(Bio-Cor Fyodorov Collagen Corneal Shield)*. This device is placed as a bandage on the cornea following surgery or injury, protecting and lubricating the cornea. Topically applied antibiotics have been used in conjunction with the shield to promote healing of corneal ulcers.

Cotton Pledgets: Small pieces of cotton can be saturated with ophthalmic solutions and placed in the conjunctival sac. These devices allow a prolonged ocular contact time with solutions that are normally administered topically into the eye. The clinical use of pledgets is usually reserved for the administration of mydriatic solutions such as cocaine or phenylephrine. This drug delivery method promotes maximum mydriasis in an attempt to break posterior synechiae or to dilate sluggish pupils.

Filter Paper Strips: Sodium fluorescein and rose bengal dyes are commercially available as drug-impregnated filter paper strips. The strips help ensure sterility of sodium fluorescein which, when prepared in solution, can become easily contaminated with *Pseudomonas aeruginosa*. These dyes are used diagnostically to disclose corneal injuries, infections such as herpes simplex, and dry eye disorders.

Artificial Tear Inserts: A rod-shaped pellet of hydroxypropyl cellulose without preservative is commercially available *(Lacrisert)*. It is inserted into the inferior conjunctival sac with a specially designed applicator. Following placement, the device absorbs fluid, swells, and then releases the nonmedicated polymer to the eye for up to 24 hours. The device is designed as a sustained-release artificial tear for the treatment of dry eye disorders.

Membrane-Bound Inserts: A membrane controlled drug delivery system *(Ocusert)* is commercially available and delivers a constant quantity of pilocarpine to the eye for up to 1 week. Placed onto the bulbar conjunctiva under the upper or lower eyelid, it is a useful substitute for pilocarpine drops or gel in glaucoma patients who cannot comply with more frequent drug instillation or in patients who have ocular or visual side effects from pilocarpine solutions.

Compliance Caps: Compliance can be improved in some glaucoma patients by dispensing pilocarpine, dipivefrin or levobunolol with *C-Cap Compliance Caps.* This dosing formulation allows the patient to keep track of daily doses of medication and can help to minimize dosing confusion in multi-drug therapy.

GENERAL CONSIDERATIONS IN
TOPICAL OPHTHALMIC DRUG THERAPY

Proper administration of a dosage form is essential to an optimal therapeutic response. In many instances, health professionals may be too casual when instructing patients on proper use of ophthalmic products. The technique used in administering such products often determines drug safety and efficacy.

♦ The normal eye can retain ≈ 10 µl of fluid (adjusted for the effect of blinking). The average dropper delivers 25 to 50 µl/drop. The value of more than one drop is questionable.

♦ Minimize systemic absorption of ophthalmic drops by compressing the lacrimal sac for 3 to 5 minutes following instillation of drops. This retards passage of drops via the nasolacrimal duct into areas of potential absorption such as nasal and pharyngeal mucosa.

♦ Because of rapid lacrimal drainage and limited eye capacity, if multiple drop therapy is indicated, the best interval between drops is 5 minutes. This ensures that the first drop is not flushed away by the second or that the second drop is not diluted by the first.

♦ Topical anesthesia will increase the bioavailability of ophthalmic agents by decreasing the blink reflex and the production and turnover of tears.

♦ Factors which may increase absorption from ophthalmic dosage forms include lax eyelids of some patients, usually the elderly, which create a greater reservoir for retention of drops, and hyperemic or diseased eyes.

♦ Use of eyecups is discouraged due to potential contamination and risk of spreading disease.

♦ Ophthalmic suspensions mix with tears less rapidly and remain in the cul-de-sac longer than solutions.

♦ Ophthalmic ointments maintain contact between the drug and ocular tissues by slowing the clearance rate to as little as 0.5% per minute. Ophthalmic ointments provide maximum contact between drug and external ocular tissues.

♦ Ophthalmic ointments may impede delivery of other ophthalmic drugs to the affected site by serving as a barrier to contact.

♦ Ointments may blur vision during the waking hours. Use with caution in conditions where visual clarity is critical (eg, operating motor equipment, reading).

♦ Monitor expiration dates closely. Do not use outdated medication.

♦ Ophthalmic solutions and ointments are frequently misused. Do not assume that patients know how to maximize safe and effective use of these agents. Appropriate patient education and counseling should accompany prescribing and dispensing of ophthalmics.

ORAL ADMINISTRATION

Although most ocular diseases respond to topical therapy, some disorders require systemic drug administration to achieve adequate therapeutic levels of drug in ocular tissue. Oral administration of certain drugs may be the most effective route of drug delivery. Examples of commonly used oral medications include: Carbonic anhydrase inhibitors for the treatment of glaucoma, corticosteroids for Graves' ophthalmopathy and optic neuritis, analgesics for the management of pain associated with ocular injury, antibiotic therapy of preseptal cellulitis and antihistamine therapy for acute allergic angioneurotic edema of the eyelids.

Some oral preparations for ocular use are available as sustained-release formulations, notably acetazolamide (eg, *Diamox Sequels*).

PARENTERAL ADMINISTRATION

Intramuscular (IM) and intravenous (IV) injections are occasionally used for the treatment of ocular disorders. Hydroxocobalamin (vitamin B_{12}; eg, *Alpha Redisol*) and some antibiotics (eg, penicillin) may be administered through the IM route. The continuous IV infusion of various antibiotics may be required for the treatment of endophthalmitis and other severe ocular infections.

PERIOCULAR ADMINISTRATION

When higher concentrations of drugs are required than can be delivered to the eye by topical, oral or parenteral administration, drugs can be injected locally into the periocular tissues. Periocular drug administration includes injections under the bulbar conjunctiva (subconjunctival), under Tenon's capsule (sub-Tenon's) and behind the globe itself (retrobulbar). Drugs most often delivered in this manner include corticosteroids and antibiotics. Local anesthetics are commonly administered via retrobulbar injection prior to cataract extraction and other intraocular surgical procedures.

INTRACAMERAL ADMINISTRATION

Intracameral administration involves placing the drug directly into the anterior chamber of the eye. This is most commonly associated with cataract extraction, during which a viscoelastic substance is injected into the anterior chamber to protect the corneal endothelium. Antibiotics are not routinely injected into the anterior chamber. This procedure is associated with a significant risk of complications as well as drug toxicity.

INTRAVITREAL ADMINISTRATION

The intravitreal injection of drugs is primarily reserved as a heroic effort to rescue eyes with severe acute intraocular inflammation or eyes that have failed to respond to more conservative therapy. Intravitreal antibiotics may be the treatment of choice for endophthalmitis; intravitreal liquid silicone is used for the treatment of complicated retinal detachment. Recently, intravitreal ganciclovir has been used with some success in treating cytomegalovirus retinitis in patients with acquired immunodeficiency syndrome (AIDS).

Jimmy D. Bartlett, OD, DOS
University of Alabama at Birmingham

For More Information

Bartlett JD, Jaanus SD, eds. Clinical Ocular Pharmacology, ed. 2. Boston, MA: Butterworth, 1989.

Feibel RM. Current concepts in retrobulbar anesthesia. *Surv Ophthalmol* 1985;30:102-10.

Fraunfelder FT. Drug-packaging standards for eye drop medications. *Arch Ophthalmol* 1988;106:1029.

Fraunfelder FT. Extraocular fluid dynamics: How best to apply topical ocular medication. *Trans Am Ophthalmol Soc* 1976;74:457-87.

Fraunfelder FT, Hanna C. Ophthalmic drug delivery systems. *Surv Ophthalmol* 1974;18:292-98.

Halberg GP, et al. Drug delivery systems for topical ophthalmic medication. *Ann Ophthalmol* 1975;7:1199-1209.

Jain MR. Drug delivery through soft contact lenses. *Br J Ophthalmol* 1988;72:150-54.

Lamberts DW. Solid delivery devices. *Int Ophthalmol Clin* 1980;20:63-77.

MacKeen DL. Aqueous formulations and ointments. *Int Ophthalmol Clin* 1980;20:79-92.

Robin JS, Ellis PP. Ophthalmic ointments. *Surv Ophthalmol* 1978;22:335-40.

Sharp J, Hanna C. Use of a spray to deliver drugs to the eye. *J Arkansas Med Soc* 1977;73:462-63.

Silbiger J, Stern GA. Evaluation of corneal collagen shields as a drug delivery device for the treatment of experimental *Pseudomonas* keratitis. *Ophthalmology* 1992;99:889-92.

Templeton WC, Eiferman RA, et al. *Serratia* keratitis by contaminated eyedroppers. *Am J Ophthalmol* 1982;93:723-26.

Zimmerman TJ, et al. Improving the therapeutic index of topically applied ocular drugs. *Arch Ophthalmol* 1984;102:551-52.

Ophthalmic Dyes

Dyes are used for a variety of diagnostic ophthalmic procedures. The ophthalmic dyes, fluorescein, fluorexon and rose bengal, are structurally similar; however, they vary slightly in their method of administration and their indications.

FLUORESCEIN SODIUM

Fluorescein sodium is a yellow water-soluble dibasic acid dye of the xanthine series that produces an intense green fluorescent color in alkaline ($>$ pH 5) solution. Fluorescein is used to demonstrate defects of corneal epithelium. It does not actually stain tissues, but is useful as an indicator dye. The normal precorneal tear film appears yellow or orange with fluorescein. The intact corneal epithelium resists penetration of water-soluble fluorescein and is not colored by it. Any break in the epithelial barrier permits rapid fluorescein penetration. Whether resulting from trauma, infection or other causes, epithelial defects of the cornea appear bright green and are easily visualized. If epithelial loss is extensive, topical fluorescein will penetrate into the aqueous and is readily visible biomicroscopically as a green flare.

Fluorescein sodium exhibits a high degree of ionization at physiologic pH. Therefore, it does not penetrate the intact corneal epithelium or form a firm bond with vital tissue. When exposed to light, fluorescein absorbs certain wavelengths and emits fluorescent light of longer wavelength. Factors which can affect its fluorescence include its concentration, the pH of the solution, the presence of other substances and the wavelength of the exciting light. At pH 8, fluorescein reaches its maximum intensity.

Ophthalmic uses of fluorescein include applanation tonometry, detection of foreign bodies, fitting of rigid contact lenses, determination of tear breakup time, Seidel's test, fluorescein angiography and vitreous fluorophotometry.

For topical ocular use, fluorescein may be administered as a solution or by fluorescein-impregnated filter paper strips (eg, *Fluorets*). Since fluorescein in solution is susceptible to bacterial contamination, multidose formulations are dispensed with a preservative such as chlorobutanol. For diagnostic purposes such as applanation tonometry, a local anesthetic is included in the formulation.

Fluorescein-impregnated filter paper strips are useful for routine office procedures such as contact lens fitting and lacrimal system evaluation. Bacterial contamination is minimized since the strips are stored in a dry state. When wetted with water or an irrigating solution, the dye is released from the strip and can be applied to the eye by gently touching the conjunctiva.

Intravenous fluorescein (fluorescein angiography) is used for detection of vascular abnormalities of the fundus. Following injection into the antecubital vein, the dye appears in the central retinal artery. Integrity of the retina and choroid, as well as arm to retina circulation time, may be determined.

Oral fluorescein can be administered by mixing fluorescein powder or several vials of 10% injectable fluorescein in a citrus drink over ice (Unlabeled use, p. 273). Time of onset of maximal fluorescence is 45 to 60 minutes as compared to seconds via the injectable route. Fasting enhances the serum concentration of the dye. Oral fluorescein can be used to study disorders characterized by late leakage of dye such as cystoid macular edema, to study retinal vascular abnormalities in young diabetic patients and to document retinal pigment epithelial detachment, central serous choroidopathy and optic disc edema.

Topical application of fluorescein has been associated with minimum adverse effects. The most common side effect of intravenous use is nausea. The oral route appears to have the clinical advantage of infrequent side effects.

FLUOREXON

With a molecular size nearly twice that of fluorescein, fluorexon penetrates hydrophilic contact lenses at a much slower rate. Upon ocular instillation, it yields a pale, yellow-brown color. These properties make it useful as an adjunct in the fitting of soft contact lenses. However, the dye can stain hydrophilic lenses if significant amounts become trapped between lens and cornea or if the dye remains in contact with the soft lens for 10 minutes or more. Fluorexon is not recommended for use with high-water content soft lenses since the possibility of discoloration is much greater and more difficult to reverse than with lower water content lenses.

Fluorexon has a lower fluorescent intensity than fluorescein. For optimum fluorescence, a special yellow filter is recommended. The dye generally causes little or no discomfort when instilled on the eye. Due to its larger molecular size, it is a less effective stain for epithelial defects, erosions and contact lens-induced effects than fluorescein. Like rose bengal, it will stain degenerated cells and mucus threads.

ROSE BENGAL

An iodine derivative of fluorescein, rose bengal stains dead or degenerated epithelial cells of the cornea and conjunctiva (including the nuclei and cell walls) a red color. It will also stain the mucus of the precorneal tear film. When applied as a solution or from a moistened filter paper strip, this dye is an effective aid in the evaluation of keratoconjunctivitis sicca, corneal abrasions and detection of foreign bodies. A correlation may exist between intensity of staining and severity of cellular defect.

Rose bengal can cause pronounced irritation and discomfort following instillation, particularly in more severely diseased eyes and with use of higher concentrations of dye. A topical anesthetic may be used to alleviate the discomfort, particularly if the solution formulation is employed. Application of dye using the commercially available filter paper strip usually results in less discomfort.

Rose bengal can stain eyelids, cheeks, fingers and clothing in a concentration-dependent manner. Keeping the amount of dye at a minimum and irrigating the eye can help circumvent this problem.

INDOCYANINE GREEN

Indocyanine green is a tricarbocyanine dye, available commercially under the trade name of *Cardio-Green,* and has been advocated for visualization of choroidal vessels with infrared absorption angiography. Toxic effects have not been associated with intravenous use of the dye when manufacturer's recommended dosage regimens have been followed. Data for routine diagnostic use are lacking since this dye is not in common clinical use.

Siret D. Jaanus, PhD
Southern California College of Optometry

For More Information

Bartlett JD, Jaanus SD, eds. Clinical Ocular Pharmacology, ed. 2. Boston, MA: Butterworth, 1989.

Duane TD, ed. Clinical Ophthalmology. Philadelphia, PA: J.B. Lippincott Company, 1988.

Flower RW, Hochheimer BF. A clinical technique and apparatus for simultaneous angiography of the separate retinal and choroidal circulation. *Invest Ophthalmol* 1973;12:248-61.

Hayashi K, et al. Indocyanine green angiography of central serous chorioretinopathy. *Int Ophthalmol Clin* 1986;9:37-41.

Kelley JS, Kincaid M. Retinal fluorography using oral fluorescein. *Arch Ophthalmol* 1979;97:2331.

Maurice DM. The use of fluorescein in ophthalmological research. *Invest Ophthalmol* 1967;6:464.

Norn MS. Rose bengal vital staining. *Acta Ophthalmol* 1970;48:546.

Refojo MF, et al. A new fluorescent stain for soft hydrophilic lens fitting. *Arch Ophthalmol* 1972;87:275.

Romanchuk KG. Fluorescein: Physiochemical factors affecting its fluorescence. *Surv Ophthalmol* 1982;26:269.

Yannuzzi LA, et al. Effective differences in the formulation of intravenous fluorescein and related side effects. *Am J Ophthalmol* 1974;78:217.

FLUORESCEIN SODIUM

Actions:

Sodium fluorescein, a yellow water-soluble dibasic acid xanthine dye, produces an intense green fluorescent color in alkaline (> pH 5) solution. Fluorescein demonstrates defects of corneal epithelium. It does not stain tissues, but is a useful indicator dye. Normal precorneal tear film will appear yellow or orange. The intact corneal epithelium resists fluorescein penetration and is not colored. Any break in the epithelial barrier permits rapid penetration. Whether resulting from trauma, infection or other causes, epithelial corneal defects appear bright green and are easily visualized. If epithelial loss is extensive, topical fluorescein penetrates into the aqueous and is readily visible biomicroscopically as a green flare.

Indications:

Topical: Used in fitting contact lenses, in applanation tonometry and for diagnosis and detection of corneal stippling, abrasions, ulcerations, herpetic lesions, foreign bodies (if not epithelialized) and contact lens pressure points. Also for making the lacrimal drainage test, wound leakage tests (Seidel Test) and for ascertaining postoperative closure of the sclerocorneal wound in delayed anterior chamber reformation.

Injection: As a diagnostic aid in ophthalmic angiography, including examination of the fundus; evaluation of the iris vasculature; distinction between viable and nonviable tissue; observation of the aqueous flow; differential diagnosis of malignant and nonmalignant tumors; determination of circulation time and adequacy.

Contraindications:

Hypersensitivity to the active ingredient or any other component.

Do not use topically with soft contact lenses; lenses may become discolored.

Topical: Not for injection. Do not use in intraocular surgery.

Warnings:

Exercise caution in administering to patients with a history of hypersensitivity, allergies or asthma. If signs of sensitivity develop, discontinue use.

Topical (Drops): Discontinue if sensitivity develops. May stain soft contact lenses. Do not touch dropper tip to any surface, as this may contaminate the solution.

Avoid extravasation during injection. The high pH of fluorescein solution can result in severe local tissue damage. Complications resulting from extravasation of fluorescein include: Sloughing of the skin, superficial phlebitis, subcutaneous granuloma and toxic neuritis along the median curve in the antecubital area. Extravasation can cause severe arm pain for up to several hours. When significant extravasation occurs, discontinue the injection and implement conservative measures to treat damaged tissue and relieve pain.

Pregnancy: (Category C). Avoid parenteral fluorescein angiography in patients who are pregnant, especially in the first trimester. There have been no reports of fetal complications during pregnancy.

Lactation: Fluorescein has been shown to be excreted in breast milk. Use caution, therefore, when administering to a nursing woman.

Children: Safety and efficacy for use in children have not been established.

Adverse Reactions:

Injection: Nausea, vomiting, headache, GI distress, syncope, hypotension and other signs and symptoms of hypersensitivity; cardiac arrest; basilar artery ischemia; thrombophlebitis at the injection site; temporary yellowish skin discoloration; severe shock; convulsions; rare cases of death. Hives, itching, bronchospasm, anaphylaxis, pyrexia, transient dyspnea, angioneurotic edema and slight dizziness may occur. A strong taste may develop with use. Urine attains a bright yellow color. Discoloration of the skin fades in 6 to 12 hours; urine fluorescence fades in 24 to 36 hours. Extravasation at the injection site causes intense pain at the site and a dull aching pain in the injected arm.

Patient Information:

May cause strong taste with use.

May cause temporary yellowish discoloration of the skin. Urine will appear a bright yellow color. Discoloration of skin fades in 6 to 12 hours; urine in 24 to 36 hours.

Soft contact lenses may become stained. Do not wear lenses while fluorescein is being used. Whenever fluorescein is used, flush the eyes with sterile normal saline solution and wait at least one hour before replacing the lenses.

Administration and Dosage:

Topical: To detect foreign bodies and corneal abrasions, instill 1 or 2 drops of 2% solution; allow a few seconds for staining. Wash out excess with sterile irrigating solution.

Strips: Moisten strip with sterile water. Place moistened strip at the fornix in the lower cul-de-sac close to the punctum. For best results, patient should close lid tightly over strip until desired amount of staining is obtained. The patient should blink several times after application.

> *For applanation tonometry strips* – Anesthetize the eyes. Retract upper lid and touch tip of strip to the bulbar conjunctiva on the temporal side until an adequate amount of stain is available for a clearly defined endpoint reading.

Injection: Inject the contents of the ampule or pre-filled syringe rapidly into the antecubital vein, *after taking precautions to avoid extravasation.* A syringe, filled with fluorescein, is attached to transparent tubing and a 25-gauge scalp vein needle for injection. Insert the needle and draw the patient's blood to the hub of the syringe so that a *small* air bubble separates the patient's blood in the tubing from the fluorescein. With the room lights on, slowly inject the blood back into the vein while watching the skin over the needle tip. If the needle has extravasated, the patient's blood will be seen to bulge the skin, and the injection should be stopped before any fluorescein is injected. When assured that extravasation has not occurred, the room light may be turned off and the fluorescein injection completed. Luminescence appears in the retina and choroidal vessels in 9 to 15 seconds and can be observed by standard viewing equipment.

If potential allergy is suspected, an intradermal skin test may be performed prior to IV administration (ie, 0.05 ml injected intradermally to be evaluated 30 to 60 minutes following injection).

In patients with inaccessible veins where early phases of an angiogram are not necessary, such as cystoid macular edema, 1 g fluorescein has been administered orally. Ten to 15 minutes are usually required before evidence of dye appears in the fundus.

Adults – 500 to 750 mg injected rapidly into the antecubital vein.

Children – 3.5 mg/lb (7.5 mg/kg) injected rapidly into the antecubital vein.

Have 0.1% epinephrine IM or IV, an antihistamine, soluble steroid, aminophylline IV and oxygen available.

Storage: Store at 46° to 86°F (8° to 30° C). Do not use if solution contains a precipitate. Discard any unused solution. Keep out of the reach of children.

				C.I.*
Rx	**AK-Fluor** (Akorn)	**Injection:** 10%	In 5 ml amps and 5 ml vials.	120
Rx	**Fluorescite** (Alcon)		In 5 ml amps and 5 ml syringes.	205
Rx	**Funduscein-10** (Iolab)		In 5 ml amps.	1701
Rx	**AK-Fluor** (Akorn)	**Injection:** 25%	In 2 ml amps and 2 ml vials.	300
Rx	**Fluorescite** (Alcon)		In 2 ml amps.	613
Rx	**Funduscein-25** (Iolab)		In 3 ml amps.	3328
Rx	**Fluorescein HCl** (Various, eg, Alcon, Iolab)	**Solution:** 2%	In 1, 2 and 15 ml.	73+
Rx	**Ful-Glo** (Sola/Barnes-Hind)	**Strips:** 0.6 mg	In 300s.	166
Rx	**Fluorets** (Akorn)	**Strips:** 1 mg	In 100s.	190
Rx	**Fluor-I-Strip-A.T.** (Wyeth-Ayerst)		In 300s.[1]	322
Rx	**Fluor-I-Strip** (Wyeth-Ayerst)	**Strips:** 9 mg	In 300s.[1]	322

FLUOREXON

Actions:

Fluorexon is a large molecular weight fluorescent solution for use as a diagnostic and fitting aid for patients with hydrogel (soft) contact lenses. Used with or without lens in place, when fluorescein is contraindicated to avoid staining lenses. It may be used for both soft and hard lenses.

Indications:

For the assessment of proper fitting characteristics of hydrogel lenses. For quickly and accurately locating the optic zone in aphakic or low-plus lenses.

For evaluating corneal integrity of patients wearing hydrogel contact lenses. In many instances, arcuate staining will show definite correlation with the edge of the optic zone, indicating improper bearing surfaces.

For use in place of sodium fluorescein when conducting the tear breakup time (B.U.T.) test.

For conducting the applanation tonometry procedure without removing the lens.

---

* Cost Index based on cost per ml or 20 strips.
[1] With polysorbate 80 and 0.5% chlorobutanol.

For locating the lathe-cut index markings (toric lenses). Use as directed for fitting contact lenses.

Contraindications:

Prior sensitivity to sodium fluorescein.

Warnings:

When used with lenses with greater than 55% hydration, some color may remain on the lens. Remove by washing repeatedly with washing solution approved for the lens. Any residual coloring will wash out with the tear flow when the lens is reinserted in the eye. Rinse with saline or water.

With highly hydrated lenses, the amount of coloring picked up will vary with exposure. Avoid unnecessary delays in examination procedure.

Precautions:

Do not use solutions containing hydrogen peroxide to clean or sterilize lenses until all traces of fluorexon are removed. Hydrogen peroxide can bind fluorexon molecules to the lens.

Administration and Dosage:

Place 1 drop on the concave surface of the lens and place the lens immediately on the eye. Alternately place 1 or 2 drops in the lower cul-de-sac and have the patient blink several times.

As the dye passes under the lens, observe a central dark zone of 6 to 9 mm in diameter (ie, a limbal fluorescent ring about 2 mm wide) which forms after each blink. If such a staining pattern cannot be observed immediately, slide the lens upward by gently pushing it with a finger, causing the dye to penetrate under the lens as it slides back into normal position. Additional drops may be used if the fluorescence starts to dissipate after prolonged examination. When the examination is completed, rinse the eye and lens with saline. The lens may be reinserted immediately, as opposed to the long waiting period required after the use of fluorescein.

Begin the examination immediately after instillation of fluorexon drops. This material tends to dissipate readily with the tear flow, leading to a progressive reduction in fluorescence. Prolonged examination may require sequential application of drops.

Applanation tonometry (without removing lens): After seating the patient at the slit lamp and instilling a drop of fluorexon along with a drop of proparacaine or similar topical anesthetic, the contact lens is displaced to one side onto the sclera with the finger and the procedure begun.

			C.I.*
Rx **Fluoresoft** (Various, eg, Akorn, Holles)	**Solution:** 0.35%	In 0.5 ml Pipettes (12s).	263+

* Cost Index based on cost per ml.

INDOCYANINE GREEN

Sterile, water soluble, tricarbocyanine dye with a peak spectral absorption at 800 to 810 nm in blood or blood plasma. Indocyanine green contains not more than 5% sodium iodide.

Actions:

Indocyanine green permits recording of indicator-dilution curves for both diagnostic and research purposes independently of fluctuations in oxygen saturation. In the performance of dye dilution curves, a known amount of dye is usually injected as a single bolus as rapidly as possible via a cardiac catheter into selected sites in the vascular system. A recording instrument (oximeter or densitometer) is attached to a needle or catheter for sampling of the blood-dye mixture from a systemic arterial sampling site.

Ear oximetry has also been used and makes it possible to monitor the appearance and disappearance of indocyanine green without the necessity of withdrawal and spectrophotometric analysis of blood samples for calibration.

Following IV injection, indocyanine green is rapidly bound to plasma protein, of which albumin is the principle carrier (95%). Indocyanine green undergoes no significant extrahepatic or enterohepatic circulation; simultaneous arterial and venous blood estimations have shown negligible renal, peripheral, lung or cerebrospinal uptake of the dye. Indocyanine green is taken up from the plasma almost exclusively by the hepatic parenchymal cells and is secreted entirely into the bile. After biliary obstruction, the dye appears in the hepatic lymph, independently of the bile, suggesting that the biliary mucosa is sufficiently intact to prevent diffusion of the dye, though allowing diffusion of bilirubin. These characteristics make indocyanine green a helpful index of hepatic function.

The peak absorption and emission of indocyanine green lie in a region (800 to 850 nm) where transmission of energy by the pigment epithelium is more efficient than in the region of visible light energy. Indocyanine green is also nearly 98% bound to blood protein, and therefore, excessive dye extravasation does not take place in the highly fenestrated choroidal vasculature. It is, therefore, useful in both absorption and fluorescence infrared angiography of the choroidal vasculature when using appropriate filters and film in a fundus camera.

Indications:

For ophthalmic angiography.

Also used for determining cardiac output, hepatic function and liver blood flow.

Warnings:

Indocyanine green powder and solution: Indocyanine green is unstable in aqueous solution and must be used within 10 hours. However, the dye is stable in plasma and whole blood so that samples obtained in discontinuous sampling techniques may be read hours later. Use sterile techniques in handling the dye solution, as well as in the performance of the dilution curves.

Use only the Aqueous Solvent (pH 5.5 to 6.5) provided, which is specially prepared Sterile Water for Injection, to dissolve indocyanine green because there have been reports of incompatibility with some commercially available Water for Injection products.

Indocyanine green powder may cling to the vial or lump together because it is freeze-dried in the vials. *This is not due to the presence of water.*

Pregnancy: (Category C). It is not known whether indocyanine green can cause fetal harm when administered to a pregnant woman or can affect reproduction capacity. This drug should be given to a pregnant woman only if clearly indicated.

Lactation: It is not known whether this drug is excreted in breast milk. Because many drugs are excreted in breast milk, exercise caution when indocyanine green is administered to a nursing woman.

Precautions:

Plasma fractional disappearance rate at the recommended 0.5 mg/kg dose has been reported to be significantly greater in women than in men, although there was no significant difference in the calculated value for clearance.

Radioactive iodine uptake studies: Do not perform for at least a week following the use of indocyanine green.

Use with caution in individuals who have a history of allergy to iodides.

Drug Interactions:

Heparin preparations containing sodium bisulfite reduce the absorption peak of indocyanine green in blood. Do not use heparin as an anticoagulant for the collection of samples for analysis.

Adverse Reactions:

Indocyanine green contains sodium iodide. Use with caution in patients who have a history of allergy to iodides. Anaphylactic or urticarial reactions have also been reported in patients without history of allergy to iodides. If such reactions occur, treat with appropriate agents (eg, epinephrine, antihistamines and corticosteroids).

Overdosage:

There are no data available describing the signs, symptoms or laboratory findings accompanying overdosage.

Administration and Dosage:

40 mg dye in 2 ml of aqueous solvent. In some patients, half of the volume has been found to produce angiograms of comparable resolution. Immediately follow the injected dye bolus with a 5 ml bolus of normal saline.

Clinically, angiograms of uniformly good quality can be assured only by taking care to optimize the contributions of all possible factors such as filter and film characteristics, film processing, camera focus, patient cooperation and dye injection. The foregoing injection regimen is designed to provide delivery of a spatially limited dye bolus of optimal concentration to the choroidal vasculature following IV injection.

Rx	**Cardio-Green (CG)** (Becton-Dickinson)	**Powder for Injection**	25 and 50 mg vials with 2 × 10 ml amps of aqueous solvent and 10 and 40 mg vials with 1 ml amps of aqueous solvent.

ROSE BENGAL

Actions:

Stains dead and degenerated epithelial cells (corneal and conjunctival); stains mucus and normally stains the line behind meibomian gland outlets. Rose bengal does not stain epithelial defects and does not pass into intercellular spaces.

Indications:

A diagnostic agent for routine ocular examinations or when superficial corneal or conjunctival tissue damage is suspected. Effective aid for diagnosis of keratitis, squamous cell carcinomas, keratoconjunctivitis sicca, corrosions or abrasions, and for the detection of foreign bodies.

Contraindications:

Known hypersensitivity to rose bengal or to any component of the formulation.

Precautions:

The solution may be irritating.

Contact lenses: Whenever rose bengal is used in patients with soft contact lenses, flush the eyes thoroughly with sterile normal saline solution and wait at least one hour before replacing the lenses.

Use appropriate care to avoid staining clothing.

Administration and Dosage:

Solution: Instill 1 or 2 drops into the conjunctival sac before examination.

Strips: Thoroughly saturate tip of strip with sterile irrigating solution. Touch bulbar conjunctiva or lower fornix with moistened strip. The patient should blink several times after application.

Keep out of the reach of children.

				C.I.*
Rx	**Rose Bengal 1%** (Akorn)	**Solution:** 1%	In 5 ml dropper bottles.	174+
Rx	**Rosets** (Akorn)	**Strips:** 1.3 mg per strip	In 100s.	265

* Cost Index based on cost per ml or 20 strips.

Local Anesthetics

Local anesthetics prevent the generation and conduction of nerve impulses by reducing sodium permeability, increasing the electrical excitation threshold, slowing the nerve impulse propagation and reducing the rate of rise of the action potential; the exact mechanism is unknown. Their action is reversible; complete recovery of nerve function occurs with no evidence of structural damage to nerve tissue. The progression of anesthesia is related to the diameter, myelination and conduction velocity of affected nerve fibers. The order of loss of nerve function is as follows: Pain, temperature, touch, proprioception and skeletal muscle tone.

With the exception of cocaine, local anesthetics are synthetic, aromatic or heterocyclic compounds. Nearly all local anesthetics in current use are weakly basic tertiary amines. The structural components consist of an aromatic lipophilic portion, an intermediate alkyl chain and a hydrophilic hydrocarbon chain containing nitrogen. The intermediate chain is linked to the aromatic group by either an ester or an amide, which determines certain pharmacologic properties of the molecule.

CLASSIFICATION

Table 1: CLASSIFICATION OF LOCAL ANESTHETICS	
Ester Linkage	**Amide Linkage** (Amides of benzoic acid)
A. Esters of benzoic acid: Cocaine	A. Lidocaine
B. Esters of meta-aminobenzoic acid: Proparacaine	B. Mepivacaine
C. Esters of para-aminobenzoic acid	C. Bupivacaine
1. Procaine	D. Etidocaine
2. Chloroprocaine	
3. Tetracaine	
4. Benoxinate	

Local anesthetics are divided into two groups: *Esters,* which are derivatives of para-aminobenzoic acid and *amides,* which are derivatives of aniline. The "ester" local anesthetics are metabolized by hydrolysis of the ester linkage by plasma esterase, probably plasma cholinesterase. The "amide" local anesthetics are metabolized in the liver, then excreted primarily in the urine as metabolites with a small fraction of unchanged drug. Biliary excretion may contribute to the disposition of lidocaine (eg, *Xylocaine*) and mepivacaine (eg, *Carbocaine*). Allergic reactions to local anesthetics occur almost exclusively to anesthetics with ester linkage (see Precautions). All commonly used topical anesthetics are of the ester type (see Table 1).

In the amine form, local anesthetics tend to be only slightly soluble in water and, therefore, are usually formulated in the form of their hydrochloride salt, which is water soluble. Since local anesthetics are weak bases, with a pK_a between 8 and 9, they ionize in solution, enhancing stability and shelf life. Upon contact with more neutral or alkaline environments (eg, tears), the nonionized form is liberated. The nonionized drug can penetrate tissues, including the cornea.

PHARMACOKINETICS

Various pharmacokinetic parameters of the local anesthetics can be significantly altered by the presence of hepatic or renal disease, addition of epinephrine, factors affecting urinary pH, renal blood flow, the route of administration and age of patient. Onset of local anesthesia is dependent on the dissociation constant (pK_a), lipid solubility, pH of the solution, protein binding and molecular size. In general, local anesthetics with high lipid solubility or low pK_a have a faster onset. The duration of action of local anesthetics is proportional to the drug's contact time with nerve tissue. To prolong contact time of injectable local anesthetics, vasoconstrictors may be added, but such adjuncts are of no benefit when used with topical anesthetics. The use of vasoconstrictors (eg, epinephrine) in conjunction with local anesthetics promotes local hemostasis, decreases systemic absorption and prolongs the duration of action.

Systemic absorption of local anesthetics affects the cardiovascular system and central nervous system. At blood concentrations achieved with normal therapeutic doses of injectable anesthetics, changes in cardiac conduction, excitability, refractoriness, contractility and peripheral vascular resistance are minimal. However, toxic blood concentrations depress cardiac conduction and excitability, which may lead to atrioventricular block and ultimately to cardiac arrest. In addition, with toxic blood concentrations, myocardial contractility may be depressed and peripheral vasodilation may occur, leading to decreased cardiac output and arterial blood pressure.

Following systemic absorption, toxic blood concentrations of local anesthetics can produce CNS stimulation, depression or both. Apparent central stimulation may be manifested as restlessness, tremors and shivering, which may progress to convulsions. Depression and coma may occur, possibly progressing ultimately to respiratory arrest. The local anesthetics have a primary depressant effect on the medulla and on higher centers. The depressed stage may occur without a prior stage of central nervous system stimulation.

Rate of systemic absorption depends on total dose and concentration of drug, vascularity of administration site and presence of vasoconstrictors. Depending on route of administration, local anesthetics are distributed to some extent to all body tissues. High concentrations are found in highly perfused organs (eg, liver, lungs, heart, brain). The rate and extent of placental diffusion is determined by plasma protein binding, ionization and lipid solubility. It is the nonionized form of the drug that crosses cellular membranes to the site of action. Fetal:maternal ratios are inversely related to degree of protein binding. Only the free, unbound drug is available for placental transfer. Drugs with the highest protein binding capacity may have the lowest fetal:maternal ratios. Lipid-soluble, nonionized drugs readily enter the fetal blood from the maternal circulation.

OPHTHALMIC USES

Anesthetics in current clinical use have relatively low systemic and ocular toxicity. They have a sufficiently long duration of action, are stable in solution and usually lack interference with the actions of other drugs. These advantages make local anesthetics useful for such ocular procedures as tonometry, foreign body and suture removal, gonioscopy and nasolacrimal irrigation and probing (see Table 2).

Table 2: OPHTHALMIC USES OF LOCAL ANESTHETICS	
Injectable	1. Facial nerve block
	2. Retrobulbar anesthesia
	3. Eyelid infiltration
Topical	1. Gonioscopy
	2. Tonometry
	3. Fundus contact lens biomicroscopy
	4. Evaluation of corneal abrasions
	5. Forced duction testing
	6. Schirmer tear testing
	7. Electroretinography
	8. Lacrimal dilation and irrigation
	9. Contact lens fitting
	10. Superficial foreign body removal
	11. Minor surgery of conjunctiva
	12. Suture removal
	13. Corneal epithelial debridement

Jimmy D. Bartlett OD, DOS
University of Alabama at Birmingham

For More Information

Bartlett JD, Jaanus SD, eds. Clinical Ocular Pharmacology, ed. 2. Boston, MA: Butterworth, 1989.

Burns RP, et al. Chronic toxicity of local anesthetics on the cornea. In: Leopold IH, Burns RP, eds. Symposium on Ocular Therapy. New York, NY: Wiley, 1977.

Bryant JA. Local and topical anesthetics in ophthalmology. *Surv Ophthalmol* 1969;13:263-83.

Chandler MJ, et al. Provocative challenge with local anesthetics in patients with a prior history of reaction. *J Allergy Clin Immunol* 1987;79:883-86.

Frayer WC, Jacoby J. Local anesthesia. In: Duane TD, Jaeger EA, eds. Clinical Ophthalmology, ed. 5. Philadelphia, PA: J.B. Lippincott, 1987.

Norden LC. Adverse reactions to topical ocular anesthetics. *J Am Optom Assoc* 1976;47:730-33.

Smith RB, Everett WG. Physiology and pharmacology of local anesthetic agents. *Int Ophthalmol Clin* 1973;13: 35-60.

Vettese T, Breslin CW. Retrobulbar anesthesia for cataract surgery: Comparison of bupivacaine and bupivacaine-lidocaine combinations. *Can J Ophthalmol* 1985;20:131-34.

Webster RB. Local anesthetics for ophthalmic use. *Aust J Optom* 1974;57:399-401.

LOCAL ANESTHETICS, INJECTABLE, General Monograph

Actions:

Pharmacology: Local anesthetics prevent the generation and conduction of nerve impulses by reducing sodium permeability, increasing the electrical excitation threshold, slowing the nerve impulse propagation and reducing the rate of rise of the action potential; the exact mechanism is unknown.

Pharmacokinetics: Various pharmacokinetic parameters of the local anesthetics can be significantly altered by the presence of hepatic or renal disease, addition of epinephrine, factors affecting urinary pH, renal blood flow, the route of administration and age of patient.

Pharmacokinetic parameters for injectable local anesthetics are summarized below:

Anesthetic	Onset (minutes)	Duration (hours)	Equivalent Anesthetic Concentration (%)	pK$_a$	Partition[1] Coefficient	Systemic Protein Binding (%)
ESTERS						
Procaine[2]	2-5	0.25-0.5	2	8.9	0.02	5
(w/Epinephrine)	nd	0.5-1.5				
AMIDES						
Lidocaine[2]	0.5-1	0.5-1	1	7.9	2.9	55-65
(w/Epinephrine)	nd	2-6				
Mepivacaine[2]	3-5	0.75-1.5	1	7.6	0.8	65-77
(w/Epinephrine)	nd	2-6				
Bupivacaine[2]	5	2-4	0.25	8.1	27.5	84-95
(w/Epinephrine)	nd	3-7				
Etidocaine[2]	3-5	2-3	0.5	7.7	141	94
(w/Epinephrine)	nd	3-7				

[1] n-Heptane/Buffer, pH 7.4.   nd – No data.
[2] Values in this line represent those for infiltrative anesthesia.

Indications:

Refer to individual product listings.

Contraindications:

Hypersensitivity to local anesthetics, drugs of similar chemical configuration, para-aminobenzoic acid derivatives or parabens.

Warnings:

Local anesthetics should only be employed by clinicians who are well versed in diagnosis and management of dose-related toxicity and other acute emergencies that may arise. Ensure the immediate availability of oxygen, other resuscitative drugs, cardiopulmonary resuscitative equipment and the personnel resources needed for proper management of toxic reactions and related emergencies. Delay in proper management of dose-related toxicity, underventilation from any cause or altered sensitivity may lead to the development of acidosis, cardiac arrest and, possibly, death (see Adverse Reactions and Precautions).

It is essential that aspiration for blood or cerebrospinal fluid be done prior to injecting any local anesthetic, both the original dose and all subsequent doses, to avoid intravascular or subarachnoid injection. However, a negative aspiration does not ensure against an intravascular or subarachnoid injection.

Do not use large doses of local anesthetics in patients with heart block.

Use with inflammation or sepsis: Use local anesthetic procedures with caution when there is inflammation or sepsis in the region of proposed injection.

Cardiovascular reactions are depressant. They may be the result of direct drug effect or the result of vasovagal reaction, particularly if the patient is in the sitting position. Failure to recognize premonitory signs such as sweating, feeling of faintness, changes in pulse or sensorium may result in progressive cerebral hypoxia and seizure, or serious cardiovascular catastrophe. Place patient in recumbent position and administer oxygen. Vasoactive drugs, such as ephedrine or methoxamine, may be administered IV.

Debilitated, elderly patients and acutely ill patients should be given reduced doses commensurate with their age and physical status. Injection of repeated doses of local anesthetics may cause significant increases in plasma levels with each repeated dose due to slow accumulation of the drug or its metabolites, or to slow metabolic degradation. Tolerance to elevated blood levels varies with the status of the patient.

Pregnancy: Category B (etidocaine, lidocaine). *Category C* (bupivacaine, mepivacaine, procaine). Safety for use in pregnant women, other than those in labor, has not been established. Local anesthetics rapidly cross the placenta.

Lactation: Safety for use in the nursing mother has not been established. It is not known whether local anesthetic drugs are excreted in breast milk.

Children: Dosages in children should be reduced to commensurate with age, body weight and physical condition. Due to lack of clinical experience, the administration of *bupivacaine* to children under 12 is not recommended.

Precautions:

Use with caution in patients with severe disturbances of cardiac rhythm, shock, heart block or hypotension.

Monitor cardiovascular and respiratory vital signs and state of consciousness after each injection. Restlessness, anxiety, incoherent speech, lightheadedness, numbness and tingling of the mouth and lips, metallic taste, tinnitus, dizziness, blurred vision, tremors, twitching, depression or drowsiness may be early signs of CNS toxicity.

Impaired hepatic function: Because amide-type local anesthetics are metabolized primarily in the liver, patients with hepatic disease, especially severe hepatic disease, may be more susceptible to potential toxicity. Use cautiously in such patients.

Renal disease: Use *mepivacaine* with caution in patients with renal disease.

Malignant hyperthermia: Many drugs used during anesthesia are considered potential triggering agents for familial malignant hyperthermia. It is not known whether local anesthetics may trigger this reaction, and the need for supplemental general anesthesia cannot be predicted in advance; therefore, have a standard protocol for management available.

Head and Neck Area: Small doses of local anesthetics injected into the head and neck area, including retrobulbar and stellate ganglion blocks, may produce adverse reactions similar to systemic toxicity seen with unintentional intravascular injections of larger doses. Fatalities have occurred. The injection procedures require the utmost care. Confusion, convulsions, respiratory depression or arrest, and cardiovascular stimulation or depression have been reported. These reactions may be due to intra-arterial injection of the local anesthetic with retrograde flow to cerebral circulation.

They also may be due to puncture of the dural sheath of the optic nerve during retro-bulbar block with diffusion of any local anesthetic along the subdural space to the midbrain. Observe and monitor patients carefully. Do not exceed dosage recommendations.

When local anesthetic solutions are employed for retrobulbar block, lack of corneal sensation should not be relied upon to determine whether or not the patient is ready for surgery since corneal sensation usually precedes clinically acceptable external ocular muscle akinesia. Therefore, presence of akinesia rather than anesthesia alone should determine readiness of the patient for surgery.

Hypersensitivity reactions including anaphylaxis may occur in a small segment of the population allergic to para-aminobenzoic acid derivatives (eg, procaine, benzocaine). Hypersensitivity reactions and anaphylaxis have occurred rarely with *lidocaine*.

Sulfite Sensitivity: Some of these products contain sulfites, which may cause allergic-type reactions (eg, hives, itching, wheezing, anaphylaxis) in certain suscep-tible persons. Although the overall prevalence of sulfite sensitivity in the general population is probably low, it is seen more frequently in asthmatics or in atopic non-asthmatic persons.

Drug Interactions:

Concurrent use: Mixtures of local anesthetics are sometimes employed to compen-sate for the slower onset of one drug and the shorter duration of action of the second drug. Toxicity is probably additive with mixtures of local anesthetics, but some experiments suggest synergism. Exercise caution regarding toxic equivalence when mixtures of local anesthetics are employed.

Chloroprocaine: Prior use may interfere with subsequent use of *bupivacaine*. Because of this, and because safety of intercurrent use of bupivacaine and chloro-procaine has not been established, such use is not recommended.

Ergot-type oxytocic drugs: Coadministration may cause severe, persistent hyperten-sion or cerebrovascular accidents. The pressor effect of epinephrine may be reversed or reduced by phenothiazines and butyrophenones (see Warnings).

Metals react with local anesthetics and cause the release of the metals' respective ions that, if injected, may cause severe local irritation. Do not use disinfecting agents containing heavy metals for skin or mucous membrane disinfection.

Sulfonamides: The para-aminobenzoic acid metabolite of procaine, chloroprocaine and tetracaine inhibits the action of sulfonamides. Despite adequate sulfonamide therapy, local infections have occurred in areas infiltrated with procaine prior to diagnostic punctures and drainage procedures. Therefore, do not use procaine, chlo-roprocaine or tetracaine in any condition in which a sulfonamide drug is employed.

Vasoconstrictors (eg, epinephrine): Serious cardiac arrhythmias may result if prepa-rations containing vasoconstrictors are administered during or immediately following the use of halothane, cyclopropane, trichloroethylene or other related agents.

Use solutions containing a vasoconstrictor with extreme caution in patients receiving drugs that produce blood pressure alterations (eg, monoamine oxidase inhibitors, tricyclic antidepressants, phenothiazines); severe and sustained hypotension or hypertension or disturbances of cardiac rhythm may occur.

Adverse Reactions:

The most common acute adverse reactions are related to the CNS and cardiovascu-lar systems. These are generally dose related and may result from rapid absorption from the injection site, from diminished tolerance or from unintentional intravascular injection.

CNS: Characterized by excitation or depression. Excitement may be transient or absent, with depression being the first manifestation of an adverse reaction. This may quickly be followed by drowsiness, merging into unconsciousness and respiratory arrest.

Restlessness, nervousness, apprehension, euphoria, confusion, chills, constriction of pupil, anxiety, drowsiness, dizziness, lightheadedness, tinnitus, blurred or double vision, sensations of heat, cold or numbness, twitching or tremors may occur, possibly proceeding to convulsions. The incidence of convulsions associated with the use of local anesthetics varies with the procedure used and the total dose administered.

Cardiovascular: High doses or inadvertent intravascular injection may lead to high plasma levels and related depression of the myocardium, decreased cardiac output, heart block, hypotension (or sometimes hypertension), bradycardia, ventricular arrhythmias and cardiac arrest.

Allergic: Allergic-type reactions are rare and may occur as a result of sensitivity to the local anesthetic or to other formulation ingredients, such as the antimicrobial preservative chlorobutanol contained in multiple-dose vials. These reactions are characterized by signs such as cutaneous lesions of delayed onset, urticaria, pruritus, erythema, angioneurotic edema (including laryngeal edema), tachycardia, sneezing, nausea, vomiting, dizziness, syncope, excessive sweating, elevated temperature, and, possibly, anaphylactoid-like symptomatology (including severe hypotension).

Cross sensitivity among members of the ester-type local anesthetic group has been reported. The usefulness of sensitivity screening has not been established.

Neurologic: The incidences of adverse neurologic reactions associated with the use of local anesthetics may be related to the total dose of local anesthetic administered, and are also dependent upon the particular drug used, the route of administration and the physical status of the patient. Many of these effects may be related to local anesthetic techniques, with or without a contribution from the drug.

Gastrointestinal: Nausea, vomiting.

Overdosage:

Acute emergencies from local anesthetics are generally related to high plasma levels encountered during therapeutic use or to unintended subarachnoid injection.

Management: The first consideration is prevention, best accomplished by careful and constant monitoring of cardiovascular and respiratory vital signs and the patient's state of consciousness after each injection. At the first sign of change, administer oxygen.

Convulsions, as well as underventilation or apnea, are due to unintentional subarachnoid injection; maintain patent airway and assist or control ventilation with oxygen and a delivery system capable of permitting immediate positive airway pressure by mask. Evaluate circulation. If convulsions persist despite respiratory support, and if the status of the circulation permits, give small increments of an ultra short-acting barbiturate (ie, thiopental or thiamylal) or a benzodiazepine (ie, diazepam) IV. Circulatory depression may require administration of IV fluids and a vasopressor.

If not treated immediately, convulsions and cardiovascular depression can result in hypoxia, acidosis, bradycardia, arrhythmias and cardiac arrest. Underventilation or apnea may produce these same signs and also lead to cardiac arrest if ventilatory support is not instituted. If cardiac arrest occurs, institute standard cardiopulmonary resuscitative measures. Endotracheal intubation may be indicated.

Dialysis is of negligible value in the treatment of acute overdosage with lidocaine or etidocaine.

Patient Information:

Avoid touching or rubbing the eye until the anesthesia has worn off because inadvertent damage may be done to the anesthetized cornea and conjunctiva.

Administration and Dosage:

The dose of local anesthetic administered varies with the procedure, vascularity of the tissues, depth of anesthesia, degree of required muscle relaxation, duration of anesthesia desired and the physical condition of the patient. Reduce dosages for children, elderly and debilitated patients and patients with cardiac or liver disease.

For specific techniques and procedures, refer to standard textbooks.

Infiltration or regional block anesthesia: Always inject slowly with frequent aspirations to avoid systemic reactions. Avoid intravascular injection.

Individual drug monographs are on the following pages.

PROCAINE HCl

For complete prescribing information see General Monograph p. 22.

Indications:

For production of local anesthesia by infiltration injection, nerve block and other peripheral blocks.

Administration and Dosage:

Do not use if solution changes color or becomes cloudy or if it contains crystals. Protect from light.

For infiltration anesthesia: 0.25% or 0.5% solution; 350 mg to 600 mg is considered to be a single safe total dose. To prepare 60 ml of a 0.5% solution (5 mg/ml), dilute 30 ml of the 1% solution with 30 ml sterile distilled water or 0.9% sodium chloride. To prepare 60 ml of a 0.25% solution (2.5 mg/ml), dilute 15 ml of the 1% solution with 45 ml sterile distilled water or 0.9% sodium chloride. An anesthetic solution of 0.5 ml to 1 ml of epinephrine 1:1,000 per 100 ml may be added for vasoconstrictive effect (1:200,000 to 1:100,000). (See Warnings and Precautions.)

For peripheral nerve block: 0.5% solution (up to 200 ml), 1% solution (up to 100 ml), or 2% solution (up to 50 ml). Limit the use of the 2% solution to cases requiring a small volume of anesthetic solution (10 ml to 25 ml). An anesthetic solution of 0.5 ml to 1 ml of epinephrine 1:1,000 per 100 ml may be added for vasoconstrictive effect (1:200,000 to 1:100,000). (See Warnings and Precautions.)

The usual initial dose should not exceed 1000 mg.

C.I.*

Rx	**Procaine HCl** (Various, eg, Abbott, Pasadena Research)	**Injection:** 1%	In 30 ml vials.	14+
Rx	**Novocain** (Sanofi Winthrop)		In 2 and 6 ml amps[1] and 30 ml multiple dose vials.[2]	57
Rx	**Procaine HCl** (Various, eg, Abbott, Pasadena Research)	**Injection:** 2%	In 30 ml vials.	14+
Rx	**Novocain** (Sanofi Winthrop)		In 30 ml multiple dose vials.[2]	57

* Cost Index based on cost per ml.
[1] With acetone sodium bisulfite.
[2] With acetone sodium bisulfite and $\leq$ 0.25% chlorobutanol.

LIDOCAINE HCl

For complete prescribing information see General Monograph p. 22.

Indications:

Infiltration:

    Percutaneous – 0.5% or 1% solution.

    IV regional – 0.5% solution.

Nerve block (eg, brachial, intercostal): 1% or 1.5% solution.

Retrobulbar or transtracheal injection: 4% solution.

Storage: Store at room temperature 59° to 86°F (15° to 30°C).

Rx				C.I.*
Rx	**Xylocaine** (Astra)	Injection: 0.5%	In 50 ml single[1] and 50 ml multiple[2] dose vials.	10
Rx	**Lidocaine HCl** (Various, eg, American Regent, Elkins-Sinn, Forest, Goldline, Steris)	Injection: 1%	In 5, 20, 30 and 50 ml vials.	7+
Rx	**L-Caine** (Century)		In 50 ml multiple dose vials.[3]	8
Rx	**Lidoject-1** (Mayrand)		In 50 ml multiple dose vials.[1]	18
Rx	**Nervocaine 1%** (Keene)		In 50 ml multiple dose vials.[3]	5
Rx	**Xylocaine** (Astra)		In 2, 5 and 30 ml amps[1], 2, 5, 10 and 30 ml single dose vials[1] and 10, 20 and 50 ml multiple dose vials.[2]	8
Rx	**Xylocaine** (Astra)	Injection: 1.5%	In 20 ml amps and 10 and 20 ml single dose vials.[1]	65
Rx	**Lidocaine HCl** (Various, eg, American Regent, Elkins-Sinn, Forest, Goldline, Schein)	Injection: 2%	In 5, 20, 30 and 50 ml vials.	7+
Rx	**Lidoject-2** (Mayrand)		In 50 ml multiple dose vials.[1]	18
Rx	**Nervocaine 2%** (Keene)		In 50 ml multiple dose vials.[4]	5
Rx	**Xylocaine** (Astra)		In 2 and 10 ml amps,[1] 2, 5 and 10 ml single dose vials[1] and 10, 20 and 50 ml multiple dose vials.[2]	10
Rx	**Lidocaine HCl** (Abbott)	Injection: 4%	In 5 ml single dose amps.	76+
Rx	**Xylocaine** (Astra)		In 5 ml amps and 5 ml disp. syringes.	141

* Cost Index based on cost per ml.
[1] With sodium chloride.
[2] With 0.1% methylparaben and sodium chloride.
[3] With 0.1% methylparaben and 0.7% sodium chloride.
[4] With 0.1% methylparaben and 0.6% sodium chloride.

LIDOCAINE COMBINATIONS   C.I.*

Rx	**Xylocaine** (Astra)	**Injection:** 0.5% with 1:200,000 epinephrine	In 50 ml multiple dose vials.[1]	10
Rx	**Xylocaine** (Astra)	**Injection:** 1% with 1:200,000 epinephrine	In 30 ml amps[2] and 5, 10 and 30 ml single dose vials.[2]	36
Rx	**Lidocaine HCl** (Various, eg, American Regent, Elkins-Sinn)	**Injection:** 1% with 1:100,000 epinephrine	In 20, 30 and 50 ml multiple dose vials.	3
Rx	**Lidoject-1** (Mayrand)		In 50 ml multiple dose vials.[3]	18
Rx	**Nervocaine 1%** (Keene)		In 50 ml multiple dose vials.[1]	5
Rx	**Xylocaine** (Astra)		In 10, 20 and 50 ml multiple dose vials.[1]	8
Rx	**Xylocaine** (Astra)	**Injection:** 1.5% with 1:200,000 epinephrine	In 5 and 30 ml amps[2] and 5, 10 and 30 ml single dose vials.[2]	41
Rx	**Xylocaine** (Astra)	**Injection:** 2% with 1:200,000 epinephrine	In 20 ml amps[2] and 5, 10 and 20 ml single dose vials.[2]	13
Rx	**Lidoject-2** (Mayrand)	**Injection:** 2% with 1:100,000 epinephrine	In 50 ml multiple dose vials.[3]	18
Rx	**Nervocaine 2%** (Keene)		In 50 ml multiple dose vials.[4]	5
Rx	**Xylocaine** (Astra)		In 10, 20 and 50 ml multiple dose vials.[1]	10

* Cost Index based on cost per ml.
[1] With 0.1% methylparaben, 0.05% sodium metabisulfite and sodium chloride.
[2] With 0.05% sodium metabisulfite and sodium chloride.
[3] With sodium metabisulfite and sodium chloride.
[4] With sodium metabisulfite, 0.1% methylparaben and 0.6% sodium chloride.

MEPIVACAINE HCl

For complete prescribing information see General Monograph p. 22.

Indications:

Nerve block (eg, cervical, brachial, caudal, epidural): 1%, 1.5% or 2% solution.

Infiltration: 1% solution.

Storage: Store at room temperature 59° to 86°F (15° to 30°C).

				C.I.*
Rx	**Mepivacaine HCl** (Various, eg, Goldline, Rugby, Schein, Steris)	**Injection:** 1%	In 50 ml multiple dose vials.	14+
Rx	**Carbocaine HCl** (Sanofi Winthrop)		In 30 ml single dose[1] and 50 ml multiple dose[2] vials.	35
Rx	**Polocaine** (Astra)		In 30 ml single dose[1] and 50 ml multiple dose[2] vials.	23
Rx	**Carbocaine** (Sanofi Winthrop)	**Injection:** 1.5%	In 30 ml single dose vials.[1]	56
Rx	**Polocaine** (Astra)		In 30 ml single dose vials.[1]	36
Rx	**Mepivacaine HCl** (Various, eg, Moore, Rugby, Schein, Steris)	**Injection:** 2%	In 50 ml multiple dose vials.	14+
Rx	**Carbocaine HCl** (Sanofi Winthrop)		In 20 ml single dose[1] and 50 ml multiple dose[3] vials.	41
Rx	**Polocaine** (Astra)		In 20 ml single dose[1] and 50 ml multiple dose[3] vials.	27

BUPIVACAINE HCl

For complete prescribing information see General Monograph p. 22.

Indications:

Local infiltration: 0.25% solution.

Nerve block (eg, peripheral): 0.25% or 0.5% solution.

Retrobulbar block: 0.75% solution.

Storage: Store at room temperature 59° to 86°F (15° to 30°C). Do not use if solution changes color or contains a precipitate. Protect from light.

---

* Cost Index based on cost per ml.
[1] With sodium chloride.
[2] With 0.1% methylparaben and 0.7% sodium chloride.
[3] With 0.1% methylparaben and 0.5% sodium chloride.

BUPIVACAINE HCl (Cont.)   C.I.*

Rx	**Bupivacaine HCl** (Abbott)	**Injection:** 0.25%	In 20, 30 and 50 ml amps, 10 and 30 ml vials, 50 ml multiple dose vials and 50 ml syringes.	25
Rx	**Marcaine HCl** (Sanofi Winthrop)		In 50 ml amps,[1] 10 and 30 ml single dose[1] and 50 ml multiple dose[2] vials.	17
Rx	**Sensorcaine** (Astra)		In 30 ml amps,[1] 10 and 30 ml single dose[1] and 50 ml multiple dose[2] vials.	19
Rx	**Bupivacaine HCl** (Abbott)	**Injection:** 0.5%	In 20 and 30 ml amps, 10 and 30 ml vials, 50 ml vials and 30 ml syringes.	27
Rx	**Marcaine HCl** (Sanofi Winthrop)		In 3 and 30 ml amps,[1] 10 and 30 ml single dose[1] and 50 ml multiple dose[2] vials.	21
Rx	**Sensorcaine** (Astra)		In 30 ml amps,[3] 10 and 30 ml single dose[1] and 50 ml multiple dose[2] vials.	21
Rx	**Bupivacaine HCl** (Abbott)	**Injection:** 0.75%	In 20 and 30 ml amps and 10 and 30 ml vials and 20 ml syringes.	32
Rx	**Marcaine HCl** (Sanofi Winthrop)		In 30 ml amps[1] and 10 and 30 ml single dose vials.[1]	24
Rx	**Sensorcaine** (Astra)		In 2 and 30 ml amps[1] and 10 ml single dose vials.[1]	51

BUPIVACAINE COMBINATIONS   C.I.*

Rx	**Bupivacaine HCl** (Abbott)	**Injection:** 0.25% with 1:200,000 epinephrine	In 20, 30 and 50 ml amps,[3] 10 and 30 ml vials[3] and 50 ml multiple dose vials.[4]	25
Rx	**Marcaine HCl** (Sanofi Winthrop)		In 50 ml amps[5], 10 and 30 ml single dose[5] and 50 ml multiple dose[6] vials.	17
Rx	**Sensorcaine** (Astra)		In 10 and 30 ml single dose[7] and 50 ml multiple dose[8] vials.	23

* Cost Index based on cost per ml.
[1] With sodium chloride.
[2] With 0.1% methylparaben and sodium chloride.
[3] With 0.01% sodium metabisulfite, 0.01% EDTA and sodium chloride.
[4] With 0.01% sodium metabisulfite, 0.01% EDTA, sodium chloride and 0.1% methylparaben.
[5] With 0.05% sodium metabisulfite, 0.01% EDTA and sodium chloride.
[6] With 0.05% sodium metabisulfite, 0.01% EDTA, 0.1% methylparaben and sodium chloride.
[7] With 0.05% sodium metabisulfite and sodium chloride.
[8] With 0.05% sodium metabisulfite, 0.1% methylparaben and sodium chloride.

BUPIVACAINE HCl COMBINATIONS (Cont.)   C.I.*

Rx	**Bupivacaine HCl** (Abbott)	**Injection:** 0.5% with 1:200,000 epinephrine	In 30 ml amps,[1] 10 and 30 ml vials[1] and 50 ml multiple dose vials.[2]	27
Rx	**Marcaine HCl** (Sanofi Winthrop)		In 3 and 30 ml amps[3], 10 and 30 ml single dose[3] and 50 ml multiple dose[4] vials.	21
Rx	**Sensorcaine** (Astra)		In 5 and 30 ml amps[5], 10 and 30 ml single dose[5] and 50 ml multiple dose[6] vials.	21
Rx	**Bupivacaine HCl** (Abbott)	**Injection:** 0.75% with 1:200,000 epinephrine	In 30 ml amps.[1]	53
Rx	**Marcaine HCl** (Sanofi Winthrop)		In 30 ml amps.[3]	36
Rx	**Sensorcaine** (Astra)		In 30 ml amps[5] and 10 and 30 ml single dose vials.[5]	34

ETIDOCAINE HCl

For complete prescribing information see General Monograph p. 22.

Indications:

Retrobulbar block: 1% or 1.5% solution.

Peripheral nerve block, central nerve block or lumbar peridural: 1% solution.

Maxillary infiltration or inferior alveolar nerve block: 1.5% solution.

Storage: Store at room temperature 59° to 86°F (15° to 30°C). Do not use if solution changes color or contains a precipitate.

				C.I.*
Rx	**Duranest** (Astra)	**Injection:** 1%	In 30 ml single dose vials.[7]	73
		1% with 1:200,000 epinephrine	In 30 ml single dose vials.[8]	79
		1.5% with 1:200,000 epinephrine	In 20 ml single dose vials.[9]	101

* Cost Index based on cost per ml.
[1] With 0.01% sodium metabisulfite, 0.01% EDTA and sodium chloride.
[2] With 0.01% sodium metabisulfite, 0.01% EDTA, sodium chloride and 0.1% methylparaben.
[3] With 0.05% sodium metabisulfite, 0.01% EDTA and sodium chloride.
[4] With 0.05% sodium metabisulfite, 0.01% EDTA, sodium chloride and 0.1% methylparaben.
[5] With 0.05% sodium metabisulfite and sodium chloride.
[6] With 0.05% sodium metabisulfite, 0.1% methylparaben and sodium chloride.
[7] With 0.71% sodium chloride.
[8] With 0.05% sodium metabisulfite and 0.71% sodium chloride.
[9] With 0.05% sodium metabisulfite and 0.62% sodium chloride.

LOCAL ANESTHETICS, TOPICAL, General Monograph

Actions:

Pharmacology: Local anesthetics stabilize the neuronal membrane so that the neuron is less permeable to ions. This prevents the initiation and transmission of nerve impulses, thereby producing the local anesthetic action.

Studies indicate that local anesthetics influence permeability of the nerve cell membrane by limiting sodium ion permeability by closing the pores through which the ions migrate in the lipid layer of the nerve cell membrane. This limitation prevents the fundamental change necessary for generation of the action potential.

Pharmacokinetics: Tetracaine and proparacaine are approximately equally potent. They have a rapid onset of anesthesia beginning within 13 to 30 seconds after instillation. The duration of action is 15 to 20 minutes.

Indications:

Corneal anesthesia of short duration (eg, tonometry, gonioscopy, removal of corneal foreign bodies and sutures); short corneal and conjunctival procedures; cataract surgery; conjunctival and corneal scraping for diagnostic purposes; paracentesis of the anterior chamber.

Contraindications:

Known hypersensitivity to similar drugs (ester-type local anesthetics), para-aminobenzoic acid or its derivatives or to any other ingredient in these preparations.

Prolonged use, especially for self-medication, is not recommended.

Warnings:

For topical use only. Prolonged use may diminish duration of anesthesia, retard wound healing and cause corneal epithelial erosions (see Adverse Reactions).

Protection of the eye from irritating chemicals, foreign bodies and rubbing during the period of anesthesia is very important. Thoroughly rinse tonometers soaked in sterilizing or detergent solutions with sterile distilled water prior to use. Advise patients to avoid touching the eye until anesthesia has worn off. Because the "blink" reflex is temporarily eliminated, it is advised that the eye be covered with a patch following instillation.

Systemic toxicity is rare with topical ophthalmic application of local anesthetics. It usually occurs as CNS stimulation followed by CNS and cardiovascular depression.

Pregnancy: Category C. Safety for use during pregnancy has not been established. Use only when clearly needed and when potential benefits outweigh potential hazards to the fetus.

Lactation: It is not known whether these drugs are excreted in human milk. Because many drugs are excreted in human milk, exercise caution when local anesthetics are administered to a nursing woman.

Children: Safety and efficacy for use in children has not been established.

Precautions:

Tolerance varies with the status of the patient. Give debilitated, elderly or acutely ill patients doses commensurate with their weight, age and physical status.

Use caution in patients with abnormal or reduced levels of plasma esterases.

Use cautiously and sparingly in patients with known allergies, cardiac disease or hyperthyroidism.

Adverse Reactions:

Prolonged ophthalmic use of topical anesthetics has been associated with corneal epithelial erosions, retardation or prevention of healing of corneal erosions and reports of severe keratitis and permanent corneal opacification with accompanying visual loss and scarring or corneal perforation. Inadvertent damage may be done to the anesthetized cornea and conjunctiva by rubbing an eye to which topical anesthetics have been applied.

Tetracaine: Transient stinging, burning and conjunctival redness may occur. A rare, severe, immediate type allergic corneal reaction has been reported characterized by acute diffuse epithelial keratitis with filament formation and sloughing of large areas of necrotic epithelium, diffuse stromal edema, descemetitis and iritis.

Rarely, local reactions including lacrimation, photophobia and chemosis have occurred.

Proparacaine: Local or systemic sensitivity occasionally occurs. At recommended concentration and dosage, proparacaine usually produces little or no initial irritation, stinging, burning, conjunctival redness, lacrimation or increased winking. However, some local irritation and stinging may occur several hours after instillation.

Rarely, a severe, immediate-type, hyperallergic corneal reaction may occur, which includes acute, intense and diffuse epithelial keratitis, a gray, ground-glass appearance, sloughing of large areas of necrotic epithelium, corneal filaments and, sometimes, iritis with descemetitis. Pupillary dilation or cycloplegic effects have rarely been observed.

Allergic contact dermatitis with drying and fissuring of the fingertips and softening and erosion of the corneal epithelium and conjunctival congestion and hemorrhage have been reported.

Patient Information:

Avoid touching or rubbing the eye until the anesthesia has worn off because inadvertent damage may be done to the anesthetized cornea and conjunctiva.

To avoid contamination, do not touch dropper tip to any surface. Replace cap after using.

Do not use if solution changes color or becomes cloudy or if it contains a precipitate. Protect from light.

Individual drug monographs are on the following pages.

TETRACAINE HCl

For complete prescribing information see General Monograph p. 33.

Administration and Dosage:

Solution: Instill 1 or 2 drops. Not for prolonged use.

Ointment: Apply ½ to 1 inch to lower conjunctival fornix. Not for prolonged use.

Storage: Store at 46° to 80°F (8° to 27°C). Protect from light.

				C.I.*
Rx	**Pontocaine** (Sanofi Winthrop)	**Ointment:** 0.5% (as base)	In 3.5 g.[1]	265
Rx	**Tetracaine HCl** (Various, eg, Alcon, Iolab, Optopics)	**Solution:** 0.5%	In 1, 2 and 15 ml.	21+
Rx	**Pontocaine HCl** (Sanofi Winthrop)		In 15 ml Mono-drop and 59 ml.[2]	134

PROPARACAINE HCl

For complete prescribing information see General Monograph p. 33.

Administration and Dosage:

Deep anesthesia as in cataract extraction: 1 drop every 5 to 10 minutes for 5 to 7 doses.

Removal of sutures: Instill 1 or 2 drops 2 or 3 minutes before removal of sutures.

Removal of foreign bodies: Instill 1 or 2 drops prior to operating.

Tonometry: Instill 1 or 2 drops immediately before measurement.

Storage: Store at 46° to 86°F (8° to 30°C). Protect from light.

				C.I.*
Rx	**Proparacaine HCl** (Various, eg, Moore, Raway, Rugby)	**Solution:** 0.5%	In 2 and 15 ml and UD 1 ml.	61+
Rx	**AK-Taine** (Akorn)		In 2 and 15 ml dropper bottles.[3,4]	51
Rx	**Alcaine** (Alcon)		In 15 ml Drop-Tainers.[3,4]	102
Rx	**Ophthaine** (Squibb)		In 15 ml dropper bottles.[5,6]	140
Rx	**Ophthetic** (Allergan)		In 15 ml dropper bottles.[4,7]	113

* Cost Index based on cost per ml or gram.
[1] With white petrolatum and light mineral oil.
[2] With 0.4% chlorobutanol and 0.75% sodium chloride.
[3] With glycerin and 0.01% benzalkonium chloride.
[4] Refrigerate when opened.
[5] With glycerin, 0.2% chlorobutanol and benzalkonium chloride.
[6] Refrigerate.
[7] With 0.01% benzalkonium chloride, glycerin and sodium chloride.

MISCELLANEOUS COMBINATIONS

For complete prescribing information see General Monograph p. 33.

Indications:

For procedures in which a topical ophthalmic anesthetic agent in conjunction with a disclosing agent is indicated: Corneal anesthesia of short duration (eg, tonometry, gonioscopy, removal of corneal foreign bodies); short corneal and conjunctival procedures.

Administration and Dosage:

Removal of foreign bodies, sutures and for tonometry: Instill 1 to 2 drops (in single instillations) in each eye before operating.

Deep ophthalmic anesthesia:

Proparacaine/fluorescein – Instill 1 drop in each eye every 5 to 10 minutes for 5 to 7 doses. Use of an eye patch is recommended.

Benoxinate/fluorescein – Instill 2 drops into each eye at 90-second intervals for 3 instillations using the 0.4% benoxinate HCl solution.

Storage: Protect from light.

				C.I.*
Rx	**Fluoracaine** (Akorn)	**Solution:** 0.5% propara- caine HCl and 0.25% fluorescein sodium	In 5 ml dropper bottles.[1,2]	204
Rx	**Fluress** (Sola/Barnes-Hind)	**Solution:** 0.4% benoxinate HCl and 0.25% fluores- cein sodium	In 5 ml with dropper.[3]	271

* Cost Index based on cost per ml.
[1] With glycerin, povidone and 0.01% thimerosal.
[2] Refrigerate.
[3] With povidone and 1% chlorobutanol.

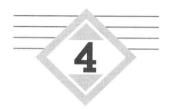

Mydriatics and Cycloplegics

Mydriatics are drugs that dilate the pupil. Adrenergic agonists are used for routine dilation of the pupil. Phenylephrine (eg, *Neo-Synephrine*) and epinephrine (eg, *Epifrin*) are the only direct-acting adrenergic agents available that produce mydriasis without cycloplegia. Epinephrine, however, is not used clinically for its mydriatic effects.

Anticholinergic agents administered topically to the eye for purposes of inhibiting accommodation are termed *cycloplegics*. Their primary use is for cycloplegic refraction and in the treatment of uveitis. Since these agents also inhibit action of the iris sphincter muscle, they are effective mydriatics. Of the cholinergic blocking agents, only tropicamide (eg, *Tropicacyl*) is used routinely for mydriasis. For most dilation procedures, the adrenergic or anticholinergic agents can be used either alone or in combination for maximum mydriasis.

MYDRIATICS

Phenylephrine

Phenylephrine is a synthetic alpha-receptor agonist that is structurally similar to epinephrine. Following topical application on the eye, it contracts the iris dilator muscle and smooth muscle of the conjunctival arterioles, causing pupillary dilation and "blanching" of the conjunctiva. Mueller's muscle of the upper lid may be stimulated, widening the palpebral fissure.

For pupillary dilation, concentrations of 2.5% and 10% are commercially available. Maximum dilation occurs within 45 to 60 minutes, depending on the concentration used or number of drops instilled. The pupil size usually returns to pre-drug levels within 4 to 6 hours. Since phenylephrine has little or no effect on the ciliary muscle, mydriasis occurs without cycloplegia.

Phenylephrine 1% solution can be used in diagnosis of Horner's syndrome. Significant mydriasis can occur in the eye with a postganglionic lesion as compared to one with a normal innervation.

The mydriatic response to phenylephrine may be affected in situations that alter corneal epithelial integrity. Corneal abrasions or trauma from such procedures as tonometry or gonioscopy, as well as prior instillation of a topical anesthetic, can enhance its pharmacologic effect. Concentrations as small as 0.125%, as present in over-the-counter decongestants, can cause mydriasis if the corneal epithelium is damaged.

Since the topical instillation of phenylephrine can be accompanied by clinically significant ocular and systemic side effects, cardiovascular effects in particular, use of the 10% concentration should be avoided if possible. The 2.5% concentration is generally recommended for routine dilation, especially in infants and the elderly. The drug should be used with caution in patients with cardiac disease, hypertension, arteriosclerosis and diabetes. It is contraindicated in patients taking tricyclic antidepressants (eg, amitriptyline), MAO inhibitors (eg, phenelzine), reserpine (eg, *Serpasil*), guanethidine (eg, *Ismelin Sulfate*) and methyldopa (eg, *Aldomet*).

Hydroxyamphetamine

Hydroxyamphetamine is an indirect-acting adrenergic agonist. Its pharmacologic effect is primarily due to release of norepinephrine from postganglionic adrenergic nerve terminals. Like phenylephrine, it has little, if any, effect on accommodation. There is a hydroxyamphetamine HBr/tropicamide combination product for use in pupillary dilation (see p. 53).

As a 1% solution, hydroxyamphetamine has a mydriatic effect comparable to 2.5% phenylephrine. Maximum pupillary dilation occurs within 45 to 60 minutes and lasts for 4 to 6 hours. Since the drug stimulates release of norepinephrine from adrenergic nerve terminals, its mydriatic effects depend on the integrity of the adrenergic innervation to the pupil. A pupil with a postganglionic sympathetic lesion will not dilate. Hydroxyamphetamine was used clinically to differentiate a postganglionic Horner's Syndrome from one that is central or preganglionic. An eye with a preganglionic or central lesion should respond with dilation since the postganglionic nerve endings should contain normal amounts of norepinephrine. Hydroxyamphetamine is a slightly weaker mydriatic in infants and young children, presumably because the adrenergic innervation to the iris is not yet fully developed in this age group.

Adverse effects from topical ocular use of hydroxyamphetamine, although not reported in the literature, could potentially be the same as for phenylephrine.

CYCLOPLEGIC MYDRIATICS

Commonly used cycloplegic mydriatics include: Atropine (eg, *Isopto Atropine*), homatropine (eg, *Isopto Homatropine*), scopolamine (eg, *Isopto Hyoscine*), cyclopentolate (eg, *Cyclogyl*) and tropicamide.

Both objective and subjective refractive procedures are employed to determine the nature of the refractive error. Under normal circumstances, this is best accomplished without interference from topically applied drugs that might adversely affect examination results. Under some conditions, however, the instillation of cycloplegics may enable a more accurate refractive examination.

Use in Esotropia

Children with strabismus, especially esotropia, should receive a cycloplegic examination. It is important to uncover the full amount of hyperopia in young patients with suspected accommodative esotropia so that plus lenses can relieve the effort placed on the accommodative-convergence system. Some clinicians use cycloplegics in children who exhibit myopia for the first time to rule out accommodative spasm (pseudomyopia) as the underlying etiology. Patients who are unresponsive or inconsistent in their responses to subjective refraction will often benefit from cycloplegia. Cycloplegic refraction is also indicated to confirm the refractive amount in patients who exhibit symptoms of malingering or conversion reaction. Refraction of young children and infants is usually more accurate and easier with cycloplegics, since these patients may fixate any distance during the examination. Patients with suspected latent hyperopia will also benefit from cycloplegic refraction.

Contraindications: Since cycloplegics cause pupillary dilation, they are contraindicated in patients with extremely narrow anterior chamber angles or a history of angle-closure glaucoma. Use atropine with caution in patients with Down's syndrome and in patients receiving systemic anticholinergic drugs. Patients allergic to atropine can usually be given scopolamine, which will enable similar examination results.

Drug Selection: Atropine provides the most effective cycloplegia of any currently available anticholinergic drug, and is indicated for the cycloplegic retinoscopy of infants and children up to 4 years of age with suspected accommodative esotropia. The use of atropine allows determination of the maximum amount of hyperopia.

Cyclopentolate has become the drug of choice for the cycloplegic refraction of strabismic patients over 4 years of age and nonstrabismic patients of any age. Although atropine is still preferred for patients under 4 years of age with suspected accommodative esotropia, there is a trend toward the use of cyclopentolate in these patients.

Clinical Procedures: The use of atropine for the refractive examination of patients with suspected accommodative esotropia requires that the medication be instilled at home for 1 to 3 days prior to the office visit. This allows time for maximum cycloplegia to occur.

Cyclopentolate is used in the practitioner's office and is instilled 30 to 60 minutes prior to refractive examination. Once maximum cycloplegia has occurred, retinoscopy or subjective refraction is performed. Considerable skill and judgment are required to interpret the findings and prescribe a useful refractive correction.

Use in Uveitis

Uveitis is an inflammation of the iris, ciliary body or choroid of the eye. The inflammation can be limited to the anterior structures or the posterior structures of the eye, or both; the clinical features depend on the site of involvement. Uveitis can be classified based on the anatomic site of inflammation. For example, uveitis involving the iris only is termed iritis. Another method to classify the uveal inflammation is based on whether it affects the anterior or posterior structures of the eye. Uveitis can also be classified as either granulomatous or nongranulomatous. Any clinical classification system has considerable overlap, but these classifications provide the opportunity to differentiate various clinical presentations and predict the natural course of the uveal inflammation.

Etiology: Uveitis is thought to be an immune-complex disease with T-cell antigen dysfunction playing a major role. Idiopathic anterior uveitis is the most common clinical presentation. Human leukocyte antigen (HLA) studies are being undertaken to identify individuals who might be predisposed to recurrent episodes of uveitis or whose uveitis might be associated with other conditions. Systemic disorders are often associated with uveitis and include collagen diseases such as rheumatoid arthritis, ankylosing spondylitis and systemic lupus erythematosus. Other systemic causes include metabolic diseases, granulomatous diseases and infectious diseases such as herpes zoster and herpes simplex.

Diagnosis: The signs and symptoms of uveitis depend largely on the anatomic site of inflammation. Anterior uveitis is characterized by conjunctival hyperemia, the distribution of which often follows a circumcorneal pattern. The pupil is frequently miotic, and there is almost always an anterior chamber reaction manifested by cells and flare. The intraocular pressure may be reduced, and there are often keratic precipitates on the corneal endothelium as seen with the slit lamp. Symptoms include ocular pain, photophobia and blurred vision. Cases of anterior uveitis that are bilateral, recurrent or resistant to treatment should be considered for more extensive diagnostic evaluation for the presence of underlying systemic disease.

Posterior uveitis is characterized by little or no pain, and although there can be some anterior chamber reaction, inflammation of the vitreous (vitritis) is most prominent. If the macula is involved or if the vitreous is sufficiently hazy to diminish vision, visual acuity will be affected.

Drug Selection: Cycloplegics are useful in the treatment of anterior uveitis because they often prevent posterior synechiae. Cycloplegia places the ciliary body and iris at rest, reducing many of the associated symptoms, and cycloplegics also reduce the anterior chamber reaction. Cyclopentolate, homatropine and atropine are the most commonly used cycloplegic agents for the treatment of uveitis.

Topical corticosteroids are usually administered in conjunction with cycloplegic therapy. In severe cases, periocular or oral steroids may also be considered; immunosuppressive agents can be used in cases where corticosteroids may not be effective. If uveitic glaucoma ensues, antiglaucoma therapy is usually initiated.

Jimmy D. Bartlett, OD, DOS
University of Alabama at Birmingham

Siret D. Jaanus, PhD
Southern California College of Optometry

Thom Zimmerman, MD, PhD
University of Louisville

For More Information

Bartlett JD. Administration of and adverse reactions to cycloplegic agents. *Am J Optom Physiol Optics* 1978;55:227-33.

Bartlett JD, Jaanus SD, eds. Clinical Ocular Pharmacology, ed 2. Boston, MA: Butterworth, 1989.

Cremer SA, et al. Hydroxyamphetamine mydriasis in Horner's Syndrome. *Am J Ophthalmol* 1990;110:71-76.

Fraunfelder FT, Scafidi AF. Possible adverse effects from topical ocular 10% phenylephrine. *Am J Ophthalmol* 1978;85:862-68.

Gambill HD, et al. Mydriatic effect of four drugs determined by pupillograph. *Arch Ophthalmol* 1967;77:740-46.

Hendly DE, et al. Changing patterns of uveitis. *Am J Ophthalmol* 1987;103:131-36.

Moore BD. Cycloplegic refraction of young children. *N Engl J Optom* 1988;41:10-15.

Schlaegel TF. Nonspecific treatment of uveitis. In: Duane TD, Jaeger EA, eds. Clinical Ophthalmology. Philadelphia, PA: J.B. Lippincott, 1987.

Schlaegel TF. Perspectives in uveitis. *Ann Ophthalmol* 1981;13:799-806.

Thompson HS, Menscher JH. Adrenergic mydriasis in Horner's Syndrome: Hydroxyamphetamine test for diagnosis of postganglionic defects. *Am J Ophthalmol* 1971;72:472-80.

PHENYLEPHRINE HCl

Actions:

Phenylephrine ophthalmic solution possesses predominantly α-adrenergic effects. In the eye, phenylephrine acts locally as a potent vasoconstrictor and mydriatic by constricting ophthalmic blood vessels and the radial muscle of the iris. The ophthalmic usefulness of phenylephrine is due to its rapid effect and moderately prolonged action.

Actions of different concentrations of phenylephrine are shown in the following table:

PHENYLEPHRINE HCl			
Strength of solution (%)	Mydriasis		Paralysis of accommodation
	Maximal (min)	Recovery time (hrs)	
2.5	15 to 60	3	trace
10	10 to 60	6	slight

Although rare, systemic absorption of sufficient quantities of phenylephrine may lead to systemic α-adrenergic effects, such as rise in blood pressure, which may be accompanied by a reflex atropine-sensitive bradycardia.

Indications:

For use as a decongestant and vasoconstrictor and for pupil dilation in uveitis (posterior synechiae), open-angle glaucoma, prior to surgery, refraction without cycloplegia, ophthalmoscopic examination and diagnostic procedures (funduscopy).

Contraindications:

Hypersensitivity to any component of the formulation; narrow-angle glaucoma or individuals with a narrow (occludable) angle who do not have glaucoma; in low birth weight infants and in some elderly adults with severe arteriosclerotic cardiovascular or cerebrovascular disease; during intraocular operative procedures when the corneal epithelial barrier has been disturbed.

Phenylephrine 10%: In infants, small children with low body weights, debilitated or elderly patients and in patients with aneurysms. The administration of phenylephrine is contraindicated in patients with long-standing insulin-dependent diabetes, hypertensive patients receiving reserpine or guanethidine, advanced arteriosclerotic changes, idiopathic orthostatic hypotension and in those patients with a known history of organic cardiac disease.

In individuals with an intraocular lens implant, the administration of 10% phenylephrine is contraindicated due to the possibility of dislodging the lens.

Warnings:

Phenylephrine 10%: There have been rare reports of the development of serious cardiovascular reactions, including ventricular arrhythmias and myocardial infarctions. These episodes, some fatal, have usually occurred in elderly patients with preexisting cardiovascular diseases.

Elderly: Use with caution. Due to the strong action of phenylephrine 2.5% to 10% on the dilator muscle, older individuals may also develop transient pigment floaters in the aqueous humor 30 to 45 minutes following administration. The appearance may be similar to anterior uveitis or microscopic hyphema.

Rebound miosis occurs in some elderly patients. Subsequent instillation of phenyl-ephrine may produce less mydriasis than the initial instillation. This may be of clini-cal importance when dilating pupils prior to retinal detachment or cataract surgery. Exercise caution not to overdose these patients.

Pregnancy: Category C. Safety for use has not been established. Use only if clearly needed and potential benefits outweigh potential hazards to the fetus.

Lactation: It is not known whether this drug is excreted in breast milk. Use caution when phenylephrine HCl is administered to a nursing woman.

Children: Safety and efficacy for use in children have not been established. Phenyl-ephrine 2.5% has been used for a "one application method" in combination with a preferred rapid-acting cycloplegic (see Administration and Dosage). Phenylephrine 10% is contraindicated in infants.

Precautions:

Systemic absorption: Exceeding recommended dosages or applying phenylephrine 2.5% to 10% to the instrumented, traumatized, diseased or postsurgical eye or adnexa, or to patients with suppressed lacrimation, as during anesthesia, may result in the absorption of sufficient quantities to produce a systemic vasopressor response.

A significant elevation in blood pressure is rare but has been reported following con-junctival instillation of recommended doses of phenylephrine 10%. Use with caution in children of low body weight, the elderly and patients with insulin-dependent dia-betes, hypertension, hyperthyroidism, generalized arteriosclerosis or cardiovascular disease. Carefully monitor the posttreatment blood pressure of these patients and any patients who develop symptoms (see Contraindications).

The hypertensive effects of phenylephrine may be treated with an α-adrenergic blocking agent such as phentolamine mesylate, 5 mg to 10 mg IV, repeated as necessary.

Narrow-angle glaucoma: Ordinarily, mydriatics are contraindicated in glaucoma patients. However, when temporary pupil dilation may free adhesions, or when intrinsic vessel vasoconstriction may lower IOP, this may temporarily outweigh danger from coincident dilation.

Corneal effects: If the corneal epithelium has been denuded or damaged, corneal clouding may occur if phenylephrine 10% is instilled. This may be especially serious following corneal epithelium removal during retinal detachment surgery or vitrec-tomy. The corneas of diabetic patients may manifest epithelial ulcerations as well as a slow rate of reepithelialization. Use of phenylephrine in such corneas may be espe-cially hazardous.

Rebound congestion may occur with extended use of ophthalmic vasoconstrictors.

Sulfite Sensitivity: Some of these products contain sulfites. Sulfites may cause allergic-type reactions (eg, hives, itching, wheezing, anaphylaxis) in certain suscep-tible persons. Although the overall prevalence of sulfite sensitivity in the general population is probably low, it is seen more frequently in asthmatics or in atopic non-asthmatic persons. Specific products containing sulfites are identified in the product listings.

Drug Interactions:

Anesthetics: Use anesthetics that sensitize the myocardium to sympathomimetics (eg, cyclopropane or halothane) cautiously. Local anesthetics can increase ocular absorption of topical drugs. Exercise caution when applying prior to use of phenylephrine.

β-adrenergic blocking agents: Systemic side effects may occur more readily in patients taking these drugs. A severe hypertensive episode and fatal intracranial hemorrhage possibly associated with ophthalmic phenylephrine 10% was reported in one patient taking *propranolol* for hypertension.

MAOIs: When given with, or up to 21 days after MAOIs, exaggerated adrenergic effects may result. Supervise and adjust dosage carefully. The pressor response of adrenergic agents may also be potentiated by *tricyclic antidepressants, propranolol, reserpine, guanethidine, methyldopa* and *anticholinergics* (see Adverse Reactions).

Adverse Reactions:

Ocular: Transitory stinging on initial instillation; irritation; headache or browache; blurred vision; transient epithelial keratitis; hypersensitivity reactions (allergic conjunctivitis, dermatitis); reactive hyperemia. May cause rebound miosis and decreased mydriatic response to therapy in older persons (see Warnings).

Cardiovascular: Palpitations; tachycardia; cardiac arrhythmias; hypertension. Ventricular arrhythmias (ie, premature ventricular contractions), reflex bradycardia, coronary occlusion, pulmonary embolism, subarachnoid hemorrhage, myocardial infarction, stroke and death associated with cardiac reactions have been reported primarily in the elderly.

> *Phenylephrine 10%:* There have been rare reports of the development of serious cardiovascular reactions, including ventricular arrhythmias and myocardial infarctions. These episodes, some fatal, have usually occurred in elderly patients with preexisting cardiovascular diseases.

Other: Occipital headache; blanching; trembling or tremor; sweating; fainting; pallor; collapse.

Patient Information:

If severe eye pain, headache, vision changes, acute eye redness or pain with light exposure occur, discontinue use and consult a physician.

Potentially hazardous tasks: May cause temporary blurred vision. Observe caution while driving or performing other hazardous tasks.

To avoid contamination, do not touch dropper tip to any surface. Replace cap after using.

Administration and Dosage:

Compress the lacrimal sac by digital pressure for 2 to 3 minutes after instillation to avoid excessive systemic absorption.

To prevent pain, a drop of topical anesthetic may be applied before using the 10% solution.

Vasoconstriction and pupil dilation: Apply a drop of topical anesthetic. Follow in a few minutes by 1 drop of the 2.5% or 10% solution on the upper limbus. The anesthetic prevents stinging and consequent dilution of solution by lacrimation. It may be necessary to repeat the instillation after 1 hour, again preceded by the use of a topical anesthetic.

Uveitis: The formation of synechiae may be prevented by using the 2.5% or 10% solution and atropine to produce wide dilation of the pupil. However, the vasoconstrictor effect of phenylephrine may be antagonistic to the increase of local blood flow in uveal infection.

To free recently formed posterior synechiae, instill 1 drop of the 2.5% or 10% solution to the upper surface of the cornea. Continue treatment the following day, if necessary. In the interim, apply hot compresses for 5 or 10 minutes, 3 times daily, using 1 drop of 1% or 2% solution of atropine sulfate before and after each series of compresses.

Glaucoma: Instill 1 drop of 10% solution on the upper surface of the cornea as often as necessary. The 2.5% and the 10% solution may be used in conjunction with miotics in patients with open-angle glaucoma. Phenylephrine reduces the difficulties experienced by the patient because of the small field produced by miosis, and permits and often supports the effect of the miotic in lowering the IOP in open-angle glaucoma. Hence, there may be marked improvement in visual acuity after using phenylephrine with miotic drugs.

Surgery: When a short-acting mydriatic is needed for wide dilation of the pupil before intraocular surgery, the 2.5% or 10% solution may be instilled from 30 to 60 minutes before the operation.

Refraction: Prior to determination of refractive errors, the 2.5% solution may be used effectively with cyclopentolate HCl, tropicamide HCl, homatropine HBr, atropine sulfate or a combination of homatropine and cocaine HCl.

> *Adults:* Instill 1 drop of the preferred cycloplegic in each eye. Follow in 5 minutes with 1 drop of phenylephrine 2.5% and in 10 minutes with another drop of the cycloplegic. In 50 to 60 minutes, the eyes are ready for refraction.

> Since adequate cycloplegia is achieved at different time intervals after the instillation of the necessary number of drops, different cycloplegics will require different waiting periods.

> *Children:* Instill 1 drop of atropine sulfate 1% in each eye. Follow in 10 to 15 minutes with 1 drop of phenylephrine 2.5% solution and in 5 to 10 minutes with a second drop of atropine sulfate 1%. In 1 to 2 hours, the eyes are ready for refraction.

> *"One application method:"* Combine 2.5% solution and a cycloplegic to elicit synergistic action. The additive effect varies depending on the patient. Therefore, it may be desirable to increase the concentration of the cycloplegic.

Ophthalmoscopic examination: Instill 1 drop of 2.5% solution in each eye. Sufficient mydriasis is produced in 15 to 30 minutes and lasts 1 to 3 hours.

Diagnostic procedures: Heavily pigmented irides may require larger doses in all the following procedures:

> *Provocative test for angle block in patients with glaucoma:* The 2.5% solution may be used as a provocative test when latent increased IOP is suspected. Measure tension before application of phenylephrine and again after dilation. A 3 to 5 mm Hg rise in pressure suggests the presence of angle block in patients with glaucoma; however, failure to obtain such a rise does not preclude the presence of glaucoma from other causes.

> *Shadow test (retinoscopy):* When dilation of the pupil without cycloplegic action is desired, the 2.5% solution may be used alone.

> *Blanching test:* Instill 1 to 2 drops of the 2.5% solution to the injected eye. After 5 minutes, examine for perilimbal blanching. If blanching occurs, the congestion is superficial and probably does not indicate iritis.

Stability: Prolonged exposure to air or strong light may cause oxidation and discoloration. Do not use if solution is brown or contains a precipitate.

PHENYLEPHRINE HCl

Storage: Store at 36° to 86°F (2° to 30°C). Keep tightly closed. Protect from light.

				C.I.*
Rx	**Phenylephrine HCl** (Various, eg, Iolab, Steris)	**Solution:** 2.5%	In 2, 5 and 15 ml.	9+
Rx	**AK-Dilate** (Akorn)		In 2 and 15 ml.[1]	12
Rx	**Mydfrin 2.5%** (Alcon)		In 3 and 5 ml Drop-Tainers.[1]	47
Rx	**Neo-Synephrine** (Sanofi Winthrop)		In 15 ml.[2]	37
Rx	**Phenoptic** (Optopics)		In 2, 5 and 15 ml.	16
Rx	**Phenylephrine HCl** (Various, eg, Iolab, Steris)	**Solution:** 10%	In 1, 2, 5 and 15 ml.	25+
Rx	**AK-Dilate** (Akorn)		In 5 ml.[1]	34
Rx	**Neo-Synephrine** (Sanofi Winthrop)		In 5 ml.[3]	107
Rx	**Neo-Synephrine Viscous** (Sanofi Winthrop)		In 5 ml.[4]	104

HYDROXYAMPHETAMINE HBr

Actions:

Hydroxyamphetamine is an indirect-acting adrenergic agonist. Its pharmacologic effect is primarily due to release of norepinephrine from postganglionic adrenergic nerve terminals. Like phenylephrine, it has little, if any, effect on accommodation.

Indications:

For dilation of the pupil.

Contraindications:

Narrow-angle glaucoma.

Precautions:

Use with caution in patients with hypertension, hyperthyroidism and diabetes.

Adverse Reactions:

Increased IOP, photophobia and blurred vision may occur.

Overdosage:

If ocular overdosage occurs, dilute pilocarpine (1%) may be administered.

Instill one drop at intervals. Repeat as necessary.

If accidentally ingested, sedation is indicated. Further treatment is symptomatic.

Symptoms of overdosage may include hypertension, palpitations, cardiac arrhythmias, substernal discomfort, headache, sweating, nausea, vomiting and GI irritation.

Administration and Dosage:

Instill 1 or 2 drops into the conjunctival sac(s).

Storage: Store at room temperature 59° to 86°F (15° to 30°C).

Rx	**Paredrine** (Pharmics)	**Solution:** 1%	In 15 ml.[5]	44

* Cost Index based on cost per ml.
[1] With 0.01% benzalkonium chloride, EDTA and sodium bisulfite.
[2] With 1:7500 benzalkonium chloride.
[3] With 1:10,000 benzalkonium chloride.
[4] With 1:10,000 benzalkonium chloride and methylcellulose.
[5] With 1:50,000 thimerosal.

CYCLOPLEGIC MYDRIATICS, General Monograph

Actions:

Anticholinergic agents block the responses of the sphincter muscle of the iris and the muscle of the ciliary body to cholinergic stimulation, producing pupillary dilation (mydriasis) and paralysis of accommodation (cycloplegia).

	CYCLOPLEGIC MYDRIATICS				
	Mydriasis		Cycloplegia		
Drug	Peak (minutes)	Recovery (days)	Peak (minutes)	Recovery (days)	Solution Available (%)
Atropine	30-40	7-12	60-180	6-12	0.5-3
Homatropine	40-60	1-3	30-60	1-3	2-5
Scopolamine	20-30	3-7	30-60	3-7	0.25
Cyclopentolate	30-60	1	25-75	0.25-1	0.5-2
Tropicamide	20-40	0.25	20-35	0.25	0.5-1

Indications:

For cycloplegic refraction and for dilation of the pupil in inflammatory conditions of the iris and uveal tract.

Contraindications:

Primary glaucoma or a tendency toward glaucoma (eg, narrow anterior chamber angle); hypersensitivity to belladonna alkaloids or any component; adhesions (synechiae) between the iris and the lens; children who have previously had a severe systemic reaction to atropine; in the elderly and others where undiagnosed glaucoma or excessive pressure in the eye may be present.

Warnings:

For topical ophthalmic use only. Not for injection.

Do not exceed recommended dosages.

Determine the intraocular tension and the depth of the angle of the anterior chamber before and during use to avoid glaucoma attacks.

Excessive use in children and in certain susceptible individuals may produce systemic toxic symptoms. Use with extreme caution in infants and small children.

Pregnancy: Category C (atropine, homatropine). Safety for use during pregnancy has not been established. Use only if clearly needed and the potential benefits outweigh the potential hazards to the fetus.

Lactation: Atropine and homatropine are absorbed systemically and are detectable, in very small amounts, in breast milk. It is not known if cyclopentolate is excreted in breast milk. Because of the potential for serious adverse reactions in nursing infants, decide whether to discontinue nursing or discontinue the drug, taking into account the importance of the drug to the mother.

Children: Do not use atropine or homatropine during the first 3 months of life, due to the possible association between the cycloplegia produced and the development of amblyopia. Increased susceptibility to cyclopentolate has been reported in infants, young children and in children with spastic paralysis or brain damage. Feeding intolerance may follow ophthalmic use of this product in neonates. It is recommended that feeding be withheld for 4 hours after examination. Do not use in concentrations higher than 0.5% in small infants.

Tropicamide may cause CNS disturbances, which may be dangerous in infants and children. Keep in mind the possibility of occurrence of psychotic reaction and behavioral disturbance due to hypersensitivity to anticholinergic drugs. Use these drugs with extreme caution.

Use these products with caution in the elderly and others where increased IOP may be encountered.

Precautions:

Avoid excessive systemic absorption by compressing the lacrimal sac by digital pressure for 1 to 3 minutes after instillation.

Down's syndrome: Use cycloplegics with caution. These patients may demonstrate a hyperreactive response to topical atropine.

Acute hypersensitivity reaction: Have epinephrine 1:1000 immediately available. Discontinue use if signs of sensitivity develop.

Potentially hazardous tasks: May produce drowsiness, loss of neuromuscular coordination, blurred vision or sensitivity to light (due to dilated pupils). Observe caution while driving or performing other tasks requiring alertness.

Sulfite Sensitivity: Some of these products contain sulfites which may cause allergic-type reactions (eg, hives, itching, wheezing, anaphylaxis) in certain susceptible persons. Although the overall prevalence of sulfite sensitivity in the general population is probably low, it is seen more frequently in asthmatics or in atopic nonasthmatic persons. Products containing sulfites are identified in the product listings.

Adverse Reactions:

Local: Increased IOP; transient stinging. Prolonged use may produce irritation characterized by allergic lid reactions, hyperemia, follicular conjunctivitis, vascular congestion, edema, exudate and eczematoid dermatitis.

Systemic: Systemic toxicity is manifested by: Flushing and dryness of the mouth and skin (a rash may be present in children), blurred vision, photophobia with or without corneal staining, punctate keratitis, synechiae, tachycardia, headache, irritability, parasympathetic stimulation, a rapid and irregular pulse, fever, bladder distention, dysarthric quality of speech, mental aberration (hallucinosis), with recovery frequently followed by retrograde amnesia; and loss of neuromuscular coordination (ataxic gait). Other toxic manifestations of anticholinergic drugs are skin rash, abdominal distention in infants, unusual drowsiness, hyperpyrexia, vasodilation, urinary retention, diminished gastrointestinal motility and decreased secretion in salivary and sweat glands, pharynx, bronchii and nasal passages. Severe manifestations of toxicity include coma, medullary paralysis and death. Severe reactions are manifested by hypotension with progressive respiratory depression.

In addition, use of cyclopentolate and tropicamide has been associated with psychotic reactions and behavioral disturbances, usually in children. CNS disturbances have occurred in children with tropicamide. Ataxia, incoherent speech, restlessness, hallucinations, hyperactivity, seizures, disorientation as to time and place and failure to recognize people have been reported with cyclopentolate.

Overdosage:

If ocular overdosage occurs, flush eye(s) with water or normal saline. Use of a topical miotic may be required. If accidentally ingested, induce emesis or gastric lavage.

Systemic – When symptoms develop (see Adverse Reactions), give physostigmine salicylate as 1 to 5 ml IV of dilution containing 1 mg in 5 ml of saline. The smaller dose is for children, and injection should take not less than 2 minutes. EKG control is advisable. Dosage can be repeated every 5 minutes up to a total dose of 2 mg in children and 6 mg in adults every 30 minutes. Physostigmine is contraindicated in hypotensive reactions. Atropine (1 mg) should be available for immediate injection if physostigmine causes bradycardia, convulsions or bronchoconstriction. In infants and small children, the body surface must be kept moist.

Cyclopentolate toxicity may produce exaggerated symptoms (see Adverse Reactions). When administration of the drug product is discontinued, the patient usually recovers spontaneously. In case of severe manifestations of toxicity the antidote of choice is physostigmine salicylate.

> *Children* – Slowly inject 0.5 mg physostigmine salicylate IV. If toxic symptoms persist and no cholinergic symptoms are produced, repeat at 5-minute intervals to a maximum cumulative dose of 2 mg.

> *Adults and adolescents* – Slowly inject 2 mg physostigmine salicylate IV. A second dose of 1 to 2 mg may be given after 20 minutes if no reversal of toxic manifestations has occurred.

Patient Information:

If eye pain occurs, discontinue use and consult a physician immediately.

To avoid contamination, do not touch dropper tip to any surface. Replace cap after using.

May cause blurred vision. Do not drive or engage in any hazardous activities while the pupils are dilated.

May cause sensitivity to light. Protect eyes in bright illumination during dilation.

Keep out of the reach of children. These drugs should not be taken orally. Wash your own hands and the child's following administration.

Individual drug monographs are on the following pages.

ATROPINE SULFATE

For complete prescribing information see General Monograph p. 46.

Indications:

A potent parasympatholytic agent for use in producing cycloplegia and mydriasis. Useful for cycloplegic refraction or for pupil dilation in acute inflammatory conditions of the iris and uveal tract.

Administration and Dosage:

Solution:

Adults:

For uveitis – Instill 1 or 2 drops into the eye(s) up to 4 times daily.

For refraction – Instill 1 or 2 drops of the 1% solution into the eye(s) 1 hour before refracting.

Children:

For uveitis – Instill 1 or 2 drops of 0.5% solution into the eye(s) up to 3 times daily.

For refraction – Instill 1 or 2 drops of 0.5% solution into the eye(s) twice daily for 1 to 3 days before examination.

Ointment: A small amount in the conjunctival sac up to 3 times daily.

Compress the lacrimal sac by digital pressure for 1 to 3 minutes after instillation.

Individuals with heavily pigmented irides may require larger doses.

Storage: Store at 46° to 86°F (8° to 30°C).

				C.I.*
Rx	**Atropisol** (Iolab)	**Solution:** 0.5%	In 1 ml Dropperettes.[1]	54
Rx	**Isopto Atropine** (Alcon)		In 5 ml Drop-Tainers.[2]	53
Rx	**Atropine Sulfate** (Various, eg, Alcon, Allergan, Bausch and Lomb, Fougera, Moore, Rugby, Schein, Steris)	**Solution:** 1%	In 2, 5 and 15 ml and UD 1 ml.	6+
Rx	**Atropine Care** (Akorn)		In 2, 5 and 15 ml.[3]	25
Rx	**Atropine-1** (Optopics)		In 2, 5 and 15 ml.	17
Rx	**Atropisol** (Iolab)		In 5[4] and 15[4] ml and 1 ml Dropperettes.[1]	36
Rx	**Isopto Atropine** (Alcon)		In 5 and 15 ml Drop-Tainers.[2]	60
Rx	**Atropine Sulfate** (Alcon)	**Solution:** 2%	In 2 ml.	53
Rx	**Atropisol** (Iolab)		In 1 ml Dropperettes.[1]	54
Rx	**Isopto Atropine** (Alcon)	**Solution:** 3%	In 5 ml Drop-Tainers.[2]	67
Rx	**Atropine Sulfate S.O.P.** (Allergan)	**Ointment:** 0.5%	In 3.5 g.[5]	64

* Cost Index based on cost per g or ml.
[1] With benzalkonium chloride.
[2] With 0.01% benzalkonium chloride and 0.5% hydroxypropyl methylcellulose.
[3] With 0.01% benzalkonium chloride and hydroxypropyl methylcellulose.
[4] With benzalkonium chloride and EDTA.
[5] With 0.5% chlorobutanol, white petrolatum, mineral oil and petrolatum (and) lanolin alcohol.

ATROPINE SULFATE (Cont.) C.I.*

				C.I.*
Rx	**Atropine Sulfate** (Various, eg, Fougera, Moore, Pharmafair, Rugby, Schein)	**Ointment:** 1%	In 3.5 g and UD 1 g.	21+
Rx	**Atropine Care** (Akorn)		In 3.5 g.[1]	72
Rx	**Atropine Sulfate S.O.P.** (Allergan)		In 3.5 g.[2]	44

HOMATROPINE HBr

For complete prescribing information see General Monograph p. 46.

Indications:

A moderately long-acting mydriatic and cycloplegic for refraction and in the treatment of inflammatory conditions of the uveal tract. For preoperative and postoperative states when mydriasis is required. As an optical aid in some cases of axial lens opacities.

Administration and Dosage:

For refraction: Instill 1 or 2 drops into the eye(s). Repeat in 5 to 10 minutes if necessary.

For uveitis: Instill 1 or 2 drops into the eye(s) up to every 3 to 4 hours.

Only the 2% strength should be used in pediatric patients.

Compress the lacrimal sac by digital pressure for 1 to 3 minutes after instillation.

Individuals with heavily pigmented irides may require larger doses.

Storage: Store at room temperature 59° to 86°F (15° to 30°C).

				C.I.*
Rx	**Homatropine HBr** (Iolab)	**Solution:** 2%	In 1 and 5 ml.	56
Rx	**Isopto Homatropine** (Alcon)		In 5 and 15 ml Drop-Tainers.[3]	63
Rx	**Homatropine HBr** (Various, eg, Alcon, Iolab)	**Solution:** 5%	In 1, 2 and 5 ml.	50+
Rx	**AK-Homatropine** (Akorn)		In 5 ml dropper bottles.[4]	34
Rx	**Isopto Homatropine** (Alcon)		In 5 and 15 ml Drop-Tainers.[5]	72

* Cost Index based on cost per g or ml.
[1] With 0.5% chlorobutanol, white petrolatum, mineral oil and anhydrous lanolin.
[2] With 0.5% chlorobutanol, white petrolatum, mineral oil and petrolatum (and) lanolin alcohol.
[3] With 0.01% benzalkonium chloride, 0.5% hydroxypropyl methylcellulose, polysorbate 80 and NaCl.
[4] With 0.01% benzalkonium chloride, hydroxyethyl cellulose and EDTA.
[5] With 0.005% benzethonium chloride, 0.5% hydroxypropyl methylcellulose and NaCl.

SCOPOLAMINE HBr (Hyoscine HBr)

For complete prescribing information see General Monograph p. 46.

Indications:

For cycloplegia and mydriasis in diagnostic procedures. For some preoperative and postoperative states in the treatment of iridocyclitis.

Administration and Dosage:

For refraction: Instill 1 or 2 drops into the eye(s) 1 hour before refracting.

For uveitis: Instill 1 or 2 drops into the eye(s) up to 4 times daily.

Compress the lacrimal sac by digital pressure for 2 to 3 minutes after instillation.

Storage: Store at 46° to 80°F (8° to 27°C). Protect from light.

C.I.*

Rx	Isopto Hyoscine (Alcon)	Solution: 0.25%	In 5 and 15 ml Drop-Tainers.[1]	63

CYCLOPENTOLATE HCl

For complete prescribing information see General Monograph p. 46.

Indications:

For mydriasis and cycloplegia in diagnostic procedures.

Administration and Dosage:

Adults: Instill 1 or 2 drops of 0.5%, 1% or 2% solution into eye(s). Repeat in 5 to 10 minutes, if necessary. Complete recovery usually occurs in 24 hours.

Children: Instill 1 or 2 drops of 0.5%, 1% or 2% solution into each eye. Follow in 5 to 10 minutes with a second application of 0.5% or 1% solution, if necessary.

> *Small infants:* Instill one drop of 0.5% solution into each eye. To minimize absorption, apply pressure over the nasolacrimal sac for 2 to 3 minutes. Observe patient closely for at least 30 minutes following instillation.

Compress the lacrimal sac by digital pressure for 1 to 2 minutes after instillation.

Individuals with heavily pigmented irides may require higher strengths.

Storage: Store at 46° to 86°F (8° to 30°C).

C.I.*

Rx	Cyclogyl (Alcon)	Solution: 0.5%	In 2, 5 and 15 ml Drop-Tainers.[2]	63
Rx	Cyclopentolate HCl (Various, eg, Bausch & Lomb, Schein, Steris)	Solution: 1%	In 2, 5 and 15 ml.	15+
Rx	AK-Pentolate (Akorn)		In 2 and 15 ml.[3]	62
Rx	Cyclogyl (Alcon)		In 2, 5 and 15 ml Drop-Tainers.[2]	73
Rx	Cyclogyl (Alcon)	Solution: 2%	In 2, 5 and 15 ml Drop-Tainers.[2]	90

* Cost Index based on cost per ml.
[1] With 0.01% benzalkonium chloride, 0.5% hydroxypropyl methylcellulose and sodium chloride.
[2] With 0.01% benzalkonium chloride and EDTA.
[3] With 0.01% benzalkonium chloride and 0.01% EDTA.

TROPICAMIDE

For complete prescribing information see General Monograph p. 46.

Indications:

For mydriasis and cycloplegia for diagnostic purposes.

Administration and Dosage:

For refraction: Instill 1 or 2 drops of 1% solution into the eye(s). Repeat in 5 minutes. If patient is not seen within 20 to 30 minutes, instill an additional drop to prolong mydriatic effect.

For examination of fundus: Instill 1 or 2 drops of 0.5% solution 15 to 20 minutes prior to examination.

Compress the lacrimal sac by digital pressure for 2 to 3 minutes after instillation to avoid excessive systemic absorption.

Individuals with heavily pigmented irides may require larger doses.

Storage: Store at 46° to 80°F (8° to 27°C). Store away from heat. Do not refrigerate.

				C.I.*
Rx	**Tropicamide** (Bausch & Lomb, Steris)	**Solution:** 0.5%	In 15 ml.	17+
Rx	**Mydriacyl** (Alcon)		In 15 ml Drop-Tainers.[1]	41
Rx	**Opticyl** (Optopics)		In 2 ml and 15 ml.	11
Rx	**Tropicacyl** (Akorn)		In 15 ml.[2]	18
Rx	**Tropicamide** (Bausch & Lomb, Steris)	**Solution:** 1%	In 15 ml.	9+
Rx	**Mydriacyl** (Alcon)		In 3 and 15 ml Drop-Tainers.[1]	44
Rx	**Opticyl** (Optopics)		In 2 ml and 15 ml.	14
Rx	**Tropicacyl** (Akorn)		In 2 and 15 ml.[2]	21

* Cost Index based on cost per ml.
[1] With 0.01% benzalkonium chloride, EDTA and sodium chloride.
[2] With 0.1% benzalkonium chloride and EDTA.

MYDRIATRIC COMBINATIONS

Phenylephrine HCl (p. 41) is used with cyclopentolate HCl (p. 46) or scopolamine HBr (p. 46) to induce mydriasis that is considerably greater than that of either drug alone.

C.I.*

Rx	**Cyclomydril** (Alcon)	**Solution:** 0.2% cyclopentolate HCl and 1% phenyl-ephrine HCl. In 2 and 5 ml Drop-Tainers.[1] **Indications:** For the production of mydriasis. **Dose:** Instill 1 drop into each eye every 5 to 10 minutes, not to exceed 3 times.	72
Rx	**Murocoll-2** (Bausch & Lomb)	**Drops:** 0.3% scopolamine HBr and 10% phenylephrine HCl. In 5 ml.[2] **Indications:** For mydriasis, cycloplegia and to break posterior synechiae in iritis. **Dose:** *For mydriasis* – 1 or 2 drops into eye(s); repeat in 5 minutes, if necessary. *Postoperatively* – 1 or 2 drops into eye(s), 3 or 4 times daily.	75
Rx	**Paremyd** (Allergan)	**Solution:** 1% hydroxyamphetamine HBr, 0.25% tropicamide. In 5 and 15 ml.[3] **Indications:** For mydriasis with partial cycloplegia. **Dose:** Instill 1 to 2 drops into the conjunctival sac(s).	NA

* Cost Index based on cost per ml.
[1] With 0.01% benzalkonium chloride and EDTA.
[2] With 0.01% benzalkonium chloride, sodium metabisulfite and EDTA.
[3] With 0.005% benzalkonium chloride, 0.015% EDTA and sodium chloride.

Antiallergy and Decongestant Agents

Histamine release can cause a variety of uncomfortable symptoms and sometimes life-threatening complications. Drug therapy is often successful in satisfactorily relieving associated signs and symptoms, especially when ocular tissues are affected.

Type I hypersensitivity reactions, also known as anaphylactic, immediate or IgE-mediated reactions, occur when an antigen such as a drug or pollen is reintroduced into an individual who has been previously exposed to the antigen. Upon initial exposure to the antigen, IgE antibodies are produced which attach to mast cells and make the cells susceptible to rupture when the patient is again exposed to the same antigen. Disruption (degranulation) of mast cells causes a release of large quantities of inflammatory mediators, including histamine, and the histamine activates H_1 receptors on blood vessels, causing vasodilation. These dilated blood vessels leak fluid, causing tissues to swell. Common symptoms and signs of local Type I reactions include redness, swelling and itching. Such reactions occur in hay fever, allergic conjunctivitis, asthma, bee stings and other chemical and toxin sensitivities (eg, penicillin). The following ocular diseases are characterized by Type I hypersensitivity reactions and may be treated with antihistamines or cromolyn sodium.

ALLERGIC CONDITIONS

Hay Fever Conjunctivitis

Allergic conjunctivitis can result from a variety of exogenous antigens and is often a component of more widespread allergic states. Airborne pollens, dust and other environmental contaminants constitute the largest single group of agents responsible for the disorder. Ophthalmic drugs and their preservatives/excipients which may cause allergic conjunctivitis include neomycin, sulfonamides, atropine and thimerosal. A careful patient history along with the typical appearance of conjunctival chemosis and hyperemia, together with itching and tearing, are necessary for the proper etiologic diagnosis.

Vernal Conjunctivitis

Affecting primarily adolescent males, vernal conjunctivitis is a bilateral inflammation involving the upper tarsal conjunctiva and sometimes the limbal conjunctiva. The disease is seasonal and has peak activity during the warm months of the year. It is characterized by the formation of large papillae having the appearance of cobblestones on the upper tarsal conjunctiva. Papillary hypertrophy can occur at the limbus and is characterized by a gelatinous thickening of the superior limbus. Tear histamine levels are significantly higher than in normal patients. Symptoms include intense itching during warm months and often a thick, ropy discharge. If the cornea becomes involved, photophobia may be marked. Significant papillary involvement of the upper lids may result in ptosis.

Atopic Keratoconjunctivitis

Atopic keratoconjunctivitis represents a hypersensitivity state caused by predispositional, constitutional or hereditary factors rather than by acquired hypersensitivity to specific antigens. Patients usually have a personal or family history of allergy, especially asthma or hay fever. Atopic dermatitis is characterized by patches of thickened, excoriated, lichenified skin which is usually dry and itchy. Ocular findings are characterized by conjunctival hyperemia and chemosis. Corneal involvement is not uncommon and may be evident as a classic shield ulcer or pannus.

Giant Papillary Conjunctivitis

Giant papillary conjunctivitis (GPC) is a specific conjunctival inflammatory reaction to materials on contact lenses (eg, protein), but has also been reported in patients wearing methylmethacrylate ocular prostheses. The condition is characterized by papillary hypertrophy and primarily affects the upper tarsal conjunctiva. Although the condition is similar in appearance to that of vernal conjunctivitis, it probably represents a chronic conjunctival inflammatory reaction to denatured proteins that are adherent to the anterior lens surface. Lens bulk (thickness and diameter) may also play a part. Once the conjunctival changes reach a certain point, itching, lens instability, mucoid discharge and contact lens intolerance occur.

DECONGESTANTS

The vasoconstrictor effect of the adrenergic agonists (ie, phenylephrine and the imidazole derivatives) makes them useful as topical ocular decongestants. Following instillation, conjunctival vessels constrict within minutes, causing the eye to whiten. Minor ocular irritation can be temporarily relieved.

Due to the relatively low concentrations required for ocular decongestion, phenylephrine and the imidazole derivatives generally do not cause systemic side effects. These products are designed for short-term use since they may mask symptoms of more serious ocular problems such as bacterial or other infections. If the condition does not respond to use within 48 hours, a more serious condition should be suspected.

Phenylephrine

Phenylephrine (eg, *Neo-Synephrine*), a synthetic amine structurally similar to epinephrine, is present in several over-the-counter products. Concentrations of 0.12% or 0.125% cause vasoconstriction with little or no pupillary dilation in eyes with intact corneal epithelium. Since a potential for mydriasis does exist at low concentration, phenylephrine is contraindicated in eyes predisposed to angle-closure glaucoma. Prolonged or excessive use can result in rebound conjunctival hyperemia. The eye may become more congested and red as the effect of the drug begins to subside.

Phenylephrine can exhibit variable effectiveness since it is subject to oxidation on exposure to air, light or heat. The solution may show no evidence of discoloration. To prolong shelf life, antioxidants such as sodium bisulfite may be added to the formulation.

Imidazole Derivatives

The imidazole derivatives, naphazoline (eg, *Naphcon*), tetrahydrozoline (eg, *Visine*) and oxymetazoline (*OcuClear*), differ structurally from phenylephrine by replacement of the benzene ring with an unsaturated ring. Concentrations used for ocular vasoconstriction do not alter pupil size or raise intraocular pressure in the normal eye.

The imidazole derivatives do not differ significantly in their ability to relieve conjunctival congestion. After instillation, the blanching effect occurs within minutes and may last up to several hours. These agents are generally more stable in solution than phenylephrine, and have a longer shelf life and duration of action. Imidazole derivatives are buffered to a pH of 6.2 and may sting upon initial instillation. Naphazoline is also available at higher concentrations as a prescription ophthalmic solution.

COMBINATION PRODUCTS

In addition to vasoconstrictor substances, ocular decongestants may also contain preservatives, antihistamines, viscosity-increasing agents, buffers and astringents. Since preservatives may induce allergic reactions in some patients, unit-dose preservative-free products are being formulated.

PHARMACOLOGIC MANAGEMENT

Since much of the symptomatic picture of Type I hypersensitivity reactions is caused by histamine release from mast cells, antihistamines are usually effective in relieving annoying symptoms. These agents are usually given with decongestants and are administered topically or orally, depending on the degree of involvement. Mast cell stabilizers such as cromolyn sodium *(Opticrom 4%)* are also effective and can even be used prophylactically. For severe reactions or when rapid relief of symptoms is warranted, topical or oral corticosteroids may be justified. In addition, ketorolac tromethamine *(Acular),* a nonsteroidal anti-inflammatory agent, is indicated for the relief of ocular itching due to seasonal allergic conjunctivitis, see p. 82.

Jimmy D. Bartlett, OD, DOS
University of Alabama at Birmingham

Siret D. Jaanus, PhD
Southern California College of Optometry

For More Information

Abelson MB, et al. Effects of ocular decongestants. *Arch Ophthalmol* 1980;98:856-58.

Allansmith MR. Vernal conjunctivitis. In: Duane TD, Jaeger EA, eds. Clinical Ophthalmology. Philadelphia, PA: J.B. Lippincott, 1987.

Allansmith MR, Ross RN. Ocular allergy and mast cell stabilizers. *Surv Ophthalmol* 1986;30:229-44.

Bartlett JD, Jaanus SD, eds. Clinical Ocular Pharmacology, ed 2. Boston, MA; Butterworth, 1989.

Bartlett JD, Ross RN. Primary care of ocular allergy. *J Am Optom Assoc* 1990;61(6) (Suppl):S3-S46.

Bartlett JD, Swanson MW. Ophthalmic products. In: Covington T, ed. Handbook of Non-Prescription Drugs, 10th ed. Washington DC: American Pharmaceutical Association, 1993.

Butler K, et al. Effects of non-prescription ocular decongestants. *Rev Optom* 1978;115:49-52.

Donshik PC, et al. Treatment of contact lens-induced giant papillary conjunctivitis. *CLAO J* 1984;10:346-50.

CROMOLYN SODIUM (Sodium Cromoglycate)

Actions:

Animal studies show that cromolyn sodium inhibits the degranulation of sensitized mast cells which occurs after exposure to specific antigens, thus inhibiting the release of histamine and SRS-A (slow-reacting substance of anaphylaxis) from the mast cell. It has no intrinsic vasoconstrictor, antihistaminic or anti-inflammatory activity.

Pharmacokinetics: Cromolyn sodium is poorly absorbed. When multiple doses are instilled into normal rabbit eyes, less than 0.07% of the administered dose is absorbed into the systemic circulation (presumably by way of the eye, nasal passages, buccal cavity and GI tract). Trace amounts (less than 0.01%) penetrate into the aqueous humor, and clearance from this chamber is virtually complete within 24 hours after treatment is stopped.

In normal volunteers, approximately 0.03% of cromolyn sodium is absorbed following administration to the eye.

Indications:

For the treatment of allergic ocular disorders including vernal keratoconjunctivitis; vernal conjunctivitis; giant papillary conjunctivitis; vernal keratitis and allergic keratoconjunctivitis.

Contraindications:

Hypersensitivity to cromolyn or to any component of the formulation.

As with all ophthalmic preparations containing benzalkonium chloride, patients are advised not to wear soft contact lenses during cromolyn sodium treatment. Wear can be resumed within a few hours after discontinuation of the drug.

Warnings:

Pregnancy: Category B. There are no adequate and well-controlled studies in pregnant women. Use during pregnancy only if clearly needed.

Lactation: It is not known whether this drug is excreted in breast milk. Exercise caution when administering to a nursing mother.

Children: Safety and efficacy in children under 4 have not been established.

Adverse Reactions:

Most frequent: Transient ocular stinging or burning upon instillation that usually regresses with continued use.

Infrequent (unclear whether attributable to the drug): Conjunctival injection; watery, itchy and puffy eyes; dryness around eyes; erythema; eye irritation and styes.

Patient Information:

A transient stinging or burning sensation may occur after instillation.

Do not wear soft contact lenses during treatment. Lenses may be worn within a few hours after discontinuation of the drug.

Administer the drug at regular intervals. Do not exceed recommended frequency of administration.

Administration and Dosage:

Symptomatic response to therapy (decreased itching, tearing, redness and discharge) is usually evident within a few days, but treatment for up to 6 weeks is sometimes required. Effect of therapy depends upon administration at regular intervals. Continue therapy as long as needed to sustain improvement. Corticosteroids may be used concomitantly.

Adults and children: Instill 1 to 2 drops in each eye 4 to 6 times daily at regular intervals. One drop contains approximately 1.6 mg cromolyn sodium.

Storage: Store below 86°F (30°C). Protect from light.

Rx **Opticrom 4%** (Fisons)	**Solution:** 40 mg per ml	In 10 ml dropper bottles.[1]

[1] With 0.01% benzalkonium chloride and 0.1% EDTA.

DECONGESTANTS, General Monograph

Actions:

Phenylephrine 0.12%, epinephrine, naphazoline and tetrahydrozoline are used as ophthalmic decongestants (vasoconstriction of conjunctival blood vessels) to relieve minor eye irritations.

OPHTHALMIC DECONGESTANTS		
Vasoconstrictor	Concentration	Duration (hr)
Epinephrine	0.1%	1 to 3
Naphazoline	0.012% 0.02% 0.025% 0.05% 0.1%	2 to 3
Oxymetazoline	0.025%	up to 6
Phenylephrine	0.12%	0.5 to 1.5
Tetrahydrozoline	0.05%	1 to 4

Phenylephrine possesses predominantly α-adrenergic effects. In the eye, it acts locally as a potent vasoconstrictor and mydriatic, by constricting blood vessels and the radial muscle of the iris. The ophthalmologic usefulness of phenylephrine HCl is due to its rapid effect and moderately prolonged action. It produces no compensatory vasodilation.

Naphazoline constricts the vascular system of the conjunctiva. It is presumed that this effect is due to direct stimulation action of the drug upon the α adrenergic receptors in the arterioles of the conjunctiva resulting in decreased conjunctival congestion. Naphazoline belongs to the imidazoline class of sympathomimetics.

Indications:

Refer to individual product listings for specific indications.

Contraindications:

Hypersensitivity to any component of the formulation; narrow-angle glaucoma.

Warnings:

Anesthetics: Discontinue prior to use of anesthetics that sensitize the myocardium to sympathomimetics (eg, cyclopropane or halothane). Local anesthetics can increase absorption of topical drugs; exercise caution when applying prior to use of phenylephrine.

Pregnancy: Category C (Epinephrine, phenylephrine, naphazoline). Safety for use has not been established. Use only if clearly needed and if the potential benefits outweigh the potential hazards to the fetus.

Lactation: It is not known whether these drugs are excreted in breast milk. Because many drugs are excreted in breast milk, use caution when epinephrine, naphazoline and/or antazoline is administered to a nursing woman.

Children: Safety and efficacy for use in children have not been established. Naphazoline use in children, especially infants, may result in CNS depression leading to coma and marked reduction in body temperature.

Elderly: Use with caution.

Precautions:

Use with caution in the presence of hypertension, diabetes, hyperthyroidism, cardiovascular abnormalities (eg, hypertensive coronary artery disease, cerebral arteriosclerosis), long-standing bronchial asthma (epinephrine), infection or injury.

Narrow-angle glaucoma: Ordinarily, mydriatics are contraindicated in glaucoma patients. However, when temporary pupil dilation may free adhesions, or when intrinsic vessel vasoconstriction may lower intraocular pressure, benefits may temporarily outweigh danger from coincident dilation. Use with caution.

Rebound congestion may occur with extended use of ophthalmic vasoconstrictors.

Systemic absorption: Exceeding recommended dosages to the instrumented, traumatized, diseased or postsurgical eye or adnexa, or to patients with suppressed lacrimation, as during anesthesia, may result in the absorption of sufficient quantities to produce a systemic vasopressor response.

Sulfite Sensitivity: Some of these products contain sulfites. Sulfites may cause allergic-type reactions (eg, hives, itching, wheezing, anaphylaxis) in certain susceptible persons. Although the overall prevalence of sulfite sensitivity in the general population is probably low, it is seen more frequently in asthmatics or in atopic nonasthmatic persons. Specific products containing sulfites are identified in the product listings.

Drug Interactions:

Anesthetics: Use anesthetics which sensitize the myocardium to sympathomimetics (eg, cyclopropane or halothane) cautiously. Local anesthetics can increase absorption of topical drugs; exercise caution when applying prior to use of phenylephrine.

β-adrenergic blocking agents: Systemic side effects may occur more readily in patients taking these drugs. A severe hypertensive episode and fatal intracranial hemorrhage associated with ophthalmic phenylephrine 10% was reported in one patient taking propranolol for hypertension.

MAOIs: When given with, or up to 21 days after MAOIs, severe hypertensive crisis may result. Supervise and adjust dosage carefully. The pressor response of adrenergic agents may also be potentiated by *tricyclic antidepressants, β-blockers, reserpine, guanethidine, methyldopa* and *anticholinergics.*

Adverse Reactions:

Ocular: Transitory stinging on initial instillation, blurring of vision. Overuse may cause increased redness of the eye. Rarely, maculopathy with a central scotoma results from use in aphakic patients; prompt reversal generally follows discontinuation.

> *Epinephrine* has been reported to cause melanin deposits in the conjunctiva and cornea after prolonged therapy. Eye pain or ache, conjunctival hyperemia, allergy and allergic lid reactions may occur.

> *Phenylephrine* may cause rebound miosis and decreased mydriatic response to therapy in older persons.

> *Naphazoline* has been reported to cause mydriasis, increased redness, irritation, discomfort, pupillary dilation, punctate keratitis, lacrimation and increased or decreased intraocular pressure.

Systemic: Dizziness, headache, nausea, sweating, decreased body temperature, nervousness, drowsiness, weakness, hypertension, cardiac irregularities and hyperglycemia.

Cardiovascular: Palpitations, tachycardia, extrasystoles, cardiac arrhythmias. Headache or browache may occur, but usually diminishes as treatment is continued. Ventricular arrhythmias (ie, premature ventricular contractions), reflex bradycardia, coronary occlusion, pulmonary embolism, subarachnoid hemorrhage, myocardial infarction, stroke and death associated with cardiac reactions have been reported.

There have been rare reports associating the use of phenylephrine 10% ophthalmic solutions with the development of serious cardiovascular reactions. These episodes, some fatal, have occurred in elderly patients with preexisting cardiovascular diseases.

Other: Occipital headache, blanching, tremor, sweating, faintness and pallor.

Patient Information:

Discontinue the drug and consult your doctor if relief is not obtained in 48 to 72 hours, if irritation, blurring or redness persists or increases, or if symptoms of systemic absorption occur (eg, dizziness, headache, nausea, decrease in body temperature or drowsiness).

To avoid contamination, do not touch tip of the container to any surface. Replace cap after using.

Potentially hazardous tasks: Phenylephrine may cause temporary blurred or unstable vision. Observe caution while driving or performing other hazardous tasks.

Keep out of the reach of children.

Remove contact lenses before using these products.

Overuse of these products may cause increased redness.

Individual drug monographs are on the following pages.

NAPHAZOLINE HCl

For complete prescribing information see General Monograph p. 60.

Indications:

For use as a topical ocular vasoconstrictor.

To soothe, refresh, moisturize and remove redness due to minor eye irritation.

Administration and Dosage:

Instill 1 or 2 drops into the conjunctival sac of affected eye(s) every 3 to 4 hours.

Storage: Store at room temperature 59° to 86° F (15° to 30° C). Protect from light. Keep tightly closed. Do not use if solution changes color or becomes cloudy.

			C.I.*
otc **Allerest Eye Drops** (Fisons)	**Solution:** 0.012%	In 15 ml.[1]	6
otc **Clear Eyes** (Ross)		In 15 and 30 ml.[2]	5
otc **Degest 2** (Sola/Barnes-Hind)		In 15 ml.[3]	12
otc **Estivin II** (Alcon)		In 7.5 ml.[4]	31
otc **Naphcon** (Alcon)		In 15 ml.[5]	22
otc **VasoClear** (Iolab)	**Solution:** 0.02%	In 15 ml.[6]	11
otc **Maximum Strength Allergy Drops** (Bausch & Lomb)	**Solution:** 0.03%	In 15 ml.[7]	NA

* Cost Index based on cost per ml.
[1] With 0.01% benzalkonium chloride and 0.1% EDTA.
[2] With benzalkonium chloride, EDTA and 0.2% glycerin.
[3] With 0.0067% benzalkonium chloride, 0.02% EDTA, hydroxyethyl cellulose and povidone.
[4] With 0.01% benzalkonium chloride, 0.1% dextran 70, 0.3% hydroxypropyl methylcellulose, EDTA and sodium chloride.
[5] With 0.01% benzalkonium chloride, EDTA and sodium chloride.
[6] With 0.01% benzalkonium chloride, 0.25% polyvinyl alcohol, PEG-400, EDTA and sodium chloride.
[7] With 0.01% benzalkonium chloride, 0.5% hydroxypropyl methylcellulose, EDTA and sodium chloride.

NAPHAZOLINE HCl (Cont.)   C.I.*

Rx	**Naphazoline HCl** (Various, eg, Major, Moore, Rugby, Schein)	**Solution:** 0.1%	In 15 ml.	10+
Rx	**AK-Con** (Akorn)		In 15 ml dropper bottles.[1]	11
Rx	**Albalon** (Allergan America)		In 15 ml.[2]	21
Rx	**Muro's Opcon** (Bausch & Lomb)		In 15 ml.[3]	18
Rx	**Naphcon Forte** (Alcon)		In 15 ml Drop-Tainers.[4]	28
Rx	**Vasocon Regular** (Iolab)		In 15 ml.[5]	19

OXYMETAZOLINE HCl

For complete prescribing information see General Monograph p. 60.

Indications:

For relief of redness of the eye due to minor irritations.

Administration and Dosage:

Adults and children 6 years and older: Instill 1 or 2 drops into the affected eye(s). This may be repeated every 6 hours.

Storage: Store at 36° to 86° F (2° to 30° C). Do not use if solution changes color or becomes cloudy.

				C.I.*
otc	**Visine L.R.** (Pfizer)	**Solution:** 0.025%	In 15 and 30 ml.[6]	7

PHENYLEPHRINE HCl

For complete prescribing information see Phenylephrine p. 41 and Decongestant General Monograph p. 60.

Indications:

A decongestant to provide relief of redness of the eye due to minor irritations.

For use as a lubricant to prevent further irritation or to relieve dryness of the eye.

Administration and Dosage:

Minor eye irritations: Instill 1 or 2 drops of the 0.12% solution into the affected eye(s) up to 4 times daily, as needed. Do not use if solution changes color or becomes cloudy.

* Cost Index based on cost per ml.
[1] With 0.01% benzalkonium chloride and 0.01% EDTA.
[2] With 0.004% benzalkonium chloride, EDTA, 1.4% polyvinyl alcohol and sodium chloride.
[3] With 0.5% hydroxypropyl methylcellulose, 0.01% benzalkonium chloride, EDTA and sodium chloride.
[4] With 0.01% benzalkonium chloride, EDTA and sodium chloride.
[5] With benzalkonium chloride, polyvinyl alcohol, EDTA, PEG-8000 and sodium chloride.
[6] With 0.01% benzalkonium chloride, 0.1% EDTA and sodium chloride.

PHENYLEPHRINE HCl (Cont.) C.I.*

otc	AK-Nefrin (Akorn)	Solution: 0.12%	In 15 ml.[1]	7
otc	Isopto Frin (Alcon)		In 15 ml.[2]	22
otc	Prefrin Liquifilm (Allergan)		In 20 ml dropper bottles.[3]	11
otc	Relief (Allergan)		Preservative free. In UD 0.3 ml.[4]	24

TETRAHYDROZOLINE HCl

For complete prescribing information see General Monograph p. 60.

Indications:

For relief of redness of the eye due to minor irritations.

For temporary relief of burning and irritation due to dryness of the eye and/or discomfort due to minor irritations or to exposure to wind or sun.

Administration and Dosage:

Instill 1 or 2 drops into the affected eye(s) up to 4 times daily.

Storage: Store at room temperature 59° to 86°F (15° to 30°C). Do not use if solution changes color or becomes cloudy.

C.I.*

otc	Tetrahydrozoline HCl (Various, eg, Moore, Rugby, Steris)	Solution: 0.05%	In 15 and 30 ml.	2+
otc	Collyrium Fresh Eye Drops (Wyeth-Ayerst)		In 15 ml.[5]	6
otc	Eyesine (Akorn)		In 15 ml.[6]	3
otc	Mallazine Eye Drops (Hauck)		In 15 ml.[7]	4
otc	Murine Plus (Ross)		In 15 and 30 ml.[8]	6
otc	Optigene 3 (Pfeiffer)		In 15 ml.[9]	4
otc	Soothe (Alcon)		In 15 ml.[10]	19
otc	Visine (Pfizer)		In 15, 22.5 and 30 ml and 15 ml with dropper.[11]	6
otc	Visine Extra (Pfizer)		In 15 and 30 ml.[12]	7

* Cost Index based on cost per ml.
[1] With 0.01% benzalkonium chloride, 0.5% hydroxyethyl cellulose, EDTA and sodium chloride.
[2] With 0.01% benzethonium chloride and 0.5% hydroxypropyl methylcellulose.
[3] With 1.4% polyvinyl alcohol, 0.004% benzalkonium chloride, EDTA and sodium thiosulfate.
[4] With 1.4% polyvinyl alcohol, EDTA and sodium thiosulfate.
[5] With 0.01% benzalkonium chloride, 0.1% EDTA and 1% glycerin.
[6] With 0.01% benzalkonium chloride, EDTA and sodium chloride.
[7] With 0.01% benzalkonium chloride, sodium borate, boric acid, sodium chloride, EDTA.
[8] With benzalkonium chloride, EDTA, 1.4% polyvinyl alcohol, 0.6% povidone, dextrose and sodium chloride.
[9] With 0.01% benzalkonium chloride, 0.1% EDTA and sodium chloride.
[10] With 0.004% benzalkonium chloride, EDTA, 1.67% povidone, PEG-90M and sodium chloride.
[11] With 0.01% benzalkonium chloride, 0.1% EDTA and sodium chloride.
[12] With 0.013% benzalkonium chloride, 1% PEG-400, 0.1% EDTA and sodium chloride.

ANTIHISTAMINE-DECONGESTANT COMBINATIONS

For complete prescribing information see General Monograph p. 60.

PHENYLEPHRINE HCl (p. 64), *NAPHAZOLINE HCl* (p. 63) and *TETRAHYDROZOLINE* (p. 65) have decongestant actions.

HYDROXYPROPYL METHYLCELLULOSE and *POLYVINYL ALCOHOL* increase the viscosity of the solution, thereby increasing contact time.

ZINC SULFATE is an astringent and antiseptic.

ANTIPYRINE is a weak local anesthetic.

PHENIRAMINE MALEATE, PYRILAMINE MALEATE and *ANTAZOLINE* are antihistamines.

Indications:

Based on a review of a related combination of drugs by the National Academy of Sciences – National Research Council and/or other information, FDA has classified the indications as follows:

"Possibly" effective for relief of ocular irritation and/or congestion or for the treatment of allergic or inflammatory ocular conditions. Final classification of the less-than-effective indication requires further investigation.

Warning:

Topical antihistamines are potential sensitizers and may produce a local sensitivity reaction. Because they may produce angle closure, use with caution in persons with a narrow angle or a history of glaucoma.

Administration and Dosage:

Administration and dosage recommendations vary. Refer to manufacturer package insert for instructions.

		Decongestant	Antihistamine	Other		C.I.*
otc	**Zincfrin** (Alcon)	phenylephrine HCl 0.12%		zinc sulfate 0.25%	In 15 ml.[1]	22
Rx	**Prefrin-A** (Allergan)	phenylephrine HCl 0.12%	pyrilamine maleate 0.1%	antipyrine 0.1%	In 15 ml.[2]	18

* Cost Index based on cost per ml.
[1] With 0.01% benzalkonium chloride and polysorbate 80.
[2] With benzalkonium chloride, EDTA and sodium bisulfite.

ANTIHISTAMINE-DECONGESTANT COMBINATIONS (Cont.)

		Decongestant	Antihistamine	Other		C.I.*
Rx	**Clear Eyes ACR** (Ross)	naphazoline HCl 0.012%		zinc sulfate 0.25%	In 15 and 30 ml.[1]	5
otc	**VasoClear A** (Iolab)	naphazoline HCl 0.02%		zinc sulfate 0.25%	In 15 ml.[2]	11
Rx	**Naphazoline Hydrochloride and Pheniramine Maleate Sterile Ophthalmic** (Various, eg, Moore, Steris)	naphazoline HCl 0.025%	pheniramine maleate 0.3%		In 15 ml.	9+
Rx	**AK-Con-A** (Akorn)				In 15 ml dropper bottles.[3]	11
Rx	**Naphcon-A** (Alcon)				In 15 ml Drop-Tainers.[3]	28
Rx	**Naphoptic-A** (Optopics)				In 15 ml dropper bottles.[4]	26
Rx	**Opcon-A** (Bausch & Lomb)				In 15 ml.[5]	18
Rx	**Naphazoline Hydrochloride and Antazoline Phosphate Ophthalmic** (Various, eg, Moore, Steris)	naphazoline HCl 0.05%	antazoline phosphate 0.5%		In 5 and 15 ml.	11+
Rx	**Albalon-A** (Allergan)				In 5 and 15 ml.[6]	21
Rx	**Antazoline-V** (Rugby)				In 15 ml.[7]	13
Rx	**Vasocon-A** (Iolab)				In 15 ml.[7]	19
otc	**Visine A.C.** (Pfizer)	tetrahydrozoline HCl 0.05%		zinc sulfate 0.25%	In 15 and 30 ml.[8]	7

* Cost Index based on cost per ml.
[1] With 0.2% glycerin, benzalkonium chloride, EDTA and sodium chloride.
[2] With 0.005% benzalkonium chloride, EDTA, 0.25% polyvinyl alcohol, PEG-400 and sodium chloride.
[3] With 0.01% benzalkonium chloride, EDTA and sodium chloride.
[4] With benzalkonium chloride, boric acid, EDTA, sodium borate.
[5] With 0.01% benzalkonium chloride, EDTA, hydroxypropyl methylcellulose and sodium chloride.
[6] With 0.004% benzalkonium chloride, EDTA, 1.4% polyvinyl alcohol, povidone and sodium chloride.
[7] With 0.01% benzalkonium chloride, PEG-8000, polyvinyl alcohol, EDTA and sodium chloride.
[8] With 0.01% benzalkonium chloride, 0.1% EDTA and sodium chloride.

Anti-inflammatory Agents

CORTICOSTEROIDS

Since their introduction into ocular therapy, corticosteroids have been useful in control of inflammatory and immunologic diseases of the eye. The anti-inflammatory effects of corticosteroids are nonspecific and they inhibit inflammation without regard to cause. In general, corticosteroids appear to be more effective in acute rather than chronic conditions. Degenerative diseases are usually completely refractory to corticosteroid therapy. Corticosteroids are generally not considered appropriate therapy for mild ocular allergies since other modalities can be effective (see Chapter 5 Antiallergy and Decongestant Agents).

The beneficial effects of these agents on inflammation are numerous and include:

- Reduction in capillary permeability and cellular exudation

- Inhibition of degranulation of mast cells, basophils and neutrophils. Stabilization of intracellular membranes of these cells inhibits release of hydrolytic enzyme and other mediators of inflammation such as histamines, bradykinins and platelet activating factor

- Suppression of lymphocyte proliferation

- Inhibition of phospholipase A synthesis, resulting in decreased synthesis of prostaglandins and leukotrienes

- Inhibition of cell-mediated immune responses

Clinical use and experimental data indicate that corticosteroids differ in their ability to suppress inflammation. This has been attributed, in part, to differences in their ability to penetrate the corneal epithelium. Acetate and alcohol formulations are sparingly soluble in water and are formulated for topical ocular use as suspensions. Phosphate derivatives are highly soluble in aqueous media and are formulated as solutions. The suspension formulations of acetate and alcohol derivatives exhibit biphasic solubility and can therefore better penetrate the lipid-rich layers of the cornea. It has also been suggested that corticosteroid particles in suspension persist in the cul-de-sac for longer periods of time and thus contact of the drug with the ocular surface is prolonged. For topical ocular use, prednisolone (eg, *AK-Pred*), fluorometholone (eg, *FML Liquifilm*) and dexamethasone (eg, *Decadron Phosphate*) can be effective in inflammations involving the lids, conjunctiva, cornea, iris and ciliary body. In severe forms of anterior uveitis, topical therapy may require supplementation with periocular injection or systemic corticosteroids. Chorioretinitis and optic neuritis are usually treated with systemic or periocular administration, or both. Medrysone (*HMS Liquifilm*) is recommended for minor reactions involving the lids and conjunctiva. Its efficacy has not been demonstrated in iritis or uveitis.

The use of corticosteroids in ocular disease remains largely empirical, but some general guidelines include the following:

- ♦ Type and location of inflammation determine which route of administration is appropriate

- ♦ Dosage is largely determined by clinical experience and should be reevaluated at frequent intervals during therapy

- ♦ Therapy should be reduced gradually, not discontinued abruptly

- ♦ The minimal effective dose should be used for the shortest time necessary

- ♦ Individualize dosage

- ♦ Maintain close supervision to assess the effects of therapy on the disease course and possible adverse effects to the patient

Patient compliance with the drug regimen is important in resolution of the inflammation. Patients should not discontinue use of medication at their own discretion. If suspensions are employed, the patient must shake the bottle sufficiently to maintain the proper concentration of drug.

Adverse effects can occur with all routes of administration and all preparations currently in use. Incidence of adverse effects appears to rise significantly as dosages are increased. Short-term topical ocular therapy usually does not produce significant ocular or systemic side effects.

NONSTEROIDAL ANTI-INFLAMMATORY AGENTS

Nonsteroidal anti-inflammatory drugs (NSAIDS), also referred to as the "aspirin-like" drugs, include the salicylates, as well as indole, pyrazolone and propionic acid derivatives and the fenamates. Following oral administration, these agents relieve discomfort associated with rheumatoid arthritis and lupus erythematosus, as well as reduce fever and alleviate pain that accompanies injury or inflammation.

The mechanism of action of the NSAIDs involves inhibition of cyclo-oxygenase, an enzyme important in synthesis of prostaglandins from their precursor, arachidonic acid. NSAIDs do not inhibit phospholipase A or the lipoxygenase enzyme, which generate the leukotrienes and related compounds that are also involved in the inflammatory response.

Prostaglandins are 20-carbon, unsaturated fatty acid derivatives which are subdivided into groups, designated by letters such as D, E and F. Evidence indicates that they also act as mediators of inflammation in ocular structures. Prostaglandins can cause vasodilation of ocular blood vessels, disrupt the blood-aqueous barrier, and induce neovascularization and miosis. Some of the prostaglandins such as $PGF_{2\alpha}$ and PGD_2 can lower intraocular pressure whereas others (eg, PGF_2) can raise it.

The primary ocular use of NSAIDs is to maintain pupillary dilation during surgery. Applied topically prior to surgery, they inhibit miosis induced during procedures such as cataract extraction. It is also possible that NSAIDs may prove topically efficacious in ocular reactions associated with surgically-induced or other nonsurgically-induced inflammatory disorders of the eye. At present, four topical ocular solution formulations are available, flurbiprofen *(Ocufen)*, suprofen *(Profenal)*, diclofenac *(Voltaren* ophthalmic) and ketorolac *(Acular)*.

Siret D. Jaanus, PhD
Southern California College of Optometry

For More Information

Bartlett JD, Jaanus SD, eds. Clinical Ocular Pharmacology, ed. 2. Boston, MA: Butterworth, 1989.

Bito LZ. Prostaglandins. Old concepts and new perspectives. *Arch Ophthalmol* 1987; 105:1036-39.

Duane TD, ed. Clinical Ophthalmology. Philadelphia, PA: J.B. Lippincott Company, 1988.

Ellis PP. Corticosteroid therapy in ophthalmology. In: Adriani J, Bernstein HN, eds. Symposium on Ocular Pharmacology and Therapy. St. Louis, MO: C.V. Mosby, 1970.

Gordon DM. Diseases of the uveal tract. In: Gordon DM, ed. Medical Management of Ocular Disease. New York, NY: Harper & Row, 1964.

Jampol LE. Non-steroidal anti-inflammatory drugs. In: Focal Points 1984: Clinical Modules for Ophthalmology. American Medical Association, 1984.

Leibowitz HM, Kupferman A. Anti-inflammatory medications. *Int Ophthalmol Clin* 1980;20:117-34.

Leopold IH. The steroid shield in ophthalmology. *Trans Am Acad Ophthalmology Otolaryngol* 1967;71:273-89.

Leopold IH, Murray D. Non-steroidal anti-inflammatory agents in ophthalmology. *Ophthalmology* 1979;86:142-55.

Neufeld AH, Sears ML. Prostaglandins and the eye. *Prostaglandins* 1973;4:157-68.

Podos SM. Prostaglandins, non-steroidal anti-inflammatory agents and eye disease. *Trans Am Ophthalmol Soc* 1976;74:637-60.

Sabiston DW, Robinson IG. An evaluation of the anti-inflammatory effects of flurbiprofen after cataract extraction. *Br J Ophthalmol* 1987;71:418-21.

CORTICOSTEROIDS, TOPICAL

Actions:

Topical corticosteroids exert an anti-inflammatory action. Aspects of the inflammatory process such as hyperemia, cellular infiltration, vascularization and fibroblastic proliferation are suppressed. Steroids cause inhibition of inflammatory response to inciting agents of mechanical, chemical or immunological nature. Topical corticosteroids are effective in acute inflammatory conditions of the anterior segment of the globe (eg, conjunctiva, sclera, cornea, lids, iris and ciliary body); they are also effective in ocular allergic conditions. In the treatment of ocular disease, the route depends on the site and extent of the disorder.

The mechanism of the anti-inflammatory action is thought to be potentiation of epinephrine vasoconstriction, stabilization of lysosomal membranes, retardation of macrophage movement, prevention of kinin release, inhibition of lymphocyte and neutrophil function, inhibition of prostaglandin synthesis and, in prolonged use, decrease of antibody production.

Indications:

For treatment of steroid responsive inflammatory conditions of the palpebral and bulbar conjunctiva, lid, cornea and anterior segment of the globe, such as: Allergic conjunctivitis; vernal conjunctivitis; episcleritis; acne rosacea; superficial punctate keratitis; herpes zoster keratitis; iritis; cyclitis; and selected infective conjunctivitis when the inherent hazard of steroid use is accepted to obtain a diminution in edema and inflammation. In difficult cases of anterior segment eye disease, systemic therapy may be required. When deeper ocular structures are involved, use systemic therapy.

For corneal injury from chemical, radiation or thermal burns or penetration of foreign bodies.

For suppression of graft reaction after keratoplasty.

Medrysone – For epinephrine sensitivity.

Contraindications:

Epithelial herpes simplex keratitis (dendritic keratitis); fungal diseases of ocular structures; acute infectious stages of vaccinia, varicella and most other viral diseases of the cornea and conjunctiva; mycobacterial infection of the eye; hypersensitivity to any component of the formulation; after uncomplicated removal of a superficial corneal foreign body.

Warnings:

Ocular damage: Prolonged use may result in glaucoma, elevated intraocular pressure (IOP), optic nerve damage, defects in visual acuity and fields of vision, posterior subcapsular cataract formation or secondary ocular infections from pathogens liberated from ocular tissues. Check IOP frequently. In diseases causing thinning of cornea or sclera, perforation has occurred with topical steroids.

Topical steroids are not effective in mustard gas keratitis or Sjogren's keratoconjunctivitis.

Infections: Acute, purulent, untreated eye infection may be masked or activity enhanced by steroids. Viral, bacterial and fungal infections of the cornea may be exacerbated by steroid application. Therefore, suspect fungal invasion in any persistent corneal ulceration where a steroid has been used, or is being used.

Treatment of herpes simplex other than epithelial herpes simplex keratitis with steroid medication (in which it is contraindicated) requires great caution; frequent slit-lamp microscopy is mandatory. Numerous cases of herpes simplex keratitis have occurred after inappropriate use of these preparations.

Medrysone is not recommended for use in iritis and uveitis as its effectiveness has not been established.

Pregnancy: Category C. There are no adequate or well-controlled studies in pregnant women. Use during pregnancy only if the potential benefits outweigh the potential hazards to the fetus. Observe infants born of mothers who have received substantial doses of corticosteroids during pregnancy carefully for signs of hypoadrenalism.

Lactation: Topically applied steroids are absorbed systemically. Therefore, because of the potential for serious adverse reactions in nursing infants, a decision should be made whether to discontinue nursing or discontinue the drug, taking into account the importance of the drug to the mother.

Children: Safety and efficacy for use in children have not been established. Safety and efficacy of fluorometholone in children under 2 have not been established.

Precautions:

Use with caution in glaucoma.

Sulfite Sensitivity: Some of these products contain sulfites that may cause allergic-type reactions (eg, hives, itching, wheezing, anaphylaxis) in certain susceptible persons. Although the overall prevalence of sulfite sensitivity in the general population is probably low, it is seen more frequently in asthmatics or in atopic nonasthmatic persons. Specific products containing sulfites are identified in the product listings.

Adverse Reactions:

Glaucoma with optic nerve damage, visual acuity and field defects; posterior subcapsular cataract formation; delayed wound healing; conjunctival erythema; secondary ocular infection from pathogens, including herpes simplex liberated from ocular tissues; perforation of globe. Viral, bacterial and fungal corneal infections may be exacerbated by steroids (see Contraindications and Warnings).

Rarely, transient stinging or burning may occur on instillation. Filtering blebs have been reported with steroid use after cataract surgery.

Ophthalmic ointments may retard corneal healing.

Systemic side effects may occur with extensive use of steroids.

Overdosage:

Overdosage will not ordinarily cause acute problems. If accidentally ingested, drink fluids to dilute.

Patient Information:

Medical supervision during therapy is recommended.

Keep out of reach of children.

To avoid contamination, do not touch applicator tip to any surface. Replace cap after using.

Do not discontinue use without consulting physician. Take care not to discontinue prematurely.

Notify physician if condition worsens or persists or if pain, itching or swelling of the eye occurs.

Discontinue use if improvement in the condition being treated does not occur within several days.

Administration and Dosage:

Treatment duration varies with type of lesion and may extend from a few days to several weeks, depending on therapeutic response. Relapse may occur if therapy is reduced too rapidly. Taper over several days. Relapses, more common in chronic active lesions than in self-limited conditions, usually respond to retreatment.

For Product Information on Steroid/Antibiotic Combinations see page 111.

Individual drug monographs are on the following pages.

DEXAMETHASONE

For complete prescribing information see p. 72.

Administration and Dosage:

Ointments: Apply a thin coating (approximately 0.5 to 1 inch) in the lower conjunctival sac 3 or 4 times a day. When a favorable response is observed, reduce the number of daily applications to 2, and later to 1 a day as a maintenance dose if sufficient to control symptoms. Ointments are particularly convenient when an eye pad is used and may be the preparation of choice when prolonged contact of drug with ocular tissues is needed.

Storage: Store at 46° to 80°F (8° to 27°C).

Suspensions and Solutions: Instill 1 or 2 drops into the conjunctival sac every hour during the day and every 2 hours during the night. When a favorable response is observed, reduce dosage to 1 drop every 4 hours. Later, 1 drop 3 or 4 times daily may suffice to control symptoms.

Shake suspension well before using. Do not freeze. Protect from light.

Storage: Store at 46° to 86°F (8° to 30°C).

			C.I.*
Rx **Dexamethasone Sodium Phosphate** (Various, eg, Bausch & Lomb, Major)	**Ointment:** 0.05% dexamethasone phosphate (as sodium phosphate)	In 3.5 g.	121+
Rx **AK-Dex** (Akorn)		In 3.5 g.[1]	135
Rx **Decadron Phosphate** (MSD)		In 3.5 g.[2]	236
Rx **Maxidex** (Alcon)		In 3.5 g.[2]	633
Rx **Dexamethasone Sodium Phosphate** (Various, eg, Bausch & Lomb, Iolab, Steris)	**Solution:** 0.1% dexamethasone phosphate (as sodium phosphate)	In 5 ml.	83+
Rx **AK-Dex** (Akorn)		In 5 ml dropper bottles.[3]	143
Rx **Decadron Phosphate** (MSD)		In 5 ml Ocumeters.[4]	404
Rx **Dexamethasone** (Steris)	**Suspension:** 0.1% dexamethasone	In 5 ml.	71
Rx **Maxidex** (Alcon)		In 5 and 15 ml Drop-Tainers.[5]	443

* Cost Index based on cost per g or ml.
[1] With lanolin anhydrous, parabens, PEG-400, white petrolatum and mineral oil.
[2] With white petrolatum and mineral oil.
[3] With 0.01% benzalkonium chloride, EDTA and hydroxyethyl cellulose.
[4] With polysorbate 80, EDTA, 0.1% sodium bisulfite, 0.25% phenylethanol and 0.02% benzalkonium chloride.
[5] With 0.01% benzalkonium chloride, 0.5% hydroxypropyl methylcellulose, NaCl, polysorbate 80 and EDTA.

FLUOROMETHOLONE

For complete prescribing information see p. 72.

Administration and Dosage:

Ointment: Apply a small amount (approximately 0.5 inch ribbon) of ointment in the conjunctival sac 1 to 3 times daily. During the initial 24 to 48 hours, the dosage may be increased to one application every 4 hours.

Storage: Store away from heat.

Suspension: Instill 1 or 2 drops into the conjunctival sac 2 to 4 times daily. During the initial 24 to 48 hours, the dosage may be safely increased to 2 drops every hour.

Shake well before using. Do not freeze.

Storage: Store at room temperature 59° to 86° F (15° to 30° C).

				C.I.*
Rx	**FML S.O.P.** (Allergan)	**Ointment:** 0.1% fluoro-metholone	In 3.5 g.[1]	659
Rx	**Fluor-Op** (Iolab)	**Suspension:** 0.1% fluorometholone	In 5, 10 and 15 ml dropper bottles.[2]	176
Rx	**FML** (Allergan)		In 1, 5, 10 and 15 ml dropper bottles.[2]	394
Rx	**Flarex** (Alcon)	**Suspension:** 0.1% fluorometholone acetate	In 2.5, 5 and 10 ml Drop-Tainers.[3]	339
Rx	**FML Forte** (Allergan)	**Suspension:** 0.25% fluorometholone	In 2, 5, 10 and 15 ml dropper bottles.[4]	356

MEDRYSONE

For complete prescribing information see p. 72.

Administration and Dosage:

Instill one drop in the conjunctival sac up to every 4 hours.

Shake well before using. Do not freeze.

				C.I.*
Rx	**HMS** (Allergan)	**Suspension:** 1% medrysone	In 5 and 10 ml dropper bottles.[5]	357

* Cost Index based on cost per g or ml.
[1] With 0.0008% phenylmercuric acetate, white petrolatum, mineral oil and petrolatum (and) lanolin alcohol.
[2] With 0.004% benzalkonium chloride, EDTA, polysorbate 80, 1.4% polyvinyl alcohol and NaCl.
[3] With 0.01% benzalkonium chloride, EDTA, hydroxyethyl cellulose, tyloxapol and NaCl.
[4] With 0.005% benzalkonium chloride, EDTA, polysorbate 80, 1.4% polyvinyl alcohol and NaCl.
[5] With 0.004% benzalkonium chloride, EDTA, 1.4% polyvinyl alcohol, hydroxypropyl methylcellulose and NaCl.

PREDNISOLONE

For complete prescribing information see p. 72.

Administration and Dosage:

Prednisolone Sodium Phosphate – Instill 1 or 2 drops into the conjunctival sac up to every hour during the day and every 2 hours during the night as necessary as initial therapy. When a favorable response is observed, reduce to 1 or 2 drops every 3 or 4 hours. Later, reduce to 1 drop 3 or 4 times daily to control symptoms.

Prednisolone Acetate – Instill 1 or 2 drops into the conjunctival sac 2 to 4 times daily. During the initial 24 to 48 hours, the dosing frequency may be increased if necessary.

Shake suspension well before using.

Storage: Store at room temperature 59° to 86°F (15° to 30°C). Do not freeze. Protect from light.

				C.I.*
Rx	**Prednisolone Sodium Phosphate** (Various, eg, Rugby, Steris)	**Solution:** 0.125% prednisolone sodium phosphate	In 5 and 15 ml.	91+
Rx	**AK-Pred** (Akorn)		In 5 ml.[1]	98
Rx	**Inflamase Mild** (Iolab)		In 5 and 10 ml with dropper.[2]	227
Rx	**Prednisolone Sodium Phosphate** (Various, eg, Bausch & Lomb, Rugby)	**Solution:** 1% prednisolone sodium phosphate	In 5 and 15 ml.	154+
Rx	**AK-Pred** (Akorn)		In 5 ml and 15 ml.[1]	134
Rx	**Inflamase Forte** (Iolab)		In 5, 10 and 15 ml with dropper.[2]	231
Rx	**Pred Mild** (Allergan)	**Suspension:** 0.12% prednisolone acetate	In 5 and 10 ml dropper bottles.[3]	272
Rx	**Econopred** (Alcon)	**Suspension:** 0.125% prednisolone acetate	In 5 and 10 ml Drop-Tainers.[4]	336
Rx	**Econopred Plus** (Alcon)	**Suspension:** 1% prednisolone acetate	In 5 and 10 ml Drop-Tainers.[4]	350
Rx	**Pred Forte** (Allergan)		In 1, 5, 10 and 15 ml dropper bottles.[3]	277

* Cost Index based on cost per ml.
[1] With 0.01% benzalkonium chloride, EDTA, hydroxypropyl methylcellulose and sodium bisulfite.
[2] With 0.01% benzalkonium chloride, EDTA and NaCl.
[3] With benzalkonium chloride, EDTA, polysorbate 80, hydroxypropyl methylcellulose, sodium bisulfite and NaCl.
[4] With 0.01% benzalkonium chloride, EDTA, polysorbate 80, hydroxypropyl methylcellulose and glycerin.

PREDNISOLONE AND ATROPINE COMBINATION

For complete prescribing information see Corticosteroids, p. 72 and Atropine, p. 46.

Actions:

The anticholinergic, atropine sulfate, blocks the responses of the sphincter muscle of the iris and the accommodative muscle of the ciliary body to cholinergic stimulation, producing pupillary dilation (mydriasis) and paralysis of accommodation (cycloplegia). Prednisolone acetate causes inhibition of the inflammatory response to inciting agents of a mechanical, chemical or immunological nature.

Indication:

For use in the treatment of anterior uveitis.

Administration and Dosage:

Adults: Instill 1 or 2 drops in the eyes up to 4 times daily.

Children: Instill 1 or 2 drops in the eyes up to 2 times daily.

Shake well before using. Carefully evaluate dosage in view of the potential toxic effects of the atropine components.

Compress the lacrimal sac by digital pressure for 1 minute after instillation.

Storage: Store upright at 46° to 80°F (8° to 27°C).

				C.I.*
Rx	**Mydrapred** (Alcon)	**Suspension:** 0.25% prednisolone acetate and 1% atropine sulfate	In 5 ml Drop-Tainers.[1]	357

* Cost Index based on cost per ml.
[1] With 0.01% benzalkonium chloride.

NONSTEROIDAL ANTI-INFLAMMATORY AGENTS

Actions:

Diclofenac sodium, flurbiprofen sodium, ketorolac tromethamine and suprofen are topical nonsteroidal anti-inflammatory agents (NSAIDs) for ophthalmic use.

NSAIDs				
Chemical Class	Generic Name	Trade Name	Manufacturer	Solution Strength
Acetic Acids	Diclofenac	*Voltaren*	Ciba Vision	0.1%
	Ketorolac	*Acular*	Allergan	0.5%
Phenylalkanoic Acids	Flurbiprofen	*Ocufen*	Allergan	0.03%
	Suprofen	*Profenal*	Alcon	1%

Pharmacology: Diclofenac is a phenylacetic acid and flurbiprofen and suprofen are phenylalkanoic acids that have analgesic, antipyretic and anti-inflammatory activity. Their mechanism of action is believed to be through inhibition of the cyclo-oxygenase enzyme that is essential in the biosynthesis of prostaglandins.

In animals, prostaglandins are mediators of certain kinds of intraocular inflammation. Prostaglandins produce disruption of the blood-aqueous humor barrier, vasodilation, increased vascular permeability, leukocytosis and increased intraocular pressure (IOP).

Prostaglandins also appear to play a role in the miotic response produced during ocular surgery by constricting the iris sphincter independently of cholinergic mechanisms. These agents inhibit the miosis induced during the course of cataract surgery.

Results from clinical studies indicate that diclofenac sodium, flurbiprofen sodium, ketorolac tromethamine and suprofen do not have a significant effect upon IOP.

Indications:

Diclofenac – For the treatment of postoperative inflammation in patients who have undergone cataract extraction.

Flurbiprofen and suprofen – For inhibition of intraoperative miosis.

Ketorolac – For the relief of ocular itching due to seasonal allergic conjunctivitis.

Contraindications:

Hypersensitivity to any component of the formulation.

Diclofenac and ketorolac – Soft contact lens wearers (see Precautions).

Flurbiprofen and suprofen – Epithelial herpes simplex keratitis (dendritic keratitis). Closely monitor patients with histories of herpes simplex keratitis.

Warnings:

Cross-sensitivity: The potential for cross-sensitivity to acetylsalicylic acid and other NSAIDs exists. Therefore, use caution when treating individuals who have previously exhibited sensitivity to these drugs.

Pregnancy: Category B (diclofenac); *Category C* (flurbiprofen, ketorolac, suprofen). There are no adequate and well-controlled studies in pregnant women. Use during pregnancy only if the potential benefits outweigh the potential hazards to the fetus.

Diclofenac – Oral doses in mice and rats cross the placental barrier. In rats, maternally toxic doses were associated with dystocia, prolonged gestation, reduced fetal weights, growth and survival. Because of the known effects of prostaglandin-inhibiting drugs on the fetal cardiovascular system (closure of the ductus arteriosus), avoid the use of ophthalmic diclofenac during late pregnancy.

Flurbiprofen is embryocidal, delays parturition, prolongs gestation, reduces weight and slightly retards fetal growth in rats at daily oral doses of greater than or equal to 0.4 mg/kg (approximately 185 times the human daily topical dose).

Ketorolac – Oral doses at 1.5 mg/kg administered after gestation day 17 caused dystocia and higher pup mortality in rats.

Suprofen – Oral doses of up to 200 mg/kg/day in animals resulted in an increased incidence of fetal resorption associated with maternal toxicity. There was an increase in stillbirths and a decrease in postnatal survival in pregnant rats treated with suprofen at 2.5 mg/kg/day and above. An increased incidence of delayed parturition occurred in rats. Because of the known effect of NSAIDs on the fetal cardiovascular system (closure of ductus arteriosus), avoid use during late pregnancy.

Lactation: It is not known whether flurbiprofen is excreted in breast milk. Because of the potential for serious adverse reactions in nursing infants, decide whether to discontinue nursing or to discontinue the drug, taking into account the importance of the drug to the mother.

Ketorolac – Exercise caution when administering to a nursing woman.

Suprofen is excreted in human milk after a single oral dose. Based on measurements of plasma and milk levels in women taking oral suprofen, the milk concentration is about 1% of the plasma level. Because systemic absorption may occur from topical ocular administration, a decision should be considered to discontinue nursing while on suprofen, since safety in human neonates has not been established.

Children: Safety and efficacy for use in children have not been established.

Precautions:

Contact lenses: Patients wearing hydrogel soft contact lenses who have been treated with diclofenac have experienced ocular irritation manifested by redness and burning.

Wound healing may be delayed with the use of diclofenac or flurbiprofen.

Closely monitor patients with histories of herpes simplex keratitis when using flurbiprofen and suprofen.

Use with caution in surgical patients with known bleeding tendencies or who are on other medications which may prolong bleeding time. Some systemic absorption occurs with drugs applied ocularly, and NSAIDs increase bleeding time by interference with thrombocyte aggregation. Diclofenac or flurbiprofen applied ocularly may cause an increased bleeding tendency of ocular tissues (including hyphemas) in conjunction with surgery.

Drug Interactions:

Acetylcholine chloride and *carbachol:* Although clinical studies with acetylcholine chloride and animal studies with acetylcholine chloride or carbachol revealed no interference and there is no known pharmacological basis for an interaction, both of these drugs have reportedly been ineffective when used in patients treated with flurbiprofen or suprofen.

Adverse Reactions:

Most frequent: Transient burning and stinging upon instillation and other minor symptoms of ocular irritation.

Diclofenac – Keratitis (28%, although most cases occurred in cataract studies prior to drug therapy); elevated IOP (15%, although most cases occurred post surgery and prior to drug therapy); anterior chamber reaction; ocular allergy; nausea, vomiting (1%); viral infections ($\leq$ 1%).

Ketorolac – Ocular irritation (3%); allergic reactions (3%); superficial ocular infections (0.5%); superficial keratitis (1%).

Suprofen – Discomfort, itching and redness have been reported. Allergy, iritis, pain, chemosis, photophobia and punctate epithelial staining occur in less than 0.5% of patients.

Some systemic absorption occurs with drugs applied ocularly, and NSAIDs increase bleeding time by interference with thrombocyte aggregation. Use with caution in surgical patients with known bleeding tendencies or who are on other medications which may prolong bleeding time (see Precautions).

Overdosage:

Overdosage will not ordinarily cause acute problems. If accidentally ingested, drink fluids to dilute.

Individual drug monographs are on the following pages.

DICLOFENAC SODIUM

For complete prescribing information see p. 79.

Administration and Dosage:

Instill one drop four times daily, beginning 24 hours after cataract surgery and continuing throughout the first 2 weeks of the postoperative period.

Storage: Store at room temperature 59° to 86° F (15° to 30° C). Protect from light.

C.I.*

Rx	**Voltaren** (Ciba Vision)	**Solution:** 0.1%	In 2.5 ml and 5 ml dropper bottles.[1]	725

FLURBIPROFEN SODIUM

For complete prescribing information see p. 79.

Administration and Dosage:

Instill 1 drop approximately every ½ hour, beginning 2 hours before surgery (total of 4 drops).

Storage: Store at room temperature 59° to 86°F (15° to 30°C).

C.I.*

Rx	**Ocufen** (Allergan)	**Solution:** 0.03%	In 2.5 ml dropper bottles.[2]	739

KETOROLAC TROMETHAMINE

For complete prescribing information see p. 79.

Administration and Dosage:

Instill 1 drop 4 times per day for ocular itching due to seasonal allergic conjunctivitis.

Storage: Store at room temperature 59° to 86°F (15° to 30°C). Protect from light.

C.I.*

Rx	**Acular** (Allergan)	**Solution:** 0.5%	In 5 ml dropper bottles.[3]	NA

SUPROFEN

For complete prescribing information see p. 79.

Administration and Dosage:

Day preceding surgery: 2 drops may be instilled into the conjunctival sac every 4 hours while awake.

Day of surgery: Instill 2 drops into the conjunctival sac at 3, 2 and 1 hour prior to surgery.

Storage: Store at room temperature 59° to 86°F (15° to 30°C).

C.I.*

Rx	**Profenal** (Alcon)	**Solution:** 1%	In 2.5 ml Drop-Tainers.[4]	404

* Cost Index based on cost per ml.
[1] With polyoxyl 35, castor oil, 0.02% sorbic acid, tromethamine and 0.01% EDTA.
[2] With 1.4% polyvinyl alcohol, 0.005% thimerosal, EDTA and NaCl.
[3] With 0.01% benzalkonium Cl, 0.1% EDTA, octoxynol 40 and sodium chloride.
[4] With 0.005% thimerosal, 2% caffeine, EDTA and NaCl.

Artificial Tear Solutions
and Ocular Lubricants

Availability of synthetic polymers suitable for ocular use has resulted in development of artificial tear solutions, ointments and other formulations to help alleviate ocular discomfort and maintain integrity of the surface epithelium. Ideally, formulations for dry eyes should be compatible with and substitute for components of the tear film, including lipid, aqueous and mucin layers.

SOLUTIONS

Lubricant preparations formulated as artificial tear solutions usually contain inorganic electrolytes, preservatives and water-soluble polymeric systems. Sodium chloride (NaCl), potassium chloride (KCl), various other ions and boric acid help maintain tonicity and pH of the formulations. Preservatives, including benzalkonium chloride, chlorobutanol, thimerosal, EDTA, methylparaben and propylparaben, are included in multi-dose preparations to prevent bacterial contamination. Methylcellulose and its derivatives, polyvinyl alcohol (PVA), povidone (PVP), dextran and propylene glycol can enhance viscosity and promote tear film stability.

In addition to polymers, lipids and vitamins have also been incorporated into ocular lubricants. One formulation, *TearGard,* contains a phospholipid derivative in an aqueous solution of hydroxyethyl cellulose and inorganic buffer. Although it has been suggested that this product can replace all layers of the tear film, these claims remain unsubstantiated due to lack of controlled clinical trials. Retinol, the alcohol form of vitamin A, is available as a solution for topical use on the eye. The formulation *Vit-A-Drops* contains vitamin A, polysorbate 80 and EDTA. *Dakrina* contains retinol palmitate, a form of vitamin A, and vitamin C. Another preparation, *NutraTear,* contains vitamin B_{12}. Definitive data on the benefits of vitamin-containing formulations in dry eye disorders are not available. Large-scale, well-controlled masked studies are lacking; however, there is some recent evidence that vitamin A (retinol) solution may be effective in superior limbic keratoconjunctivitis and some forms of severe dry eye syndromes.

Artificial tear solutions should be administered at dosage frequencies of 4 to 6 hours. However, depending on the severity of the clinical signs and symptoms, they may be used as often as hourly or only occasionally. It is highly recommended that the prescriber of the artificial tear product recommend a specific dosage schedule for the patient, particularly at the start of therapy.

OINTMENTS

Petrolatum, lanolin and mineral oil ointments are the second most frequent approach for ocular lubrication. When placed on the eye, they dissolve at the temperature of the ocular tissue and disperse with the tear fluid. A major advantage is that ointments appear to be retained in the cul-de-sac longer than artificial tear solutions.

Ointments are usually applied directly to the inferior conjunctival sac as a 0.25 to 0.5-inch ribbon. An alternative method is to place the ointment on a cotton-tipped applicator and apply it to the lid margins and lashes. Both blurring of vision and possible irritation are minimized with this method of instillation. Recently, manufacturers have begun to formulate preservative-free ointment preparations. These preparations are less toxic and less allergenic than those containing preservatives.

Ophthalmic lubricant ointments are generally preferred for bedtime use. Depending on the clinical signs and patient symptoms, they may also be used as often as necessary during the day. Since ointments may block access of solution to the ocular surface, solutions should be instilled prior to ointment application.

SOLID DEVICES

Another approach to relief of dry eye symptoms is use of a preservative-free, water-soluble, polymeric insert (*Lacrisert*). The cylindrical rod, which contains 5 mg hydroxypropyl cellulose, is placed in the lower cul-de-sac. It then imbibes fluid and swells. As it dissolves, the polymer is released to the ocular surface for 12 to 24 hours.

The device can be beneficial in dry eye syndromes such as keratitis sicca. It is comfortable and well accepted, but some disadvantages are associated with its use. Manual dexterity is required for placement in the cul-de-sac and the cost to the patient is considerably greater than use of solutions and ointments. A common patient complaint is blurred vision as the rod dissolves, causing the tear film to thicken. Adding fluid drops (eg, isotonic saline) can reduce viscosity and minimize visual complaints.

PUNCTAL PLUGS

Mechanical occlusion of the lacrimal puncta has become an accepted method to block tear drainage and thereby prolong action of natural tears as well as artificial tear preparations. Two types of punctal plugs are currently used: a silicone-based plug and a temporary absorbable collagen implant.

The Freeman Punctal Plug is usually inserted directly into the inferior puncta. The procedure requires topical anesthesia and punctal dilation prior to placement.

The Temporary Intracanalicular Collagen Implant consists of 0.2, 0.3 or 0.4 mm diameter collagen inserts, packaged at the edge of a foam strip. The implants are placed halfway into the punctal opening and advanced into the horizontal canaliculus with the aid of a jeweler's forceps and magnification. The procedure can be done with or without an anesthetic. Following placement, the implant swells, impeding tear flow up to 14 days before the implants are totally absorbed.

Punctal occlusion can benefit patients whose symptoms are not relieved by topical therapy alone. Although rare, punctal occlusion can lead to epiphora.

Siret D. Jaanus, PhD
Southern California College of Optometry

For More Information

Bartlett JD, Jaanus SD, eds. Clinical Ocular Pharmacology, ed. 2. Boston, MA: Butterworth, 1989.

Duane TD, ed. Clinical Ophthalmology. Philadelphia, PA: J.B. Lippincott Company, 1988.

Holly FJ. Tear film physiology. *Int Ophthalmol Clin* 1987;27:2-6.

Holly FJ, Lemp MA. Tear physiology and dry eyes. *Surv Ophthalmol* 1977;22:69-87.

Jaanus SD. Managing the Dry Eye. Part I and II. *Clinical Eye and Vision Care* 1990;2(1):38-45 (Part II in press).

Lemp MA. Recent developments in dry eye management. *Surv Ophthalmol* 1987;94:1299-1304.

Norn MS, Opauszki A. Effects of ophthalmic vehicles on the stability of the precorneal tear film. *Acta Ophthalmol* 1977;55:23-34.

Ohashi Y, et al. Vitamin A eye drops for superior limbic keratoconjunctivitis. *Am J Ophthalmol* 1988;105:523-27.

Pfister RR, Burnstein N. The effects of ophthalmic drugs, vehicles and preservatives on corneal epithelium: A scanning electron microscope study. *Invest Ophthalmol* 1976;15:246-59.

Stenbeck A, Ostholm I. Ointments for ophthalmic use. *Acta Ophthalmol* 1954;43:405-23.

Tseng SCG. Topical retinoid treatment for dry eye disorders. *Trans Ophthalmol Soc UK* 1985;104:489-95.

Tuberville AW, et al. Punctal occlusion in tear deficiency syndromes. *Ophthalmology* 1982;89:1170-72.

Werblin TP, et al. The use of slow-release artificial tears in the long-term management of keratitis sicca. *Ophthalmol* 1981;88:78-81.

ARTIFICIAL TEAR SOLUTIONS AND OCULAR LUBRICANTS

Actions:

Artificial tear solutions contain electrolytes to maintain ocular tonicity and pH, preservatives to prevent bacterial contamination and water-soluble polymeric systems to increase viscosity. By increasing the viscosity, the water-soluble polymers increase the bioavailability of the drug by lengthening the amount of time the drug is in contact with the eye. Examples of electrolytes, preservatives and water-soluble polymers include:

Buffers – Boric acid, hydrochloric acid, sodium bicarbonate, sodium borate, sodium citrate, sodium hydroxide, sodium phosphate.

Tonicity Agents – Dextran 40, Dextran 70, dextrose, potassium chloride, propylene glycol, sodium chloride.

Preservatives – Benzalkonium chloride, chlorobutanol, thimerosal.

Water-soluble polymers – Methylcellulose, hydroxyethyl cellulose, hydroxypropyl cellulose, hydroxypropyl methylcellulose, carboxymethylcellulose, polyvinyl alcohol.

Ocular lubricants contain emollients, which lubricate and protect the eye. They are also used as vehicles in other ophthalmic preparations. Examples of emollients include petrolatum, mineral oil and lanolin derivatives.

Indications:

For use as a lubricant to prevent further irritation or to relieve dryness of the eye.

For temporary relief of burning, dryness and discomfort due to minor irritations of the eye or to exposure to wind or sun.

Patient Information:

Keep out of the reach of children.

Wash hands thoroughly.

If headache, eye pain, vision changes, continued redness or irritation occurs, or if condition worsens or persists for more than 3 days, discontinue use and consult a physician.

To avoid contamination, do not touch tip of container or dropper to any surface. Replace cap after using. If solution changes color or becomes cloudy, do not use.

Allergy to thimerosal: Do not use products containing thimerosal or any other ingredient containing mercury.

Do not use some of these products with contact lenses (refer to individual products).

Individual drug monographs are on the following page

ARTIFICIAL TEAR SOLUTIONS

For complete prescribing information see General Monograph p. 86.

Administration and Dosage:

Instill 1 to 2 drops into eye(s) 3 times daily, as needed.

Storage: Store at 46° to 86°F (8° to 30°C). Protect from light.

				C.I.*
otc	**Adsorbotear** (Alcon)	Solution: Hydroxyethyl cellulose, 1.67% povidone, water soluble polymers, 0.004% thimerosal and 0.1% EDTA	In 15 ml.	49
otc	**Akwa Tears** (Akorn)	Solution: Polyvinyl alcohol, sodium chloride, 0.01% benzalkonium chloride and EDTA	In 15 ml.	21
otc	**Artificial Tears** (Rugby)		In 15 ml.	19
otc	**Artificial Tears** (Various, eg, Steris, United Research)	Solution: 1.4% polyvinyl alcohol, 0.01% benzalkonium chloride, EDTA and sodium chloride	In 15 and 30 ml.	11+
otc	**Teargen** (Goldline)		In 15 ml.	17
otc	**AquaSite** (Ciba Vision)	Solution: 0.2% PEG-400, 0.1% dextran 70, polycarbophil, sodium chloride, EDTA and sodium hydroxide	Preservative free. In 0.6 ml (single use 24s).	NA
otc	**Artificial Tears Plus** (Various, eg, Rugby, Steris)	Solution: 1.4% polyvinyl alcohol, 0.6% povidone, 0.5% chlorobutanol and sodium chloride	In 15 ml.	12+
otc	**Cellufresh** (Allergan)	Solution: 0.5% carboxymethylcellulose sodium and sodium chloride	Preservative free. In 0.3 ml (single use 4s and 30s).	57
otc	**Celluvisc** (Allergan)	Solution: 1% carboxymethylcellulose sodium and sodium chloride	Preservative free. In 0.3 ml (UD 30s and 50s.)	74
otc	**Dakrina** (Dakryon)	Solution: 5% povidone, 0.6% polyvinyl alcohol, 350 IU vitamin A palmitate, vitamin C, 0.2% potassium sorbate and 0.05% EDTA	In 15 ml.	20
otc	**Dry Eye Therapy** (Bausch & Lomb)	Solution: 0.3% glycerin and sodium chloride	Preservative free. In 0.3 ml (single use 32s).	50
otc	**Dwelle** (Dakryon)	Solution: Polyvinyl alcohol, poly (N-glucose), 0.2% potassium sorbate and 0.05% EDTA	In 15 ml.	NA
otc	**Eye-Lube-A** (Optopics)	Solution: 0.25% Glyercin, EDTA, sodium chloride, benzalkonium chloride	In 15 ml.	21
otc	**Hypo Tears** (Iolab)	Solution: 1% polyvinyl alcohol, PEG-400, dextrose, benzalkonium chloride and EDTA	In 15 and 30 ml.	31
otc	**Hypo Tears PF** (Iolab)	Solution: 1% polyvinyl alcohol, PEG-400, dextrose and EDTA	Preservative free. In 0.6 ml (UD 30s).	27

* Cost Index based on cost per ml.

ARTIFICIAL TEAR SOLUTIONS (Cont.)   C.I.*

otc	**Isopto Alkaline** (Alcon)	**Solution:** 1% hydroxypropyl methylcellulose, 0.01% benzalkonium chloride and sodium chloride	In 15 ml Drop-Tainers.	88
otc	**Ultra Tears** (Alcon)		In 15 ml.	88
otc	**Isopto Plain** (Alcon)	**Solution:** 0.5% hydroxypropyl methylcellulose, 0.01% benzalkonium chloride and sodium chloride	In 15 ml Drop-Tainers.	49
otc	**Isopto Tears** (Alcon)		In 15 and 30 ml.	49
otc	**Just Tears** (Blairex)	**Solution:** 1.4% polyvinyl alcohol, benzalkonium chloride, EDTA and sodium chloride	In 15 ml.	14
otc	**Lacril** (Allergan)	**Solution:** 0.5% hydroxypropyl methylcellulose, 0.01% gelatin A, 0.5% chlorobutanol, sodium chloride, polysorbate 80 and dextrose	In 15 ml dropper bottles.	46
otc	**Liquifilm Forte** (Allergan)	**Solution:** 3% polyvinyl alcohol, 0.002% thimerosal, sodium chloride and EDTA	In 15 and 30 ml dropper bottles.	46
otc	**Liquifilm Tears** (Allergan)	**Solution:** 1.4% polyvinyl alcohol, 0.5% chlorobutanol and sodium chloride	In 15 and 30 ml dropper bottles.	44
otc	**Moisture Drops** (Bausch & Lomb)	**Solution:** 0.5% hydroxypropyl methylcellulose, 0.1% dextran 70, 0.2% glycerin, NaCl, 0.01% benzalkonium chloride and EDTA	In 15 and 30 ml.	26
otc	**Murine** (Ross)	**Solution:** 1.4% polyvinyl alcohol, 0.6% povidone, benzalkonium chloride, dextrose, EDTA and sodium chloride	In 15 and 30 ml dropper bottles.	16
otc	**Murocel** (Bausch & Lomb)	**Solution:** 1% methylcellulose, propylene glycol, sodium chloride, 0.023% methylparaben and 0.01% propylparaben	In 15 ml.	53
otc	**Nature's Tears** (Rugby)	**Solution:** 0.3% Hydroxypropyl methylcellulose 2906, 0.1% dextran 70, sodium chloride, potassium chloride and EDTA	In 15 ml.	29
otc	**Nu-Tears II** (Optopics)	**Solution:** 1% polyvinyl alcohol, 1% PEG-400, EDTA and benzalkonium chloride	In 15 ml.	21
otc	**NutraTear** (Dakryon)	**Solution:** 0.05% vitamin B_{12}, polyvinyl alcohol, 0.004% benzalkonium chloride and 0.08% EDTA	In 15 ml.	16
otc	**Refresh** (Allergan)	**Solution:** 1.4% polyvinyl alcohol, 0.6% povidone and sodium chloride	Preservative free. In 0.3 ml (UD 30s and 50s).	57
otc	**Tear Gard** (Medtech)	**Solution:** Hydroxyethyl cellulose, 0.25% sorbic acid and 0.1% EDTA	Thimerosal free. In 15 ml.	NA
otc	**Tearisol** (Iolab)	**Solution:** 0.5% hydroxypropyl methylcellulose, benzalkonium chloride and EDTA	In 15 ml.	37

* Cost Index based on cost per ml.

ARTIFICIAL TEAR SOLUTIONS (Cont.) C.I.*

otc	**Tears Naturale Free** (Alcon)	**Solution:** 0.3% hydroxypropyl methyl-cellulose, 0.1% dextran 70 and sodium chloride	In 0.6 ml single-use containers.	42
otc	**Tears Naturale II** (Alcon)	**Solution:** 0.1% dextran 70, 0.3% hy-droxypropyl methylcellulose, 0.001% polyquarternium-1 and sodium chloride	In 15 and 30 ml Drop-Tainers.	45
otc	**Tears Plus** (Allergan)	**Solution:** 1.4% polyvinyl alcohol, 0.6% povidone, 0.5% chlorobutanol and sodium chloride	In 15 and 30 ml dropper bottles.	35
otc	**Tears Renewed** (Akorn)	**Solution:** Dextran 70, sodium chloride, hydroxypropyl methylcellulose, 0.01% benzalkonium chloride and 0.05% EDTA	In 15 ml.	26
otc	**Vit-A-Drops** (Vision Pharm)	**Solution:** Vitamin A, polysorbate 80, 0.05% EDTA and sodium chloride	In 10 and 15 ml.	43

* Cost Index based on cost per ml.

OCULAR LUBRICANTS

For complete prescribing information see General Monograph p. 86.

Administration and Dosage:

Pull down the lower lid of affected eye(s) and apply a small amount (0.25 inch) of ointment to the inside of the eyelid.

Storage: Store at room temperature 59° to 86°F (15° to 30°C). Store away from heat. Do not freeze.

			C.I.*
otc **Akwa Tears** (Akorn)	**Ointment:** White petrolatum, mineral oil and lanolin	Preservative free. In 3.5 g.	91
otc **Dry Eyes** (Bausch & Lomb)		In 3.5 g and UD 0.7 g (24s).	104
otc **Artificial Tears** (Rugby)	**Ointment:** White petrolatum, anhydrous liquid lanolin and mineral oil	In 3.5 g.	93
otc **Duratears Naturale** (Alcon)		In 3.5 g.	221
otc **Hypo Tears** (Iolab)	**Ointment:** White petrolatum and light mineral oil	In 3.5 g.	141
otc **Puralube** (Fougera)		In 3.5 g.	33
otc **Tears Renewed** (Akorn)		Preservative free. In 3.5 g.	121
otc **Lacril** (Allergan)	**Ointment:** 0.5% hydroxypropyl methylcellulose, 0.01% gelatin A, 0.5% chlorobutanol, dextrose, magnesium chloride, polysorbate 80, sodium borate and sodium chloride	In 15 ml dropper bottles.	46
otc **Lacri-Lube NP** (Allergan)	**Ointment:** 55.5% white petrolatum, 42.5% mineral oil, 2% petrolatum and lanolin alcohol	Preservative free. In UD 0.7 g (24s).	216
otc **Lacri-Lube S.O.P.** (Allergan)	**Ointment:** 56.8% white petrolatum, 42.5% mineral oil, 0.5% chlorobutanol and lanolin alcohols	In 3.5 and 7 g and UD 0.7 g (24s).	165
otc **Refresh PM** (Allergan)	**Ointment:** 56.8% white petrolatum, 41.5% mineral oil, sodium chloride and lanolin alcohols	Preservative free. In 3.5 g.	169

* Cost Index based on cost per g.

ARTIFICIAL TEAR INSERT

Actions:

The artificial tear insert is sterile, translucent, rod-shaped, water soluble and is made of hydroxypropyl cellulose. It acts to stabilize and thicken the precorneal tear film and prolong the tear film breakup time, which is usually accelerated in patients with dry eye states. The insert also acts to lubricate and protect the eye.

Signs and symptoms resulting from moderate to severe dry eye syndromes, such as conjunctival hyperemia, corneal and conjunctival staining with rose bengal, exudation, itching, burning, foreign body sensation, smarting, photophobia, dryness and blurred or cloudy vision are reduced. Progressive visual deterioration may be retarded, halted or sometimes reversed.

In a multicenter crossover study the 5 mg insert administered into the inferior cul-de-sac once a day during the waking hours was compared to artificial tears used four or more times daily. There was a prolongation of tear film breakup time and a decrease in foreign body sensation associated with dry eye syndrome in patients during treatment with inserts as compared to artificial tears. Improvement, as measured by amelioration of symptoms, by slit-lamp examination and by rose bengal staining of the cornea and conjunctiva, was greater in most patients.

During studies in healthy volunteers, a thickened precorneal tear film was usually observed through the slit-lamp while the insert was present in the conjunctival sac.

Pharmacokinetics: Hydroxypropyl cellulose is a physiologically inert substance. Dissolution studies in rabbits showed that the inserts became softer within 1 hour after they were placed in the conjunctival sac. Most dissolved completely in 14 to 18 hours; with a single exception, all had disappeared by 24 hours after insertion. Similar dissolution of the inserts was observed during prolonged administration (up to 54 weeks).

Indications:

For moderate to severe dry eye syndromes including keratoconjunctivitis sicca; exposure keratitis; decreased corneal sensitivity; recurrent corneal erosions.

Contraindications:

Hypersensitivity to hydroxypropyl cellulose.

Adverse Reactions:

The following adverse reactions have been reported, but in most instances were mild and transient: Blurring of vision; ocular discomfort or irritation; matting or stickiness of eyelashes; photophobia; hypersensitivity; edema of the eyelids; hyperemia.

Patient Information:

Do not rub the eye(s) containing the insert.

May produce transient blurring of vision; exercise caution while operating hazardous machinery or driving.

If improperly placed, corneal abrasion may result. The patient should practice insertion and removal of insert while in physician's office until proficiency is achieved.

Illustrated instructions are included in each package.

If symptoms worsen, remove insert and notify physician.

Administration:

Once daily, inserted into the inferior cul-de-sac beneath the base of the tarsus, not in apposition to the cornea nor beneath the eyelid at the level of the tarsal plate. Individual patients may require twice-daily use for optimal results.

If not properly positioned, the insert will be expelled into the interpalpebral fissure, and may cause symptoms of a foreign body.

Occasionally, the insert is inadvertently expelled from the eye, especially in patients with shallow conjunctival fornices. Caution the patient against rubbing the eye(s), especially upon awakening, so as not to dislodge or expel the insert. If required, another insert may be used. If transient blurred vision develops, the patient may want to remove the insert a few hours after insertion to avoid this.

Storage: Store below 86°F (30°C).

				C.I.*
Rx	**Lacrisert** (MSD)	**Insert:** 5 mg hydroxypropyl cellulose	Preservative free. In 60s with applicator.	79

* Cost Index based on cost per insert.

PUNCTAL PLUGS

These flexible silicone plugs block the puncta and canaliculus and eliminate tear loss by this route.

Indications:

For the treatment of keratitis sicca (dry eye).

Contraindications:

Hypersensitivity to silicone; eye infection.

Precautions:

If injecting an anesthetic agent in the region of the canaliculus, maintain approximately a 5 mm distance between the injection path and the angular vessels.

Do not dilate punctual opening more than 1.2 mm.

If irritation caused by plug insertion persists longer than several days, re-examine the patient and consider plug removal.

Patient Information:

Do not press fingers on or near the eyelid. Use a cotton-tipped swab to remove "sleep" from the corner of eyes.

Do not attempt to replace a plug that has fallen out.

Relief may not occur immediately after insertion; some discomfort and tearing may occur for a few days.

Administration:

Plugs must be inserted by a physician.

Herrick Lacrimal Plug (Lacrimedics):

> *Insertion* – Using a pair of fine-tipped jeweler's forceps, insert one tip of the forceps into the large hollow end of the plug.

> While magnifying the punctum, evert the eyelid to fully expose. Insert the small end of the plug into the punctum.

> Advance the plug down out of sight. Insertion may be made easier by applying lateral traction to the eyelid. This straightens the bend between the vertical and horizontal canaliculus and clears the way for placement into the horizontal canaliculus. As the plug passes the punctum, the large hollow end will fold in upon itself. Once past the punctum it will re-open and regain original shape.

> Once the plug is down out of sight, withdraw the forceps from the punctum. The friction from the walls of the canaliculus will cause the plug to detach from the forceps and remain within the canaliculus.

> After placement, the blink mechanism and the pressure from the tear fluid passing through the tear drainage system will cause the plug to migrate into the distal end of the horizontal canaliculus.

> *Removal* – Should removal be required (due to epiphora, irritation or infection), irrigation or probing of the canaliculus will propel the plug into the nasolacrimal sac; it is then flushed down into the nose.

Punctum Plug (Eagle Vision):

Pretreatment – Anesthetize the eye with a topical anesthetic solution such as proparacaine HCl 0.5% or cocaine 1% to 4%. Apply several drops and wait a few minutes for maximum anesthesia. The concomitant use of an anesthetic-wetted cotton pledget may be helpful. Alternatively, anesthetic solutions may be applied to the inner lid by means of a cotton-tipped applicator.

Highly nervous patients can be given either appropriate sedation or pre-op treatment. If needed, xylocaine can be injected in the area of the canaliculus (inject about 5 mm from the angular vessels).

Insertion – Normally, this is an outpatient procedure done with the aid of an operating microscope, but a loupe is adequate. Plug only the lower punctum of one eye and let the fellow eye serve as a control. If necessary, plug the upper punctum. Plug the fellow eye based on results with the first eye.

Two methods of lid immobilization are recommended: 1.) Retract the lid by pressure applied with the hand. 2.) Grasp the lid with curved non-toothed forceps or cotton-tip applicator forceps. Moisten the cotton, which contacts the conjunctiva with saline or anesthetic drops.

Prepare the punctum plug by loading it on the inserter or on an appropriate diameter blunt-ended needle or cannula. Insert the blunt end into the opening in the center of the dome head.

Lean the patient back and gently dilate the punctum using *only* a 1.2 mm controlled punctum dilator. This should provide adequate dilation without the danger of fracturing the punctal ring. If fractured, the punctal ring will heal but may not be as tight.

Do not insert the dilator tip more than 2 to 3 mm into the vertical canaliculus.

Withdraw the dilator from the punctal opening, *quickly* flip the inserter (if used), aim the plug at the punctal opening and swiftly insert the punctum plug into the punctum down to the base of the domed head. The punctal ring will quickly reconstrict the opening after the dilator is retracted. If unsuccessful, redilate.

After the plug has been inserted, withdraw the inserter from the plug while holding down the exposed dome with the outside sleeve of the inserter, or by pressing the domehead gently with small forceps. Assure that the plug is fully inserted. The base of the dome should appear to be flush with the surface of the punctal opening.

Removal – If necessary, grasp underneath the dome with suitable small forceps and gently pull the plug along the plug axis from the punctal opening.

Rx **Herrick Lacrimal Plug** (Lacrimedics)	**Plug:** Silicone plug	In 0.3 and 0.5 mm sizes. Available in packs of 2 plugs.
Rx **Punctum Plug** (Eagle Vision)		In 1.6, 2 and 2.8 mm sizes. Available in packs of 2, 10 and 20 plugs. Contains one inserter tool.

COLLAGEN IMPLANTS

These absorbable implants block the puncta, eliminating tear loss by this route.

Indications:

For the relief of dry eyes and secondary abnormalities such as conjunctivitis, corneal ulcer, pterygium, blepharitis, keratitis, red lid margins, recurrent chalazion, recurrent corneal erosion, filamentary keratitis and other non-infectious external eye diseases.

To temporarily enhance the effect of ocular medications.

Contraindications:

Tearing secondary to chronic dacryocystitis with mucopurulent discharge.

Patient Information:

Relief may not occur immediately after insertion.

No removal is necessary; implants dissolve within 4 to 7 days.

Re-examination is usually required within 3 to 14 days.

Successful treatment may indicate a need for permanent treatment (eg, nondissolvable silicone plugs).

Administration:

Implants must be inserted by a physician. Placement of implants in all four canaliculi is recommended to prevent a false negative response.

Rx **Collagen Implant** (Lacrimedics)	**Implant:** Collagen implant	In 0.2, 0.3, 0.4, 0.5 and 0.6 mm sizes (12s).
Rx **Temporary Intracanalicular Collagen Implant** (Eagle Vision)		In 0.2, 0.3 and 0.4 mm sizes (12s).

CLEANING/LUBRICANT FOR ARTIFICIAL EYES

Action:

The cleaning/lubricant solution is a sterile, buffered isotonic solution formulated especially for artificial eye wearers. It contains the antibacterial agent benzalkonium chloride to kill most germs which are commonly found in the eye socket of artificial eye wearers. Tyloxapol, a detergent, liquifies the solid matter so that it is less irritating. Benzalkonium chloride, in addition to its germ-killing action, aids tyloxapol in wetting the artificial eye so that it is completely covered.

Indication:

To lubricate, clean and wet the artificial eye to increase wearing comfort.

Contraindication:

Hypersensitivity to any component of the formulation.

Patient Information:

If irritation persists or increases, discontinue use and consult your physician. Keep container tightly closed. Keep out of the reach of children.

To avoid contamination, do not touch dropper tip to any surface. Replace cap after using.

Administration and Dosage:

Use drops just as ordinary eye drops are used. With the artificial eye in place, apply 1 or 2 drops to it, 3 or 4 times daily. The artificial eye may be removed periodically if advised by your physician, and 2 or 3 drops applied to remove oily or mucous materials. The artificial eye is then rubbed between the fingers and rinsed with tap water. Then 1 or 2 drops may be applied to the artificial eye, either prior to or after reinsertion.

Storage: Store at 46° to 80°F (8° to 27°C).

otc	**Enuclene** (Alcon)	**Solution:** 0.25% tyloxapol and 0.02% benzalkonium chloride	In 15 ml Drop-Tainers.

Anti-infective Agents

ANTIBIOTIC AGENTS

Topical and systemic antibiotics may be utilized in the treatment of ocular infections. The most common ocular infections include blepharitis, conjunctivitis, dacryoadenitis, dacryocystitis, keratitis, orbital cellulitis, endophthalmitis, attendant sinusitis and superficial erysipelas of the skin.

The indigenous flora of the eyelids and conjunctiva are primarily *Staphylococcus aureus* and *Staphylococcus epidermidis,* which can overwhelm the ocular defenses and produce infection. Staphylococcal species are most commonly associated with acute papillary conjunctivitis, chronic blepharitis, dacryocystitis, impetigo, blepharoconjunctivitis, superficial keratitis and endophthalmitis.

A purulent discharge and papillary conjunctivitis are associated with a bacterial infection. A serous discharge with conjunctival chemosis and itching is more frequently associated with conjunctival allergy. Hazing of the anterior chamber, hypopyon, infiltrative keratitis in the visual axis or decreased vision are harbingers of imminent visual loss and require prompt microbiologic studies for organism identification and proper antibiotic selection. Similar fastidious cultures of the lids or conjunctiva are important for any chronic conjunctivitis.

The table on page 98 reflects the sensitivity studies of the Department of Ophthalmology, University of Oklahoma. Individual laboratory sensitivities may vary. See individual product inserts for more information on susceptible microorganisms.

TOPICAL OPHTHALMIC ANTIBIOTIC PREPARATIONS

Organism/Infection	Bacitracin	Gramicidin	Polymyxin B	Erythromycin	Chloramphenicol	Trimethoprim	Quino-lones: Norfloxacin	Ciprofloxacin	Amino-glycosides: Neomycin	Gentamicin	Tobramycin	Tetra-cyclines: Tetracycline	Chlortetracycline	Oxytetracycline	Sulfon-amides: Sodium Sulfacetamide	Sulfisoxazole
Gram-Positive																
Staphylococci sp	✓	✓					✓	✓		✓	✓					
S aureus	✓	✓		✓	✓	✓	✓	✓	✓	✓	✓	✓	✓		✓	
Streptococcus sp	✓	✓			✓			✓				✓	✓		✓	
S pneumoniae	✓	✓		✓	✓	✓	✓	✓		✓*	✓	✓	✓			
α-hemolytic streptococci (viridans group)				✓												
β-hemolytic streptococci	✓									✓*	✓					
S pyogenes	✓			✓		✓		✓		✓			✓			
Corynebacterium sp	✓	✓		✓						✓	✓	✓				
Gram-Negative																
Escherichia coli			✓		✓	✓	✓	✓	✓	✓	✓	✓	✓	✓	✓	✓
Hemophilus aegyptius (Koch-Weeks bacillus)					✓	✓	✓			✓	✓				✓	✓
H ducreyi					✓			✓		✓	✓		✓	✓		
H influenzae				✓	✓	✓	✓	✓	✓	✓	✓		✓	✓		
Klebsiella sp					✓		✓	✓	✓					✓		
K pneumoniae			✓				✓	✓		✓	✓			✓		
Neisseria sp	✓				✓				✓	✓	✓	✓				
N gonorrhoeae	✓			✓‡			✓	✓		✓		✓‡	✓		✓	
Proteus sp						✓	✓	✓	✓	✓	✓					
Acinetobacter calcoaceticus							✓	✓		✓	✓					
Enterobacter aerogenes			✓				✓	✓	✓	✓	✓			✓		
Enterobacter sp					✓		✓	✓	✓	✓	✓					
Serratia marcescens							✓	✓		✓	✓					
Moraxella lacunata					✓					✓	✓					
Chlamydia trachomatis				✓‡				✓				✓‡‡	✓‡‡		✓**	✓
Pasturella tularensis													✓	✓		
Pseudomonas aeruginosa			✓		✓		✓	✓		✓*	✓					
Bartonella bacilliformis															✓	
Bacteroides sp				✓									✓	✓	✓	
Vibrio sp					✓		✓	✓		✓	✓				✓	
Yersinia pestis													✓	✓		

‡ For prophylaxis
‡‡ In conjunction with oral therapy
* Increasing resistance has been seen.
** Adjunct in systemic sulfonamide therapy.

ANTIFUNGAL AGENT

Natamycin (*Natacyn*) is the only topical ophthalmic antifungal agent available commercially. It is a tetraene polyene antibiotic derived from *Streptomyces natalensis*. It possesses in vitro activity against a variety of yeasts and filamentous fungi, including *Candida, Aspergillus, Cephalosporium, Fusarium* and *Penicillium*.

ANTIVIRAL AGENTS

The topical ophthalmic antiviral preparations appear to interfere with viral reproduction by altering DNA synthesis. Idoxuridine, vidarabine and trifluridine are effective treatment for herpes simplex infections of the conjunctiva and cornea. Ganciclovir is indicated for use in immunocompromised patients with cytomegalovirus (CMV) retinitis and for prevention of CMV retinitis in transplant patients. Foscarnet is indicated for use only in AIDS patients with CMV retinitis.

OPHTHALMIC ANTIVIRAL PREPARATIONS			
Generic Name	Trade Name (Manufacturer)	Preparations	Indications
Foscarnet Sodium	*Foscavir* (Astra)	Solution for Injection (24 mg/ml)	Cytomegalovirus (CMV) Retinitis
Ganciclovir Sodium	*Cytovene* (Syntex)	Reconstituted Powder (500 mg/vial)	Cytomegalovirus (CMV) Retinitis
Idoxuridine	*Herplex* (Allergan)	Solution 0.1%	Herpes simplex
Vidarabine	*Vira-A* (Parke-Davis)	Ointment 3%	Herpes simplex types 1 and 2 Idoxuridine-resistant herpes
Trifluridine	*Viroptic* (Burroughs Wellcome)	Solution 1%	Herpes simplex types 1 and 2 Idoxuridine and vidarabine-resistant herpes

Viral infection, especially epidemic keratoconjunctivitis (EKC), is more often associated with a follicular conjunctivitis, a serous conjunctival discharge and preauricular lymphadenopathy. The exceptionally contagious organism causing EKC is not susceptible to antiviral therapy at this time. Pustular lesions of the nose and face, and spade-shaped fascicular keratitis in association with chronic blepharitis, suggesting acne rosacea, warrants a trial of systemic tetracycline (eg, *Achromycin V*) or doxycycline (eg, *Vibramycin*) as both an antibiotic and potentially anti-inflammatory regimen.

J. James Rowsey, MD
University of South Florida

For More Information

Bartlett JD, Jaanus SD, eds. Clinical Ocular Pharmacology, ed. 2. Boston, MA: Butterworth, 1989.

Duane TD, ed. Clinical Ophthalmology. Philadelphia, PA: J.B. Lippincott Company, 1988.

Kucers A, Bennett NM. The Use of Antibiotics, ed. 4. Philadelphia, PA: J.B. Lippincott Company, 1987.

ANTIBIOTICS

Indications:

For the treatment of superficial ocular infections involving the conjunctiva or cornea (eg, conjunctivitis, keratitis, keratoconjunctivitis, corneal ulcers, blepharitis, blepharoconjunctivitis, acute meibomianitis and dacryocystitis) due to strains of microorganisms susceptible to antibiotics.

Refer to individual product listings for specific indications.

For a listing of the microorganisms usually susceptible to these agents, refer to page 98.

Contraindications:

Hypersensitivity to any component of the formulation.

Epithelial herpes simplex keratitis (dendritic keratitis), vaccinia, varicella, mycobacterial infections or fungal diseases of the ocular structure.

Steroid combinations: After uncomplicated removal of a corneal foreign body.

Warnings:

Neomycin: Allergic cross-reactions may occur which could prevent the use of any or all of the following antibiotics for the treatment of future infections: *Kanamycin, paromomycin, streptomycin* and possibly *gentamicin*.

Neomycin sulfate-containing products may cause cutaneous sensitization (10%).

Chloramphenicol: Hematopoietic toxicity has occurred occasionally with the systemic use of chloramphenicol and rarely with topical administration. It is generally a dose-related toxic effect on bone marrow, and is usually reversible on cessation of therapy. Rare cases of aplastic anemia, bone marrow hypoplasia and death have been reported with prolonged (months to years) or frequent intermittent (over months and years) use of ocular chloramphenicol.

Ophthalmic ointments may retard corneal epithelial healing.

Pregnancy: Category B (tobramycin). *Category C* (ciprofloxacin, gentamicin, norfloxacin). Safety for use during pregnancy has not been established. Use only when clearly needed and when the potential benefits outweigh the potential hazards to the fetus.

Lactation: It is not known whether ciprofloxacin or norfloxacin appears in breast milk. Caution should be exercised when ciprofloxacin is administered to a nursing mother. Because of the potential for adverse reactions in nursing infants from norfloxacin and tobramycin, decide whether to discontinue nursing or discontinue the drug, taking into account the importance of the drug to the mother.

Children: Safety and efficacy of ciprofloxacin in children under 12 and norfloxacin in infants under 1 have not been established. Tobramycin has been found safe and effective in children.

Precautions:

Ciprofloxacin and norfloxacin: Serious and occasionally fatal hypersensitivity (anaphylactoid or anaphylactic) reactions, some following the first dose, have been reported in patients receiving systemic quinolone therapy. Some reactions were accompanied by cardiovascular collapse, loss of consciousness, tingling, pharyngeal or facial edema, dyspnea, urticaria and itching. Only a few patients had a history of hypersensitivity reactions. Serious anaphylactoid or anaphylactic reactions require immediate emergency treatment with epinephrine and other resuscitation measures.

Sulfite Sensitivity: Some of these products contain sulfites which may cause allergic-type reactions (eg, hives, itching, wheezing, anaphylaxis) in certain suscepti- ble persons. Although the overall prevalence of sulfite sensitivity in the general pop- ulation is probably low, it is seen more frequently in asthmatics or in atopic nonasth- matic persons. Specific products containing sulfites are identified in the product listings.

Laboratory tests: Perform culture and susceptibility testing during treatment.

Do not use topical antibiotics in deep-seated ocular infections or in those that are likely to become systemic. The prolonged use may result in overgrowth of nonsus- ceptible organisms, particularly fungi. Institute an appropriate antibiotic or chemo- therapy if new infections develop during treatment.

Superinfection: Use of antibiotics (especially prolonged or repeated therapy) may result in bacterial or fungal overgrowth of nonsusceptible organisms. Such over- growth may lead to a secondary infection. Take appropriate measures if superinfec- tion occurs.

Systemic antibiotics: In all except very superficial infections, supplement the topical use of antibiotics by appropriate systemic medication. Systemic aminoglycoside anti- biotics require monitoring of the total serum concentration (peak and trough).

Crystalline precipitate: A white crystalline precipitate located in the superficial por- tion of the corneal defect was observed in ≈ 17% of patients with bacterial corneal ulcer on ciprofloxacin. Onset was within 1 to 7 days after starting therapy. The pre- cipitate resolved in most patients within 2 weeks, and did not preclude continued use nor adversely affect the clinical course or outcome.

Drug Interactions:

Chymotrypsin: Concomitant use of *chloramphenicol* may inhibit the enzyme.

Specific drug interaction studies have not been conducted with ophthalmic ciproflox- acin or norfloxacin. However, the systemic administration of some quinolones has been shown to elevate plasma concentrations of theophylline, interfere with the metabolism of caffeine, enhance the effects of the oral anticoagulant warfarin and its derivatives and has been associated with transient elevations in serum creatinine and cyclosporine in patients receiving cyclosporine concomitantly.

Adverse Reactions:

Sensitivity reactions such as transient irritation, burning, stinging, itching, inflamma- tion, angioneurotic edema, urticaria, vesicular and maculopapular dermatitis have occurred in some patients.

Chloramphenicol: Hematological events (including aplastic anemia) have been reported (see Warnings).

Ciprofloxacin: White crystalline precipitates; lid margin crusting; crystals/scales; for- eign body sensation; itching; conjunctival hyperemia; bad taste in mouth; corneal staining; keratopathy/keratitis; allergic reactions; lid edema; tearing; photophobia; corneal infiltrates; nausea; decreased vision.

Norfloxacin: Conjunctival hyperemia; chemosis; photophobia; bitter taste in mouth.

Tetracycline and *chlortetracycline:* Dermatitis has been reported with the use of these antibiotics.

Topical aminoglycosides: Localized ocular toxicity and hypersensitivity, lid itching, lid swelling and conjunctival erythema have occurred (< 3%) with tobramycin; mydriasis and conjunctival paresthesia have occurred with gentamicin. Similar reactions may occur with the topical use of other aminoglycoside antibiotics.

Overdosage:

Ciprofloxacin: If ocular overdosage occurs, flush eye(s) with warm tap water.

Tobramycin: Symptoms of overdosage include punctate keratitis, erythema, increased lacrimation, edema and lid itching. These may be similar to adverse reactions.

Patient Information:

Tilt head back, place medication in conjunctival sac and close eyes. Apply light finger pressure on lacrimal sac for 1 minute following instillation.

May cause temporary blurring of vision or stinging following administration. Notify physician if stinging, burning or itching becomes pronounced, or if redness, irritation, swelling or pain persists or increases.

Ciprofloxacin and norfloxacin: Discontinue use and notify physician at the first sign of a skin rash or other allergic reaction.

To avoid contamination, do not touch tip of container to any surface. Replace cap after using.

Keep out of the reach of children.

Individual drug monographs are on the following pages.

BACITRACIN

For complete prescribing information see General Monograph p. 100.

Administration and Dosage:

Apply directly to conjunctival sac(s) 1 to 3 times daily.

Blepharitis: Carefully remove all scales and crusts and then spread ointment uniformly over lid margins.

Storage: Store at room temperature 59° to 86°F (15° to 30°C).

			C.I.*
Rx **Bacitracin** (Various, eg, Bausch & Lomb, Fougera, Goldline, Major, Rugby, Schein, United Research)	**Ointment:** 500 units bacitracin/g	In 3.5 and 3.75 g.	97+
Rx **AK-Tracin** (Akorn)		Preservative free. In 3.5 g.	102

POLYMYXIN B SULFATE

For complete prescribing information see General Monograph p. 100.

Indication:

For treatment of infections of the eye caused by susceptible strains of *Pseudomonas aeruginosa.*

Administration and Dosage:

Dissolve 500,000 units polymyxin B sulfate in 20 to 50 ml sterile distilled water (Sterile Water for Injection, USP) or sterile physiologic saline (Sodium Chloride Injection, USP) for a 10,000 to 25,000 units per ml concentration.

For the treatment of P aeruginosa infections of the eye: Administer a concentration of 0.1% to 0.25% (10,000 to 25,000 units per ml) 1 to 3 drops every hour, increasing the intervals as response indicates.

Subconjunctival injection of up to 100,000 units/day may be used for the treatment of *P aeruginosa* infections of the cornea and conjunctiva.

Avoid total systemic and ophthalmic instillations of over 25,000 units/kg/day.

			C.I.*
Rx **Polymyxin B Sulfate Sterile** (Roerig)	**Powder for solution:** 500,000 units polymyxin B sulfate	In 20 ml vials.	38

* Cost Index based on cost per g or ml.

ERYTHROMYCIN

For complete prescribing information see General Monograph p. 100.

Indications:

For the treatment of superficial ocular infections involving the conjunctiva or cornea caused by organisms susceptible to erythromycin.

For prophylaxis of ophthalmia neonatorum due to *Neisseria gonorrhoeae* or *Chlamydia trachomatis*. The Centers for Disease Control and the Committee on Drugs, the Committee on Infectious Diseases of the American Academy of Pediatrics and the Committee on Fetus and Newborn recommend 1% silver nitrate solution in single-use ampules or single-use tubes of an ophthalmic ointment containing 0.5% erythromycin or 1% tetracycline as "effective and acceptable regimens for prophylaxis of gonococcal ophthalmia neonatorum." (For infants born to mothers with clinically apparent gonorrhea, give IV or IM injections of aqueous crystalline penicillin G: A single dose of 50,000 units for term infants or 20,000 units for infants of low birth weight. Topical prophylaxis alone is inadequate for these infants.)

For the prevention of neonatal conjunctivitis due to *C trachomatis*, a condition that may develop 1 to several weeks after delivery in infants of mothers whose birth canals harbor the organism.

Administration and Dosage:

External ocular infections: Apply directly to the infected area 1 or more times daily depending on the severity of the infection.

Prophylaxis of neonatal gonococcal or chlamydial conjunctivitis: Instill a thin line of ointment approximately 0.5 to 1 cm in length into each conjunctival sac. Do not flush the ointment from the eye following application. Use a new tube for each infant. Administer to infants born by cesarian section and those delivered vaginally.

Storage: Store at room temperature 59° to 86°F (15° to 30°C).

			C.I.*
Rx	**Erythromycin** (Various, eg, Bausch & Lomb, Fougera, Rugby)	**Ointment:** 5 mg erythromycin/g	In 3.5 and 3.75 g and UD 1 g. 80+
Rx	**AK-Mycin** (Akorn)		Preservative free. In 3.75 g.[1] 107
Rx	**Ilotycin** (Dista)		In 3.5 and UD 1 g.[2] 196

* Cost Index based on cost per g.
[1] With white petrolatum and mineral oil.
[2] With white petrolatum, mineral oil and parabens.

CHLORAMPHENICOL

For complete prescribing information see General Monograph p. 100.

Use only in those serious infections for which less potentially dangerous drugs are ineffective or contraindicated (see Warnings).

Administration and Dosage:

Ointment: Place a small amount in the conjunctival sac(s) every 3 hours, or more often if required, day and night for the first 48 hours. Intervals between applications may be increased after the first 2 days. Since chloramphenicol is primarily bacteriostatic, continue therapy for 48 hours after an apparent cure has been obtained.

Storage: Store at room temp 59° to 86°F (15° to 30°C). Store away from heat.

Solution (reconstituted): Instill 2 drops into the affected eye(s) every 3 hours or more frequently if deemed advisable. Continue administration day and night for the first 48 hours, after which the interval between applications may be increased. Continue treatment for at least 48 hours after the eye appears normal.

SOLUTION PREPARATION	
Strength of solution desired	Add sterile distilled water
0.5%	5 ml
0.25%	10 ml
0.16%	15 ml

Storage: Store below 86°F (30°C). Reconstituted solutions remain stable at room temperature for 10 days.

Solution: Instill 1 or 2 drops 4 to 6 times a day for the first 72 hours, depending upon the severity of the condition. Intervals between applications may be increased after the first 2 days. Since the action of the drug is primarily bacteriostatic, continue therapy for 48 hours after an apparent cure has been attained.

Storage: Refrigerate at 36° to 46°F (2° to 8°C) until dispensed. Protect from light. Remove from refrigerator for dispensing; discard 21 days thereafter. **C.I.***

Rx				C.I.*
Rx	**Chloramphenicol** (Various, eg, Bausch & Lomb)	**Ointment:** 10 mg chloramphenicol/g	In 3.5 g.	98+
Rx	**AK-Chlor** (Akorn)		In 3.5 g.[1]	184
Rx	**Chloromycetin** (Parke-Davis)		Preservative free. In 3.5 g.[2]	430
Rx	**Chloroptic S.O.P.** (Allergan)		In 3.5 g.[3]	502
Rx	**Chloromycetin** (Parke-Davis)	**Powder for solution:** 25 mg chloramphenicol/vial	Preservative free. In 15 ml. With diluent.	145
Rx	**Chloramphenicol** (Various, eg, Bausch & Lomb)	**Solution:** 5 mg chloramphenicol/ml[4]	In 7.5 and 15 ml.	58+
Rx	**AK-Chlor** (Akorn)		In 7.5 and 15 ml.[5]	80
Rx	**Chloroptic** (Allergan)		In 2.5 and 7.5 ml.[6]	239

* Cost Index based on cost per g or ml.
[1] In a white petrolatum base with mineral oil and polysorbate 60.
[2] In a liquid petrolatum and polyethylene base.
[3] With white petrolatum, mineral oil, polyoxyl 40 stearate, petrolatum (and) lanolin alcohol, PEG-300 and 0.5% chlorobutanol.
[4] Refrigerate until dispensed.
[5] With 0.5% chlorobutanol, polyethylene glycol and polyoxyl 40 stearate.
[6] With 0.5% chlorobutanol, PEG-300 and polyoxyl 40 stearate.

GENTAMICIN

For complete prescribing information see General Monograph p. 100.

Administration and Dosage:

Solution: Instill 1 or 2 drops into the affected eye(s) every 4 hours. In severe infections, dosage may be increased to 2 drops once every hour.

This solution is not for injection. Do not inject subconjunctivally. Do not directly introduce into the anterior chamber.

Storage: Store at 36° to 86°F (2° to 30°C). Store away from heat.

Ointment: Apply a small amount to affected eye(s) 2 to 3 times daily.

Storage: Store at 36° to 86°F (2° to 30°C). Store away from heat.

			C.I.*
Rx **Gentamicin** (Various, eg, Bausch & Lomb, Goldline, Major, Moore, Parmed, Rugby, Schein)	**Ointment:** 3 mg gentamicin (as sulfate)/g	In 3.5 g.	148+
Rx **Garamycin** (Schering)		In 3.5 g.[1]	508
Rx **Genoptic S.O.P.** (Allergan)		In 3.5 g.[1]	529
Rx **Gentacidin** (Iolab)		In 3.5 g.[2]	269
Rx **Gentak** (Akorn)		In 3.5 g.[3]	191
Rx **Gentamicin** (Various, eg, Bausch & Lomb, Geneva, Goldline, Major, Moore, Parmed, Rugby, Schein, Steris, United Research)	**Solution:** 3 mg gentamicin (as sulfate)/ml	In 5 and 15 ml.	140+
Rx **Garamycin** (Schering)		In 5 ml dropper bottles.[4]	355
Rx **Genoptic** (Allergan)		In 1 and 5 ml dropper bottles.[5]	371
Rx **Gentacidin** (Iolab)		In 5 ml dropper bottles.[4]	189
Rx **Gentak** (Akorn)		In 5 and 15 ml dropper bottles.[6]	130

* Cost Index based on cost per g or ml.
[1] In a white petrolatum base with parabens.
[2] With mineral oil and white petrolatum.
[3] With anhydrous liquid lanolin, white petrolatum, mineral oil and parabens.
[4] With benzalkonium chloride and sodium chloride.
[5] With benzalkonium chloride, 1.4% polyvinyl alcohol, EDTA and sodium chloride.
[6] With 0.1% benzalkonium chloride and sodium chloride.

TOBRAMYCIN

For complete prescribing information see General Monograph p. 100.

Administration and Dosage:

Solution: Mild to moderate disease – Instill 1 or 2 drops into the affected eye(s) every 4 hours.

> *Severe infections* – Instill 2 drops into the eye(s) hourly until improvement. Reduce treatment prior to discontinuation.

> Not for injection into the eye.

Ointment: Mild to moderate disease – Apply 0.5 inch ribbon into the affected eye(s) 2 or 3 times daily.

> *Severe infections* – Instill 0.5 inch ribbon into the affected eye(s) every 3 to 4 hours until improvement. Reduce treatment prior to discontinuation.

Storage: Store at 46° to 80°F (8° to 27°C).

				C.I.*
Rx	**Tobrex** (Alcon)	**Ointment:** 3 mg tobramycin/g	In 3.5 g.[1]	633
Rx	**Tobrex** (Alcon)	**Solution:** 3 mg tobramycin/ml	In 5 ml Drop-Tainers.[2]	443

TETRACYCLINE

For complete prescribing information see General Monograph p. 100.

Indications:

For the treatment of superficial ocular infections susceptible to tetracycline HCl.

For prophylaxis of ophthalmia neonatorum due to *Neisseria gonorrhoeae* or *Chlamydia trachomatis*. The Centers for Disease Control and the Committee on Drugs, the Committee on Infectious Diseases of the American Academy of Pediatrics and the Committee on Fetus and Newborn recommend 1% silver nitrate solution in single-use ampules or single-use tubes of an ophthalmic ointment containing 0.5% erythromycin or 1% tetracycline as "effective and acceptable regimens for prophylaxis of gonococcal ophthalmia neonatorum." (For infants born to mothers with clinically apparent gonorrhea, give IV or IM injections of aqueous crystalline penicillin G. A single dose of 50,000 units for term infants or 20,000 units for infants of low birth weight. Topical prophylaxis alone is inadequate for these infants.)

Administration and Dosage:

Suspension: Shake well, then instill 2 drops into the affected eye(s) 2 to 4 times daily, or more frequently, depending upon the severity of the infection. Very severe infections may require several days of treatment. Other cases may be cured by instillation with much less frequency for 48 hours.

> *Acute or chronic trachoma* – Instill 2 drops into the affected eye(s) 2 to 4 times daily. Continue for 1 to 2 months. Certain individual or complicated cases may require a longer duration. Concomitant oral tetracycline is helpful.

---

* Cost Index based on cost per g or ml.
[1] With mineral oil, white petrolatum and 0.5% chlorobutanol.
[2] With 0.01% benzalkonium chloride, tyloxapol and sodium chloride.

For unit-dose administration – Immediately prior to use, simultaneously roll, invert and squeeze dispenser between thumb and fingers. Repeat several times to mix contents well. Use aseptic technique to cut the tip of the dispenser. Discard first 2 drops before instilling drops in eye(s). Instill 2 drops in eye(s), then discard.

Ointment: Apply directly to the affected area every 2 hours or more often, as the severity of the infection and the degree of response indicate. Severe or stubborn ocular infections may require treatment for many days, and may also require oral therapy. Mild infections may respond within 48 hours.

Storage: Store at room temperature 59° to 86°F (15° to 30°C).

				C.I.*
Rx	**Achromycin** (Storz/Lederle)	**Ointment:** 10 mg tetracycline HCl/g	In 3.75 g.[1]	362
Rx	**Achromycin** (Storz/Lederle)	**Suspension:** 10 mg tetracycline HCl/ml	In 4 ml.[2]	505

CHLORTETRACYCLINE

For complete prescribing information see General Monograph p. 100.

Administration and Dosage:

Apply to the affected eye(s) every 2 hours or more often as the condition and response indicate. Severe or stubborn infections may require treatment for many days, and may also require oral therapy. Mild infections may respond in as little as 48 hours.

				C.I.*
Rx	**Aureomycin** (Storz/Lederle)	**Ointment:** 10 mg chlortetracycline HCl/g	In 3.5 g.[3]	396

CIPROFLOXACIN

For complete prescribing information see General Monograph p. 100.

Administration and Dosage:

Not for injection into the eye.

For the treatment of corneal ulcers: Instill 2 drops into the affected eye(s) every 15 minutes for the first 6 hours and then 2 drops every 30 minutes for the remainder of the first day. On the second day, instill 2 drops every hour. On the third through the fourteenth day, instill 2 drops every 4 hours. Treatment may be continued after 14 days if corneal re-epithelialization has not occurred.

For the treatment of bacterial conjunctivitis: Instill 1 or 2 drops into the conjunctival sac(s) every 2 hours while awake for 2 days, and 1 or 2 drops every 4 hours while awake for the next 5 days.

Storage: Store at 36° to 86°F (2° to 30°C). Protect from light.

Rx	**Ciloxan** (Alcon)	**Solution:** 3.5 mg ciprofloxacin HCl/ml (equivalent to 3 mg base)	In 2.5 and 5 ml DropTainers.[4]	500

* Cost Index based on cost per g or ml.
[1] With white petrolatum, light mineral oil and anhydrous lanolin.
[2] With plastibase 50W and light mineral oil.
[3] With petrolatum and anhydrous lanolin.
[4] With 0.006% benzalkonium chloride, 4.6% mannitol and 0.05% EDTA.

NORFLOXACIN

For complete prescribing information see General Monograph p. 100.

Administration and Dosage:

Instill 1 or 2 drops into the affected eye(s) 4 times daily for up to 7 days. Depending on the severity of the infection, the dosage for the first day of therapy may be 1 or 2 drops every 2 hours during the waking hours.

Storage: Store at room temperature 59° to 86°F (15° to 30°C). Protect from light.

Rx **Chibroxin** (MSD)	**Solution:** 3 mg norfloxacin/ml	In 5 ml Ocumeters.[1]	375

COMBINATION ANTIBIOTIC PRODUCTS

For complete prescribing information see General Monograph p. 100 and individual product monographs.

Precautions:

Neomycin: Allergic cross-reactions may occur which could prevent the use of any or all of the following antibiotics for the treatment of future infections: *Kanamycin, paromomycin, streptomycin* and possibly *gentamicin.*

Administration and Dosage:

Solution: Instill 1 to 2 drops into the lower conjunctival sac(s) 3 or more times daily as required.

Ointment: Instill 0.5 inch ribbon into the conjunctival sac(s) up to 5 times daily.

For complete dosage instructions, see individual manufacturer inserts.

Product and Distributor	Polymyxin B Sulfate (units/g or ml)	Neomycin as Sulfate (mg/g or ml)	Bacitracin Zinc (units/g)	Oxytetracycline as HCl (mg/g)	Gramicidin (mg/ml)	Trimethoprim (mg/ml)	How Supplied	C.I.*
Rx **Neotal Ophthalmic Ointment** (Hauck)	5000	5	400				In 3.5 g.[2]	76
Rx **Triple Antibiotic Ointment** (Various, eg, Rugby)							In 3.5 g.	80+
Rx **Terramycin w/Polymyxin B Ointment** (Roerig)	10,000			5			In 3.5 g.[3]	313

* Cost Index based on cost per g or ml.
[1] With 0.0025% benzalkonium chloride, EDTA and sodium chloride.
[2] In a white petrolatum and mineral oil base.
[3] In a white and liquid petrolatum base.

COMBINATION ANTIBIOTIC PRODUCTS C.I.*

	Product and Distributor	Polymyxin B Sulfate (units/g or ml)	Neomycin as Sulfate (mg/g or ml)	Bacitracin Zinc (units/g)	Oxytetracycline as HCl (mg/g)	Gramicidin (mg/ml)	Trimethoprim (mg/ml)	How Supplied	C.I.*
Rx	**AK-Poly-Bac Ointment** (Akorn)	10,000		500				Preservative free. In 3.5 g.[1]	184
Rx	**Polysporin Ophthalmic Ointment** (Burroughs Wellcome)							In 3.5 g.[2]	571
Rx	**Polytrim Ophthalmic Solution** (Allergan)	10,000					1	In 10 ml dropper bottles.[3]	216
Rx	**Neomycin Sulfate-Polymyxin B Sulfate-Gramicidin Solution** (Various, eg, Iolab, Rugby, Steris)	10,000	1.75			0.025		In 10 ml.	56+
Rx	**AK-Spore Solution** (Akorn)							In 2 and 10 ml.[4]	64
Rx	**Neosporin Ophthalmic Solution** (Burroughs Wellcome)							In 10 ml Drop Dose.[4]	200
Rx	**Ocutricin Ophthalmic Solution** (Bausch & Lomb)							In 10 ml dropper bottles.[1]	62
Rx	**Statrol Ointment** (Alcon)	10,000	3.5					In 3.5 g.[5]	459
Rx	**Bacitracin-Neomycin-Polymyxin B Ophthalmic Ointment** (Various, eg, Fougera, Major)	10,000	3.5	400				In 3.5 g.	103+
Rx	**AK-Spore Ointment** (Akorn)							Preservative free. In 3.5 g.[1]	161
Rx	**Neosporin Ophthalmic Ointment** (Burroughs Wellcome)							In 3.5 g.[2]	571
Rx	**Ocutricin Ointment** (Bausch & Lomb)							In 3.5 g.[1]	98
Rx	**Statrol Solution** (Alcon)	16,250	3.5					In 5 ml Drop-Tainers.[6]	321

* Cost Index based on cost per g or ml.
[1] With white petrolatum and mineral oil.
[2] In white petrolatum base.
[3] With 0.004% benzalkonium chloride and sodium chloride.
[4] With 0.001% thimerosal, 0.5% alcohol, propylene glycol, polyoxyethylene, polyoxypropylene and sodium chloride.
[5] With 0.05% methylparaben and 0.01% propylparaben, white petrolatum and anhydrous liquid lanolin.
[6] With 0.004% benzalkonium chloride, 0.5% hydroxypropyl methylcellulose and sodium chloride.

STEROID AND ANTIBIOTIC COMBINATIONS

For complete prescribing information see Steroid Preparations p. 72 and Antibiotic Preparations p. 100.

Indications:

For steroid-responsive inflammatory ocular conditions for which a corticosteroid is indicated and where bacterial infection or a risk of bacterial ocular infection exists.

For inflammatory conditions of the palpebral and bulbar conjunctiva, cornea and anterior segment of the globe where the inherent risk of steroid use in certain infective conjunctivitides is accepted to obtain a diminution in edema and inflammation. For chronic anterior uveitis and corneal injury from chemical, radiation or thermal burns, or penetration of foreign bodies.

STEROID AND ANTIBIOTIC SOLUTIONS AND SUSPENSIONS

Administration and Dosage:

Store suspensions upright and shake well before using.

Instill 1 or 2 drops into the affected eye(s) every 3 or 4 hours, or more frequently as required.

Not more than 20 ml should be prescribed initially, and the prescription should not be refilled without further evaluation. For complete dosage instructions, see individual manufacturer inserts.

Product and Distributor	Steroid (per ml)	Antibiotic (per ml)	Other Content	How Supplied	C.I.*
Rx **Chloromycetin Hydro-cortisone for Suspen-sion** (Parke-Davis)	0.5% hydrocortisone acetate† (2.5% as powder)	0.25% chloramphenicol† (1.25% as powder)	Cholesterol, methylcellulose, 0.01% benzethonium chloride and NaCl	In 5 ml with diluent and dropper.	600

* Cost Index based on cost per ml.
† As a prepared solution.

STEROID AND ANTIBIOTIC SOLUTIONS AND SUSPENSIONS (Cont.)

For complete prescribing information see Steroid Preparations p. 72 and Antibiotic Preparations p. 100.

	Product and Distributor	Steroid (per ml)	Antibiotic (per ml)	Other Content	How Supplied	C.I.*
Rx	**Neomycin and Polymyxin B Sulfate and Hydrocortisone Ophthalmic Suspension** (Various, eg. Iolab, Steris)	1% hydrocortisone	Neomycin sulfate equivalent to 0.35% neomycin base and 10,000 units polymyxin B sulfate	0.001% thimerosal or 0.01% benzalkonium chloride, cetyl alcohol, glyceryl monostearate, polyoxyl 40 stearate, propylene glycol and mineral oil	In 7.5 ml.	113+
Rx	**AK-Spore H.C.** (Akorn)				In 7.5 ml.	136
Rx	**Bacticort Suspension** (Rugby)				In 7.5 ml with dropper.	178
Rx	**Ocutricin HC Suspension** (Bausch & Lomb)				In 7.5 ml.	62
Rx	**Cortisporin Suspension** (Burroughs Wellcome)				In 7.5 ml Drop Dose.	270
Rx	**Terra-Cortril Suspension** (Roerig)	1.5% hydrocortisone acetate	0.5% oxytetracycline (as HCl)	Mineral oil and aluminum tristearate	In 5 ml with dropper.	545
Rx	**Poly-Pred Suspension** (Allergan)	0.5% prednisolone acetate	Neomycin sulfate equivalent to 0.35% neomycin base and 10,000 units polymyxin B sulfate	1.4% polyvinyl alcohol, 0.001% thimerosal, polysorbate 80 and propylene glycol	In 5 and 10 ml dropper bottles.	447

* Cost Index based on cost per ml.

STEROID AND ANTIBIOTIC SOLUTIONS AND SUSPENSIONS (Cont.)

For complete prescribing information see Steroid Preparations p. 72 and Antibiotic Preparations p. 100.

	Product and Distributor	Steroid (per ml)	Antibiotic (per ml)	Other Content	How Supplied	C.I.*
Rx	**Pred-G Suspension** (Allergan)	1% prednisolone acetate	Gentamicin sulfate equivalent to 0.3% gentamicin base	1.4% polyvinyl alcohol, 0.005% benzalkonium chloride, EDTA, hydroxypropyl methylcellulose, polysorbate 80 and NaCl	In 2, 5 and 10 ml dropper bottles.	454
Rx	**Neomycin Sulfate-Dexamethasone Sodium Phosphate Ophthalmic Solution** (Various, eg, Rugby, Steris)	0.1% dexamethasone phosphate (as sodium phosphate)	Neomycin sulfate equivalent to 0.35% neomycin base	Polysorbate 80, EDTA, 0.02% benzalkonium chloride and 0.1% sodium bisulfite	In 5 ml.	161+
Rx	**NeoDecadron Solution** (MSD)				In 5 ml Ocu-meters.	404
Rx	**Neo Dexair** (Bausch & Lomb)				In 5 ml.	198
Rx	**AK-Neo-Dex Solution** (Akorn)			0.01% benzalkonium chloride, EDTA, polysorbate 80 and sodium bisulfite	In 5 ml bottles with applicator.	182
Rx	**TobraDex Suspension** (Alcon)	0.1% dexamethasone	0.3% tobramycin	0.01% benzalkonium chloride, tyloxapol, EDTA, hydroxyethyl cellulose, sodium sulfate and NaCl	In 2.5 and 5 ml Drop-Tainers.	529

* Cost Index based on cost per ml.

STEROID AND ANTIBIOTIC SOLUTIONS AND SUSPENSIONS (Cont.)

For complete prescribing information see Steroid Preparations p. 72 and Antibiotic Preparations p. 100.

Product and Distributor	Steroid (per ml)	Antibiotic (per ml)	Other Content	How Supplied	C.I.*
Rx **Neomycin and Polymyxin B Sulfates and Dexamethasone Ophthalmic Suspension** (Various, eg, Moore, Schein, Steris)	0.1% dexamethasone	Neomycin sulfate equivalent to 0.35% neomycin base and 10,000 units polymyxin B sulfate	Hydroxypropyl methylcellulose, polysorbate 20, benzalkonium chloride and NaCl	In 5 and 10 ml.	129+
Rx **Dexacidin Suspension** (Iolab)				In 5 ml dropper bottles.	157
Rx **AK-Trol Suspension** (Akorn)			0.01% benzalkonium chloride, polysorbate 20, NaCl and hydroxypropyl methylcellulose	In 5 ml dropper bottles.	154
Rx **Maxitrol Suspension** (Alcon)			0.5% hydroxypropyl methylcellulose, polysorbate 20, 0.004% benzalkonium chloride and NaCl	In 5 ml Drop-Tainers.	471
Rx **Dexasporin Suspension** (Various, eg, Rugby, United Research)				In 5 ml.	163+

* Cost Index based on cost per ml.

STEROID AND ANTIBIOTIC OINTMENTS

For complete prescribing information see Steroid Preparations p. 72 and Antibiotic Preparations p. 100.

Administration and Dosage:

Apply ointment to the affected eye(s) every 3 or 4 hours, depending on the severity of the condition.

Not more than 8 g should be prescribed initially, and the prescription should not be refilled until further evaluation. For complete dosage instructions, see individual manufacturer inserts.

	Product and Distributor	Steroid (per g)	Antibiotic (per g)	Other Content	How Supplied	C.I.*
Rx	**Ophthocort** (Parke-Davis)	0.5% hydrocortisone acetate	1% chloramphenicol and 10,000 units polymyxin B (as sulfate)	Liquid petrolatum and polyethylene	Preservative free. In 3.5 g.	549
Rx	**Bacitracin Zinc-Neomycin Sulfate-Polymyxin B Sulfate-Hydrocortisone Ophthalmic** (Various, eg. Fougera)	1% hydrocortisone	Neomycin sulfate equivalent to 0.35% neomycin base, 400 units bacitracin zinc and 10,000 units polymyxin B sulfate	White petrolatum and mineral oil base	In 3.5 g.	150+
Rx	**AK-Spore H.C.** (Akorn)				In 3.5 g.	184
Rx	**Cortisporin** (Burroughs Wellcome)			White petrolatum	In 3.5 g.	578
Rx	**Coracin** (Hauck)	1% hydrocortisone acetate	0.5% neomycin sulfate, 400 units bacitracin zinc and 10,000 units polymyxin B sulfate	White petrolatum and mineral oil base	In 3.5 g.	89
Rx	**Pred-G S.O.P.** (Allergan)	0.6% prednisolone acetate	Gentamicin sulfate equivalent to 0.3% gentamicin base	0.5% chlorobutanol, white petrolatum, mineral oil and petrolatum (and) lanolin alcohol	In 3.5 g.	694

* Cost Index based on cost per g.

STEROID AND ANTIBIOTIC OINTMENTS (Cont.)

For complete prescribing information see Steroid Preparations p. 72 and Antibiotic Preparations p. 100.

	Product and Distributor	Steroid (per g)	Antibiotic (per g)	Other Content	How Supplied	C.I.*
Rx	**NeoDecadron** (MSD)	0.05% dexamethasone phosphate (as sodium phosphate)	Neomycin sulfate equivalent to 0.35% neomycin base	White petrolatum and mineral oil	In 3.5 g.	236
Rx	**TobraDex** (Alcon)	0.1% dexamethasone	0.3% tobramycin	0.5% chlorobutanol, white petrolatum and mineral oil	In 3.5 g.	633
Rx	**Neomycin and Polymyxin B Sulfate and Dexamethasone Ophthalmic** (Various, eg, Fougera, Moore)	0.1% dexamethasone	Neomycin sulfate equivalent to 0.35% neomycin base and 10,000 units polymyxin B sulfate	White petrolatum, anhydrous liquid lanolin, mineral oil and parabens	In 3.5 g.	235+
Rx	**AK-Trol** (Akorn)			White petrolatum, anhydrous liquid lanolin, mineral oil, 0.05% methylparaben and 0.01% propylparaben	In 3.5 g.	217
Rx	**Dexacidin** (Iolab)			White petrolatum and mineral oil	In 3.5 g.	214
Rx	**Dexasporin** (Various, eg, Bausch & Lomb, Rugby)			White petrolatum, anhydrous liquid lanolin, mineral oil, 0.05% methylparaben and 0.01% propylparaben	In 3.5 and 5.0 g.	230+
Rx	**Maxitrol** (Alcon)			White petrolatum, anhydrous liquid lanolin, 0.05% methylparaben and 0.01% propylparaben	In 3.5 g.	673

* Cost Index based on cost per g.

SULFONAMIDES

Actions:

Sulfonamides exert a bacteriostatic effect against a wide range of susceptible gram-positive and gram-negative microorganisms. Through competition with para-aminobenzoic acid (PABA), they restrict the synthesis of folic acid, which bacteria require for growth.

Indications:

For conjunctivitis, corneal ulcer and other superficial ocular infections due to susceptible microorganisms.

As an adjunct to systemic sulfonamide therapy in the treatment of trachoma.

Contraindications:

Hypersensitivity to sulfonamides or to any component of the formulation.

Infants less than 2 months of age. In epithelial herpes simplex keratitis (dendritic keratitis), vaccinia, varicella and many other viral diseases of the cornea and conjunctiva. Mycobacterial infection or fungal diseases of the ocular structures.

Oral sulfonamides: In pregnancy at term and during the nursing period because sulfonamides pass the placenta, are excreted in the milk and may cause kernicterus.

Steroid combinations: After uncomplicated removal of a corneal foreign body.

Warnings:

Staphylococcus sp: A significant percentage of isolates are resistant to sulfa drugs.

Severe sensitivity reactions have been identified in individuals with no prior history of sulfonamide hypersensitivity (see Adverse Reactions).

Pregnancy: Category C (sulfisoxazole diolamine, sodium sulfacetamide/phenylephrine HCl). Safety for use during pregnancy has not been established. Use only when clearly needed and when the potential benefits outweigh the potential hazards to the fetus.

Lactation: Sulfonamides are excreted in breast milk (see Contraindications).

Children: Safety and efficacy for use in children have not been established. Sulfonamides are contraindicated in infants less than 2 months (see Contraindications).

Precautions:

For topical use only. Not for injection.

Superinfection: Use of antibiotics (especially prolonged or repeated therapy) may result in bacterial or fungal overgrowth of nonsusceptible organisms. Such overgrowth may lead to a secondary infection. Take appropriate measures if superinfection occurs.

Ophthalmic ointments may retard corneal epithelial healing.

Sensitization may occur when a sulfonamide is readministered, regardless of the route of administration. Cross-sensitivity between different sulfonamides may occur. If signs of sensitivity or other untoward reactions occur, discontinue use of the preparation.

PABA present in purulent exudates inactivates sulfonamides.

Use with caution in patients with severe dry eye.

Sulfite sensitivity: May cause allergic-type reactions (eg, hives, itching, wheezing, anaphylaxis) in certain susceptible persons. Although the overall prevalence of sulfite sensitivity in the general population is probably low, it is seen more frequently in asthmatics or in atopic nonasthmatic persons. Specific products containing sulfites are identified in the product listings.

Drug Interactions:

Silver preparations are incompatible with these solutions.

Adverse Reactions:

Headache or browache, blurred vision, local irritation, itching, transient epithelial keratitis, reactive hyperemia, conjunctival edema, burning and transient stinging. Rarely, sensitization reactions to sulfacetamide sodium may occur. As with all sulfonamide preparations, severe sensitivity reactions include rare occurrences of Stevens-Johnson syndrome, exfoliative dermatitis, toxic epidermal necrolysis, photosensitivity, fever, skin rash, GI disturbance and bone marrow depression.

A single instance of local hypersensitivity was reported which progressed to a fatal syndrome resembling systemic lupus erythematosus.

Patient Information:

For topical use only.

Do not discontinue use without consulting physician. Take care not to discontinue prematurely.

To avoid contamination, do not touch tip of container to any surface. Replace cap after using.

Keep bottle tightly closed when not in use. Do not use if solution has darkened or contains a precipitate.

May cause sensitivity to bright light; this may be minimized by wearing sunglasses.

Notify physician if improvement is not seen after 7 to 8 days, if condition worsens, or if pain, increased redness, itching or swelling of the eye occurs.

Administration and Dosage:

Solutions:

Conjunctivitis or corneal ulcer – Instill 1 to 2 drops into the lower conjunctival sac(s) every 1 to 3 hours according to severity of infection.

Trachoma (30%) – 2 drops every 2 hours. Concomitant systemic sulfonamide therapy is indicated.

Storage – Store at 46° to 86°F (8° to 30°C). Protect from light. Do not use solution if it is discolored (dark brown).

Ointments: Apply a small amount (0.5 inch) into the lower conjunctival sac(s) 1 to 4 times daily and at bedtime. Or apply 0.5 to 1 inch into the conjunctival sac(s) at night in conjunction with the use of drops during the day, or before an eye is patched.

Storage – Store at 46° to 86°F (8° to 30°C). Store away from heat.

SULFONAMIDES (Cont.)

C.I.*

Rx	Drug	Form	Size	C.I.
Rx	**Sodium Sulfacetamide** (Various, eg, Bausch & Lomb, Fougera, Major, Moore, Schein, United Research)	**Ointment:** 10% sodium sulfacetamide	In 3.5 g.	96+
Rx	**AK-Sulf** (Akorn)		In 3.5 g.[1]	97
Rx	**Bleph-10** (Allergan)		In 3.5 g.[2]	481
Rx	**Cetamide** (Alcon)		In 3.5 g.[3]	490
Rx	**Sodium Sulamyd** (Schering)		In 3.5 g.[4]	508
Rx	**Sodium Sulfacetamide** (Various, eg, Bausch & Lomb, Major, Moore, Parmed, Rugby, Steris, United Research)	**Solution:** 10% sodium sulfacetamide	In 2 and 15 ml.	24+
Rx	**AK-Sulf** (Akorn)		In 2, 5 and 15 ml dropper bottles.[5]	28
Rx	**Bleph-10** (Allergan)		In 2.5, 5 and 15 ml dropper bottles.[6]	158
Rx	**Ocusulf-10** (Optopics)		In 2 and 15 ml.[7]	28
Rx	**Sodium Sulamyd** (Schering)		In 5 and 15 ml dropper bottles.[8]	145
Rx	**Sulf-10** (Iolab)		In 1 ml Dropperettes[9] and 15 ml dropper bottles.[10]	61

* Cost Index based on cost per g or ml.
[1] With 0.05% methylparaben and 0.01% propylparaben in a petrolatum base.
[2] With 0.0008% phenylmercuric acetate, white petrolatum, mineral oil and petrolatum (and) lanolin alcohol.
[3] With 0.05% methylparaben, 0.01% propylparaben, white petrolatum, anhydrous liquid lanolin and mineral oil.
[4] With 0.05% methylparaben, 0.01% propylparaben and 0.025% benzalkonium chloride.
[5] With 0.35% hydroxyethyl cellulose, 0.2% sodium thiosulfate, 0.2% chlorobutanol and 0.015% methyl and propyl parabens.
[6] With 1.4% polyvinyl alcohol, 0.005% thimerosal, polysorbate 80, sodium thiosulfate and EDTA.
[7] With methyl and propyl parabens, 1.4% polyvinyl alcohol and sodium thiosulfate.
[8] With 0.31% sodium thiosulfate, 0.5% methylcellulose, 0.05% methylparaben and 0.01% propylparaben.
[9] With sodium thiosulfate and 0.005% thimerosal.
[10] With 0.1% hydroxypropyl methylcellulose, sodium thiosulfate and 0.01% thimerosal.

SULFONAMIDES (Cont.)   C.I.*

Rx	Sodium Sulfacetamide (Various, eg, Alcon, Bausch & Lomb, Moore)	Solution: 15% sodium sulfacetamide	In 2 and 15 ml.	45+
Rx	Isopto Cetamide (Alcon)		In 5 and 15 ml Drop-Tainers.[1]	138
Rx	Sodium Sulfacetamide (Various, eg, Bausch & Lomb, Rugby, Schein, Steris)	Solution: 30% sodium sulfacetamide	In 15 ml.	56+
Rx	Sodium Sulamyd (Schering)		In 15 ml dropper bottles.[2]	154
Rx	Gantrisin (Roche)	Solution: 4% sulfisoxazole (as diolamine)	In 15 ml with dropper.[3]	85

SULFONAMIDE DECONGESTANT COMBINATION

In this combination, *phenylephrine HCl,* an alpha sympathetic receptor agonist, produces vasoconstriction.

For complete prescribing information see Sulfonamide General Monograph p. 117 and phenylephrine HCl p. 60.

Administration and Dosage:

Instill 1 or 2 drops into the lower conjunctival sac(s) every 2 or 3 hours during the day, less often at night.

Storage: Store at room temperature 59° to 86°F (15° to 30°C). Keep tightly closed. Protect from light.

                                                                          C.I.*

Rx	Vasosulf (Iolab)	Solution: 15% sodium sulfacetamide and 0.125% phenylephrine HCl	In 5 and 15 ml dropper bottles.[4]	85

* Cost Index based on cost per ml.
[1] With 0.05% methylparaben, 0.01% propylparaben, 0.5% hydroxypropyl methylcellulose and 0.3% sodium thiosulfate.
[2] With 0.15% sodium thiosulfate, 0.05% methylparaben and 0.01% propylparaben.
[3] With 1:100,000 phenylmercuric nitrate.
[4] With sodium thiosulfate, poloxamer 188 and methyl and propyl parabens.

STEROID AND SULFONAMIDE COMBINATIONS

For complete prescribing information see Steroid Preparations p. 72 and Sulfonamide Preparations p. 117.

Indications:

For steroid-responsive inflammatory ocular conditions for which a corticosteroid is indicated and where superficial bacterial ocular infection or a risk of bacterial ocular infection exists.

For inflammatory conditions of the palpebral and bulbar conjunctiva, cornea and anterior segment of the globe where the inherent risk of steroid use in certain infective conjunctivitides is accepted to obtain a diminution in edema and inflammation. They are also indicated in chronic anterior uveitis and corneal injury from chemical, radiation or thermal burns, or penetration of foreign bodies.

STEROID AND SULFONAMIDE SOLUTIONS AND SUSPENSIONS

Administration and Dosage:

Instill 1 to 3 drops into the conjunctival sac(s) every 1 to 2 hours during the day and at bedtime until a favorable response is obtained.

Not more than 20 ml should be prescribed initially, and the prescription should not be refilled without further evaluation.

For complete dosage instructions, see individual manufacturer inserts.

Storage: Store at room temperature 59° to 86°F (15° to 30°C). Protect from light. Do not freeze. Shake suspensions well before using. Do not use if solution or suspension has darkened.

	Product and Distributor	Steroid	Sulfonamide	Other Content	How Supplied	C.I.*
Rx	**FML-S Suspension** (Allergan)	0.1% fluorometholone	10% sodium sulfacetamide	1.4% polyvinyl alcohol, 0.006% benzalkonium chloride, EDTA, polysorbate 80, povidone, sodium thiosulfate and NaCl	In 5 and 10 ml dropper bottles.	244

* Cost Index based on cost per ml.

STEROID AND SULFONAMIDE SOLUTIONS AND SUSPENSIONS (Cont.)

For complete prescribing information see Steroid Preparations p. 72 and Sulfonamide Preparations p. 117.

Product and Distributor	Steroid	Sulfonamide	Other Content	How Supplied	C.I.*
Rx **Blephamide Suspension** (Allergan)	0.2% prednisolone acetate	10% sodium sulfacetamide	EDTA, 1.4% polyvinyl alcohol, polysorbate 80, sodium thiosulfate and benzalkonium chloride	In 5 and 10 ml dropper bottles.	271
Rx **Sulfacort Suspension** (Rugby)			0.5% hydroxypropyl methylcellulose, 0.01% benzalkonium chloride, polysorbate 80 and sodium thiosulfate pentahydrate	In 5 ml bottles.	255
Rx **Isopto Cetapred Suspension** (Alcon)	0.25% prednisolone acetate	10% sodium sulfacetamide	0.5% hydroxypropyl methylcellulose, EDTA, polysorbate 80, sodium thiosulfate, 0.025% benzalkonium chloride, 0.05% methylparaben and 0.01% propylparaben	In 5 and 15 ml Drop-Tainers.	221
Rx **Metimyd Suspension** (Schering)	0.5% prednisolone acetate	10% sodium sulfacetamide	0.5% phenylethyl alcohol, 0.025% benzalkonium chloride, sodium thiosulfate, EDTA and tyloxapol	In 5 ml dropper bottles.	605

* Cost Index based on cost per ml.

STEROID AND SULFONAMIDE SOLUTIONS AND SUSPENSIONS (Cont.)

For complete prescribing information see Steroid Preparations p. 72 and Sulfonamide Preparations p. 117.

	Product and Distributor	Steroid	Sulfonamide	Other Content	How Supplied	C.I.*
Rx	**Predsulfair Suspension** (Bausch & Lomb)	0.5% prednisolone acetate	10% sodium sulfacetamide	0.5% hydroxypropyl methylcellulose, polysorbate 80, sodium thiosulfate and 0.01% benzalkonium chloride	In 5 and 15 ml dropper bottles.	20
Rx	**Sulphrin Suspension** (Bausch & Lomb)			0.5% hydroxypropyl methylcellulose, EDTA, polysorbate 80, sodium metabisulfite, propylene glycol, sodium thiosulfate, 0.05% methylparaben and 0.01% propylparaben	In 5 ml dropper bottles.	164
Rx	**Vasocidin Solution** (Iolab)	0.25% prednisolone sodium phosphate	10% sodium sulfacetamide	EDTA, 0.01% thimerosal and poloxamer 407	In 5 and 10 ml dropper bottles.	189
Rx	**Optimyd Solution** (Schering)	0.5% prednisolone phosphate (as sodium phosphate)	10% sodium sulfacetamide	EDTA, sodium thiosulfate, tyloxapol, 0.025% benzalkonium chloride and 0.5% phenylethyl alcohol	In 5 ml dropper bottles.	605

* Cost Index based on cost per ml.

STEROID AND SULFONAMIDE OINTMENTS

For complete prescribing information see Steroid Preparations p. 72 and Sulfonamide Preparations p. 117.

Administration and Dosage:

Apply a small amount into the conjunctival sac(s) 3 or 4 times daily and once at bedtime until a favorable response is obtained.

Not more than 8 g should be prescribed initially, and the prescription should not be refilled without further evaluation.

For complete dosage instructions, see individual manufacturer inserts.

Storage: Store at 36° to 86°F (2° to 30°C). Keep tightly closed. Store away from heat.

	Product and Distributor	Steroid	Sulfonamide	Other Content	How Supplied	C.I.*
Rx	**Blephamide S.O.P.** (Allergan)	0.2% prednisolone acetate	10% sodium sulfacetamide	0.0008% phenylmercuric acetate, mineral oil, white petrolatum and petrolatum (and) lanolin alcohol	In 3.5 g.	519
Rx	**Cetapred** (Alcon)	0.25% prednisolone acetate	10% sodium sulfacetamide	Mineral oil, white petrolatum, anhydrous liquid lanolin, 0.05% methylparaben and 0.01% propylparaben	In 3.5 g.	551
Rx	**AK-Cide** (Akorn)	0.5% prednisolone acetate	10% sodium sulfacetamide	Mineral oil, white petrolatum, lanolin, 0.05% methylparaben and 0.01% propylparaben	In 3.5 g.	189
Rx	**Sulphrin** (Bausch & Lomb)				In 3.5 g.	117
Rx	**Metimyd** (Schering)			Mineral oil, white petrolatum, 0.05% methylparaben and 0.01% propylparaben	In 3.5 g.	760
Rx	**Vasocidin** (Iolab)			Mineral oil and white petrolatum	In 3.5 g.	421

* Cost Index based on cost per g.

ANTISEPTIC PREPARATIONS

BORIC ACID

Indications:

For the treatment of irritated and inflamed eyelids.

Warnings:

If irritation persists or increases, discontinue use and consult physician.

Administration and Dosage:

Apply a small quantity to the inner surface of the lower eyelid 1 or 2 times daily or as directed.

Do not use if metal edge of tube is not fully rolled over cap edge. Contamination may have occurred.

Storage: Store at room temperature 59° to 86°F (15° to 30°C). Keep tightly closed.

C.I.*

otc	**Boric Acid** (Various, eg, Bausch & Lomb, Major)	**Ointment:** 5%	In 3.5 g.	55+
otc	**Boric Acid** (Various, eg, Fougera, Major, Rugby)	**Ointment:** 10%	In 3.5 and 30 g.	4+

SILVER NITRATE

Actions:

Silver nitrate ophthalmic solution is an anti-infective. In weak solutions, it is used as a germicide and astringent to mucous membranes. The germicidal action is due to precipitation of bacterial proteins by liberated silver ions.

Indications:

For prevention of gonorrheal ophthalmia neonatorum.

Silver nitrate has not been effective for the prevention of neonatal chlamydial conjunctivitis.

Contraindications:

Hypersensitivity to any component of the formulation.

Warnings:

A 1% solution is considered optimal. Use with caution, since cauterization of the cornea and blindness may result, especially with repeated applications.

Silver nitrate is caustic and irritating to the skin and mucous membranes.

---

* Cost Index based on cost per g.

Precautions:

Handle solutions carefully, since they tend to stain skin and utensils. Stains may be removed from linen by applications of iodine tincture followed by sodium thiosulfate solution.

Drug Interactions:

Sulfacetamide preparations are incompatible with silver preparations.

Adverse Reactions:

A mild chemical conjunctivitis should result from a properly performed Credé prophylaxis using silver nitrate. A more severe chemical conjunctivitis occurs in 20% or less of cases.

Overdosage:

When ingested, silver nitrate is highly toxic to the GI tract and CNS. Swallowing can cause severe gastroenteritis that may be fatal. Sodium chloride may be used by gastric lavage to remove the chemical.

When a solution of 2% or higher silver nitrate concentration is used in the eye, conjunctivitis may be produced. Irrigate the eye with an isotonic solution of sodium chloride after solutions of silver nitrate stronger than 1% are instilled.

Administration and Dosage:

Immediately after birth, clean the child's eyelids with sterile absorbent cotton or gauze and sterile water. Use a separate pledget for each eye; wash unopened lids from the nose outward until free of blood, mucus or meconium. Next, separate the lids and instill 2 drops of 1% solution. Elevate lids away from the eyeball so that a lake of silver nitrate may lie for at least 30 seconds between them, contacting the entire conjunctival sac.

The American Academy of Pediatrics has endorsed a statement from the Committee on Ophthalmia Neonatorum of the National Society for the Prevention of Blindness, which does NOT recommend irrigation of the eyes following instillation of the silver nitrate.

Storage: Store ampoules at room temperature 59° to 86°F (15° to 30°C). Do not freeze. Do not use ampoules when cold. Protect from light.

C.I.*

Rx	**Silver Nitrate** (Lilly)	**Solution:** 1% with acetic acid and sodium acetate	In 100s (wax ampoules). 178

* Cost Index based on cost per wax ampoule.

SILVER PROTEIN, MILD

Actions:

Instilled prior to eye surgery, it stains and coagulates mucus. It has antimicrobial action at low doses against gram-positive and gram-negative organisms.

Indications:

For treatment of eye infections and preoperatively in eye surgery.

Contraindications:

Hypersensitivity to any component of the formulation.

Warnings:

Pregnancy: Category C. Safety for use during pregnancy has not been established. Use only when clearly needed and when the potential benefits outweigh the potential hazards to the fetus.

Lactation: It is not known whether this drug is excreted in breast milk. Safety for use in the nursing mother has not been established. Use caution.

Children: Safety and efficacy in children have not been established.

Precautions:

Not for prolonged use. When used preoperatively, remove all stained material before entering the eye. This may reduce the incidence of postoperative infection.

Drug Interactions:

Sulfacetamide preparations are incompatible with silver preparations.

Adverse Reactions:

Uninterrupted or too frequent use over a long period may result in a permanent discoloration of the skin and conjunctiva (argyria).

Administration and Dosage:

Preoperatively: Instill 2 or 3 drops into eye(s). Rinse out with sterile irrigating solution.

Infections: Instill 1 to 3 drops into eye(s) every 3 or 4 hours for several days.

				C.I.*
otc	**Argyrol S.S. 10%** (Iolab)	**Solution:** 10%	In 15 and 30 ml.	75
Rx	**Argyrol S.S. 20%** (Iolab)	**Solution:** 20% with EDTA	In 1 ml Dropperettes.	230

* Cost Index based on cost per ml.

YELLOW MERCURIC OXIDE

Indications:

For treatment of irritation and minor infections of the eyelids.

For the relief of discomfort of styes.

Warnings:

If irritation or rash develops or if condition persists, discontinue use and consult physician.

Frequent or prolonged use may cause serious mercury poisoning.

Administration and Dosage:

Apply a small quantity to inner surface of lower eyelid once daily, at bedtime, or as directed.

			C.I.*
otc **Stye** (Del Pharm.)	**Ointment:** 1%	In 3.5 g.[1]	176

ZINC SULFATE SOLUTION

Indications:

A mild astringent for temporary relief of minor eye irritation.

Warnings:

If irritation persists or increases or if eye pain or a change in vision occurs, discontinue use and consult physician.

Administration and Dosage:

Instill 1 to 2 drops into the affected eye(s) up to 4 times daily. If solution discolors or becomes cloudy, do not use.

			C.I.*
otc **Eye-Sed** (Scherer)	**Solution:** 0.25%	In 15 ml.[2]	24

* Cost Index based on cost per g or ml.
[1] With light mineral oil, microcrystalline wax, wheat germ oil and white petrolatum.
[2] With 0.05% tetrahydrozoline hydrochloride, EDTA, benzalkonium chloride and sodium chloride.

NATAMYCIN

Actions:

Pharmacology: Natamycin, a tetraene polyene antibiotic, is derived from *Strepto-myces natalensis.* It possesses in vitro activity against a variety of yeast and fila-mentous fungi, including *Candida, Aspergillus, Cephalosporium, Fusarium* and *Penicillium.* Mechanism of action appears to be through binding of the molecule to the fungal cell membrane. The polyenesterol complex alters membrane permeability, depleting essential cellular constituents. Although activity against fungi is dose-related, natamycin is predominantly fungicidal. It is not effective in vitro against bacteria.

Pharmacokinetics: Topical administration appears to produce effective concentra-tions within the corneal stroma, but not in intraocular fluid. Absorption from the GI tract is very poor. Systemic absorption should not occur after topical administration.

Indications:

For fungal blepharitis, conjunctivitis and keratitis caused by susceptible organisms. Natamycin is the initial drug of choice in *Fusarium solani* keratitis.

The effectiveness of topical natamycin as a single agent in fungal endophthalmitis has not been established.

Contraindications:

Hypersensitivity to any component of the formulation.

Warnings:

Pregnancy: Safety for use during pregnancy has not been established. Use only when clearly needed and when the potential benefits outweigh the potential hazards to the fetus.

Precautions:

For topical use only. Not for injection.

Failure of keratitis to improve following 7 to 10 days of administration suggests that the infection may be caused by a microorganism not susceptible to natamycin. Base continuation of therapy on clinical reevaluation and additional laboratory studies.

Adherence of the suspension to areas of epithelial ulceration or retention in the for-nices occurs regularly. Should suspicion of drug toxicity occur, discontinue the drug.

Laboratory tests: Determine initial and sustained therapy of fungal keratitis by the clinical diagnosis, laboratory diagnosis by smear and culture of corneal scrapings and by response to the drug. Whenever possible, determine the in vitro activity of natamycin against the responsible fungus. Monitor tolerance of natamycin at least twice weekly.

Adverse Reactions:

One case of conjunctival chemosis and hyperemia, thought to be allergic in nature, was reported.

Administration and Dosage:

Fungal keratitis: Instill 1 drop into the conjunctival sac(s) at 1- or 2-hour intervals. The frequency of application can usually be reduced to 1 drop 6 to 8 times daily after the first 3 to 4 days. Continue therapy for 14 to 21 days, or until there is resolution of active fungal keratitis. In many cases, it may help to reduce the dosage gradually at 4- to 7-day intervals to assure that the organism has been eliminated.

Fungal blepharitis and conjunctivitis: 4 to 6 daily applications may be sufficient.

Storage: Store at room temperature 46° to 75°F (8° to 24°C) or refrigerate 36° to 46°F (2° to 8°C). Do not freeze. Avoid exposure to light and excessive heat. Shake well before each use.

Rx	**Natacyn** (Alcon)	**Suspension:** 5% with 0.02% benzalkonium chloride	In 15 ml with dropper.

IDOXURIDINE (IDU)

Actions:

Idoxuridine (IDU) blocks reproduction of herpes simplex virus by altering normal DNA synthesis.

In chemical structure, IDU closely approximates the configuration of thymidine, one of the four building blocks of DNA. As a result, IDU replaces thymidine in the enzymatic step of viral replication. The consequent production of faulty DNA results in a pseudostructure which cannot infect or destroy tissue.

Indications:

For the treatment of herpes simplex keratitis. Epithelial infections (especially initial attacks), characterized by the presence of a dendritic figure, respond better than stromal infections. Recurrences are common. IDU will often control the infection, but will have no effect on accumulated scarring, vascularization or resultant progressive loss of vision.

Contraindications:

Hypersensitivity to IDU or any component of the formulation.

Warnings:

Recurrence may be seen if medication is not continued for 5 to 7 days after the epithelial lesion is apparently healed.

Sensitization: IDU may be sensitizing; this is more common with dermal rather than ocular use.

Corticosteroids can accelerate the spread of a viral infection and are usually contraindicated in herpes simplex epithelial keratitis.

Oncogenic potential: Regard this cytotoxic drug as potentially carcinogenic, although data are inadequate for assessment. It can inhibit DNA synthesis or function, and is incorporated into the DNA of mammalian cells as well as into the genome of DNA viruses. IDU induces RNA tumor virus production from mouse cells and has caused in vitro cell transformation and induction of specific neoplasms (lymphatic leukemias and carcinomas) upon inoculation into syngeneic mice.

Pregnancy: Category C. IDU crosses the placental barrier and produces fetal malformations when administered topically to the eyes of pregnant rabbits in clinical doses and when administered by various routes in high doses to other rodents. Safety for use during pregnancy has not been established. Use only if clearly needed and when the potential benefits outweigh the potential hazards to the fetus.

Lactation: It is not known whether IDU is excreted in breast milk. Because of the potential for tumorigenicity shown for IDU in animal studies, decide whether to discontinue nursing or to discontinue the drug, taking into account the importance of the drug to the mother.

Children: Safety and efficacy in children have not been established.

Precautions:

Resistance: Some strains of herpes simplex appear to be resistant. If there is no lessening of fluorescein staining in 14 days, another form of therapy should be undertaken.

Do not exceed the recommended frequency and duration of administration.

Drug Interactions:

Boric acid-containing solutions: Coadministration may result in a precipitate formation which may cause irritation.

Adverse Reactions:

Occasional irritation, pain, pruritus, inflammation, edema of the eyes or lids; allergic reactions; photophobia; occasional corneal clouding; stippling; punctate defects in the corneal epithelium. The punctate defects may be a manifestation of the infection, since healing usually takes place without interruption of therapy. These defects have been observed in untreated herpes simplex keratitis.

Overdosage:

Local: Overdosage due to frequent administration is possible and may result in small defects on the epithelium of the cornea. Discontinue therapy, either temporarily or permanently, as indicated after close observation of the progress of the infection.

Accidental ingestion: Animal data indicate that the minimum systemic dose that will produce toxic effects is many times greater than the quantity in a commercial bottle or tube. Also, metabolic breakdown and excretion take place very rapidly. Thus, no untoward consequences should be expected from accidental ingestion of even an entire bottle of the solution or tube of ointment. No treatment is indicated.

Patient Information:

May cause sensitivity to bright light; this may be minimized by wearing sunglasses.

Notify physician if improvement is not seen after 14 days, if condition worsens or if pain, decreased vision, itching or swelling of the eye occurs.

Administration and Dosage:

For optimal results, keep infected tissues saturated with IDU.

Examine patients at frequent intervals. In epithelial infections, improvement is usually seen within 7 to 8 days. If the patient continues to improve, continue therapy, usually not longer than 21 days.

Solution: Initially, instill 1 drop into affected eye(s) every hour during the day and every 2 hours at night. Continue until definite improvement has taken place, as evidenced by loss of staining with fluorescein. Then reduce dosage to 1 drop every 2 hours during the day and every 4 hours at night. To minimize recurrences, continue therapy at this reduced dosage for 3 to 7 days after healing appears complete.

> *Alternate dosing schedule:* Instill 1 drop every minute for 5 minutes. Repeat every 4 hours, day and night.

Concomitant therapy: In the management of herpes simplex with stromal lesions, corneal edema or iritis, *topical corticosteroids* may be used with IDU. Use such combined therapy for as long as the condition warrants. It is important to continue IDU therapy a few days after the steroid has been withdrawn (see Warnings).

Antibiotics may be used with IDU to control secondary infections, and *atropine* preparations may be employed adjunctively as indicated.

Stability: Do not mix with other medications.

Storage: Store at room temperature 59° to 86°F (15° to 30°C). Protect from light.

C.I.*

Rx **Herplex** (Allergan)	**Solution:** 0.1%	In 15 ml dropper bottles.[1]	126

* Cost Index based on cost per ml.
[1] With 1.4% polyvinyl alcohol, benzalkonium chloride, EDTA and sodium chloride.

VIDARABINE (Adenine Arabinoside; Ara-A)

Actions:

Microbiology: Vidarabine possesses in vitro and in vivo antiviral activity against herpes simplex types 1 and 2, varicella-zoster and vaccinia viruses. Except for rhabdovirus and oncornavirus, it does not display antiviral activity against other RNA or DNA viruses, including adenovirus.

Pharmacology: The mechanism of action has not been established. Vidarabine appears to interfere with the early steps of viral DNA synthesis. It is rapidly deaminated to arabinosylhypoxanthine (Ara-Hx), the principal metabolite. Ara-Hx possesses in vitro antiviral activity less than vidarabine's. In contrast to topical *idoxuridine* (IDU), vidarabine demonstrated less cellular toxicity in regenerating corneal epithelium of rabbits.

Pharmacokinetics: Absorption – Systemic absorption is not expected to occur following ocular administration and swallowing lacrimal secretions. In laboratory animals, vidarabine is rapidly deaminated in the GI tract to Ara-Hx.

> *Distribution* – Because of its low solubility, trace amounts of both vidarabine and Ara-Hx can be detected in the aqueous humor only if there is an epithelial defect in the cornea. If the cornea is normal, only trace amounts of Ara-Hx can be recovered from the aqueous humor.

Indications:

For the treatment of acute keratoconjunctivitis and recurrent epithelial keratitis due to herpes simplex virus types 1 and 2. It is also effective in superficial keratitis caused by herpes simplex virus which has not responded to topical IDU, or when toxic or hypersensitivity reactions to IDU have occurred. Effectiveness against stromal keratitis and uveitis due to herpes simplex virus has not been established.

Vidarabine is not effective against RNA virus, adenoviral ocular infections, bacterial, fungal or chlamydial infections of the cornea, or trophic ulcers.

Contraindications:

Hypersensitivity to vidarabine; sterile trophic ulcers.

Warnings:

Corticosteroids alone are normally contraindicated in herpes simplex virus eye infections. If vidarabine is coadministered with topical corticosteroid therapy, consider corticosteroid-induced ocular side effects such as glaucoma or cataract formation and progression of bacterial or viral infection.

Temporary visual haze may be produced with vidarabine.

Mutagenic potential: In vitro vidarabine can be incorporated into mammalian DNA and can induce mutation. In vivo studies have not been conclusive; however, vidarabine may be capable of producing mutagenic effects in male germ cells.

Vidarabine has caused chromosome breaks and gaps when added to human leukocytes in vitro. While the significance is not fully understood, there is a well-known correlation between the ability of various agents to produce such effects and their ability to produce heritable genetic damage.

Oncogenic potential: In mice, there was an increase in liver tumor incidence among the vidarabine-treated (IM) females; some male mice developed kidney neoplasia. In rats, intestinal, testicular and thyroid neoplasia occurred with greater frequency among the vidarabine-treated animals.

Pregnancy: Category C. A 10% ointment applied to 10% of the body surface during organogenesis induced fetal abnormalities in rabbits. The possibility of embryonic or fetal damage in pregnant women is remote. The topical ophthalmic dose is small, and the drug is relatively insoluble. Its ocular penetration is very low. However, a safe dose for a human embryo or fetus has not been established. Therefore, use only if the potential benefits outweigh the potential hazards to the fetus.

Lactation: It is not known whether vidarabine is excreted in breast milk, although it is unlikely because the drug is rapidly deaminated in the GI tract. However, it is recommended that either nursing or the drug be discontinued, taking into account the importance of the drug to the mother.

Precautions:

Viral resistance to vidarabine has not been observed, although this possibility exists.

Adverse Reactions:

Lacrimation; foreign body sensation; conjunctival injection; burning; irritation; superficial punctate keratitis; pain; photophobia; punctal occlusion; sensitivity.

The following have also been reported, but appear disease-related: Uveitis; stromal edema; secondary glaucoma; trophic defects; corneal vascularization; hyphema.

Overdosage:

The rapid deamination to Ara-Hx should preclude any difficulty. No untoward effects should result from ingestion of the entire contents of a tube. Overdosage by ocular instillation is unlikely because any excess should be quickly expelled from the conjunctival sac. Avoid too frequent administration.

Patient Information:

May cause sensitivity to bright light; this may be minimized by wearing sunglasses.

Do not discontinue use without consulting physician.

Notify physician if improvement is not seen after 7 days, if condition worsens or if pain, decreased vision, burning or irritation of the eye occurs.

Administration and Dosage:

Apply approximately 0.5 inch of ointment into the lower conjunctival sac(s) 5 times daily at 3-hour intervals. If there are no signs of improvement after 7 days, or if complete reepithelialization has not occurred in 21 days, consider other forms of therapy. Some severe cases may require longer treatment.

After reepithelialization has occurred, treat for an additional 7 days at a reduced dosage (such as twice daily) to prevent recurrence.

Concomitant therapy: Topical *antibiotics* (eg, gentamicin, erythromycin) or *steroids* (eg, prednisolone) have been used with vidarabine without an increase in adverse reactions. Consider their advantages and disadvantages (see Warnings).

C.I.*

Rx	Vira-A (Parke-Davis)	**Ointment:** 3% vidarabine monohydrate (equivalent to 2.8% vidarabine)	In a petrolatum base. In 3.5 g.	714

* Cost Index based on cost per g.

TRIFLURIDINE (Trifluorothymidine)

Actions:

Pharmacology: A fluorinated pyrimidine nucleoside with in vitro and in vivo activity against herpes simplex virus types 1 and 2 and vaccinia virus. Some strains of adenovirus are also inhibited in vitro. Trifluridine interferes with DNA synthesis in cultured mammalian cells. However, its antiviral mechanism of action is not completely known.

Absorption: Intraocular penetration occurs after topical instillation. Decreased corneal integrity or stromal or uveal inflammation may enhance the penetration into the aqueous humor. Systemic absorption following therapeutic dosing appears negligible.

Indications:

For the treatment of primary keratoconjunctivitis and recurrent epithelial keratitis due to herpes simplex virus types 1 and 2. Also effective in the treatment of epithelial keratitis that has not responded clinically to the topical administration of idoxuridine, or when ocular toxicity or hypersensitivity to idoxuridine has occurred. In a smaller number of patients resistant to topical vidarabine, trifluridine was also effective.

The clinical efficacy in the treatment of stromal keratitis and uveitis due to herpes simplex virus or ophthalmic infections caused by vaccinia virus and adenovirus, or in the prophylaxis of herpes simplex virus keratoconjunctivitis and epithelial keratitis has not been established by well-controlled clinical trials.

Not effective against bacterial, fungal or chlamydial infections of the cornea, or trophic lesions.

Contraindications:

Hypersensitivity reactions or chemical intolerance to trifluridine.

Warnings:

Do not exceed the recommended dosage or frequency of administration.

Mutagenic potential: Trifluridine has exerted mutagenic, DNA-damaging and cell-transforming activities in various standard in vitro test systems. Although the significance of these test results is not clear or fully understood, it is possible that mutagenic agents may cause genetic damage in humans.

Pregnancy: Safety for use during pregnancy has not been established. Use only when clearly needed and when the potential benefits outweigh the potential hazards to the fetus.

Based upon animal findings, it is unlikely that trifluridine would cause embryonic or fetal damage if given in the recommended ophthalmic dosage to pregnant women. A safe dose, however, has not been established for the human embryo or fetus.

Lactation: It is unlikely that trifluridine is excreted in breast milk after ophthalmic instillation because of the relatively small dosage (less than or equal to 5 mg/day), its dilution in body fluids and its extremely short half-life (approximately 12 minutes). However, do not prescribe to nursing mothers unless the potential benefits outweigh the potential risks.

Precautions:

Although documented in vitro, viral resistance has not been reported following multiple exposure to trifluridine; this possibility may exist.

Adverse Reactions:

The most frequent adverse reactions reported are mild, transient burning or stinging
upon instillation (4.6%) and palpebral edema (2.8%). Other adverse reactions in
decreasing order of reported frequency were: Superficial punctate keratopathy;
epithelial keratopathy; hypersensitivity reaction; stromal edema; irritation; keratitis
sicca; hyperemia and increased intraocular pressure.

Overdosage:

Overdosage by ocular instillation is unlikely because any excess solution should be
quickly expelled from the conjunctival sac.

No untoward effects are likely to result from ingestion of the entire contents of a bottle. Single IV doses of 15 to 30 mg/kg/day in children and adults with neoplastic
disease produce reversible bone marrow depression as the only potentially serious
toxic effect and only after three to five courses of therapy.

Patient Information:

Do not discontinue use without consulting physician.

Transient stinging may occur upon instillation.

Notify physician if improvement is not seen after 7 days, if condition worsens or if
irritation occurs.

Administration and Dosage:

Instill 1 drop onto the cornea of the affected eye(s) every 2 hours while awake for a
maximum daily dosage of 9 drops until the corneal ulcer has completely reepithelial-
ized. Following reepithelialization, treat for an additional 7 days with 1 drop every 4
hours while awake for a minimum daily dosage of 5 drops.

If there are no signs of improvement after 7 days, or if complete reepithelialization
has not occurred after 14 days, consider other forms of therapy. Avoid continuous
administration for periods exceeding 21 days because of potential ocular toxicity.

Storage: Refrigerate at 36° to 46°F (2° to 8°C).

C.I.*

Rx **Viroptic** (Burroughs Wellcome)	**Solution:** 1%	In 7.5 ml Drop-Dose.[1]	798

* Cost Index based on cost per ml.
[1] In aqueous solution with 0.001% thimerosal and NaCl.

GANCICLOVIR SODIUM (DHPG)

> **Warning:**
>
> The clinical toxicity of ganciclovir includes granulocytopenia and thrombocytopenia. In animal studies, the drug was carcinogenic, teratogenic and caused aspermatogenesis. Ganciclovir is indicated for use *only* in immunocompromised patients with cytomegalovirus (CMV) retinitis and for the prevention of CMV disease in transplant patients at risk for CMV disease.

Actions:

Pharmacology: Ganciclovir sodium is an antiviral drug active against cytomegalovirus (CMV). It is a synthetic nucleoside analogue of 2'-deoxyguanosine. Sensitive human viruses include CMV, herpes simplex virus -1 and -2 (HSV-1, HSV-2), Epstein-Barr virus and varicella zoster virus. Clinical studies have been limited to assessment of efficacy in patients with CMV infection.

Median effective inhibitory doses (ED_{50}) of ganciclovir for human CMV isolates tested in vitro in several cell lines ranged from 0.2 to 3 mcg/ml. The relationship between in vitro sensitivity of CMV to ganciclovir and clinical response has not been established. Ganciclovir inhibits mammalian cell proliferation in vitro at higher concentrations (10 to 60 mcg/ml) with bone marrow colony-forming cells being the most sensitive (ID_{50} greater than or equal to 10 mcg/ml) of those cell types tested.

Upon entry into host cells, CMVs induce one or more cellular kinases that phosphorylate ganciclovir to its triphosphate. There is approximately a tenfold greater concentration of ganciclovir-triphosphate in CMV-infected cells than in uninfected cells, indicating a preferential phosphorylation of ganciclovir in virus-infected cells. In vitro, ganciclovir-triphosphate is catabolized slowly, with 60% to 70% of the original level remaining in the infected cells 18 hours after removal of ganciclovir from the extracellular medium. The antiviral activity of ganciclovir-triphosphate is believed to be the result of inhibition of viral DNA synthesis by two known modes: Competitive inhibition of viral DNA polymerases and direct incorporation into viral DNA, resulting in eventual termination of viral DNA elongation. The cellular DNA polymerase alpha is inhibited, but at a higher concentration than required for viral DNA polymerase.

Pharmacokinetics: Twenty-two immunocompromised patients with serious CMV disease and normal renal function received ganciclovir 5 mg/kg, each dose infused IV over 1 hour. The mean plasma level of ganciclovir at the end of the first 1 hour infusion (C_{max}) was 8.3 ± 4 mcg/ml and the plasma level 11 hours after the start of infusion (C_{min}) was 0.56 ± 0.66 mcg/ml. The plasma half-life was 2.9 ± 1.3 hours and the systemic clearance was 3.64 ± 1.86 ml/kg/min (approximately 250 ml/ 1.73m²/min). Dose-independent kinetics were demonstrated over the range of 1.6 to 5 mg/kg. Multiple-dose kinetics were measured in eight patients with normal renal function who received ganciclovir 5 mg/kg twice daily for 12 to 14 days. After the first dose and after multiple dosing, plasma levels at the end of infusion were 7.1 mcg/ml (3.1 to 14 mcg/ml) and 9.5 mcg/ml (2.7 to 24.2 mcg/ml), respectively. At 7 hours after infusion, plasma levels after the first dose were 0.85 mcg/ml (0.2 to 1.8 mcg/ml) and were 1.2 mcg/ml (0.6 to 1.8 mcg/ml) after multiple dosing.

Renal excretion of unchanged drug by glomerular filtration is the major route of elimination. In patients with normal renal function, more than 90% of the administered ganciclovir was recovered unmetabolized in the urine. In four patients with mild renal impairment (creatinine clearance [Ccr] 50 to 79 ml/1.73m²/min), the systemic clearance of ganciclovir was 128 ± 63 ml/1.73m²/min, and the plasma half-life was 4.6 ± 1.4 hours. In three patients with moderate renal impairment (Ccr 25 to 49 ml/1.73m²/min), the systemic clearance of ganciclovir was 57 ± 8 ml/ 1.73m²/min, and the plasma half-life was 4.4 ± 0.4 hours. In three patients with severe renal impairment (Ccr less than 25 ml/1.73m²/min) the systemic clearance was 30 ± 13 ml/1.73m²/min, and the plasma half-life was 10.7 ± 5.7 hours. There was a positive correlation between systemic clearance of ganciclovir and Ccr.

Data from four patients with severe renal impairment showed that hemodialysis reduced plasma drug levels by approximately 50%. Binding of ganciclovir to plasma proteins is 1% to 2%. Drug interactions involving binding site displacement are not expected.

There is limited evidence to suggest that ganciclovir crosses the blood brain barrier. Cerebrospinal fluid (CSF) concentrations have been measured in three patients:

GANCICLOVIR CSF CONCENTRATIONS				
Patient	CSF Conc. (mcg/ml)	Plasma Conc. (mcg/ml)	Hr after dose	CSF/Plasma Ratio
1	0.62	0.92	5.67	0.67
	0.68	2.20	3.50	0.31
	0.51	1.96	2.75	0.26
2	0.50	2.05	0.25	0.24
3	0.31	0.44	5.50	0.70

Clinical Pharmacology: Clinical Trials – Of 314 immunocompromised patients enrolled in an open label study of the treatment of life- or sight-threatening CMV disease, 121 patients had a positive culture for CMV within 7 days prior to treatment.

VIROLOGIC RESPONSE TO GANCICLOVIR TREATMENT			
Culture Source	No. Patients Cultured	No. (%) Patients Responding	Median Days to Response
Urine	107	93 (87)	8
Blood	41	34 (83)	8
Throat	21	19 (90)	7
Semen	6	6 (100)	15

Emergence of viral resistance has been reported. The prevalence of resistant isolates is unknown, and some patients may be infected with strains of CMV resistant to ganciclovir. Therefore, consider the possibility of viral resistance in patients who show poor clinical response or experience persistent viral excretion during therapy.

Indications:

For the treatment of *CMV retinitis* in immunocompromised individuals, including patients with acquired immunodeficiency syndrome (AIDS). It also is indicated for the prevention of CMV disease in transplant patients at risk for CMV disease. Safety and efficacy of ganciclovir have not been established for: Congenital or neonatal CMV disease; treatment of other CMV infections (eg, pneumonitis, colitis); use in non-immunocompromised individuals.

> *Diagnosis of CMV retinitis* is ophthalmologic and should be made by indirect ophthalmoscopy. The diagnosis of CMV retinitis may be supported by culture of CMV from urine, blood, throat, etc, but a negative CMV culture does not rule out CMV retinitis.

Contraindications:

Hypersensitivity to ganciclovir or acyclovir.

Warnings:

Hematologic: Granulocytopenia – Approximately 40% of 522 immunocompromised patients with serious CMV infections who received IV ganciclovir developed granulocytopenia (neutropenia, ie, neutrophil count less than 1,000 cells/mm³). Therefore, use with caution in patients with preexisting cytopenias, or with a history of cytopenic reactions to other drugs, chemicals or irradiation. Granulocytopenia usually occurs during the first or second week of treatment, but may occur at any time during treatment. Cell counts usually begin to recover within 3 to 7 days of discontinuing drug. Do not administer if the absolute neutrophil count is less than 500 cells/mm³ or the platelet count is less than 25,000/mm³.

Thrombocytopenia (platelet count less than 50,000/mm³) was observed in approximately 20% of the same 522 patients treated with ganciclovir. Patients with iatrogenic immunosuppression were more likely to develop thrombocytopenia than patients with AIDS (46% versus 14% of cases).

Renal function impairment: Use with caution because the plasma half-life and peak plasma levels of ganciclovir will be increased due to reduced renal clearance (see Administration and Dosage).

Transplant recipients: There is a high frequency of impaired renal function in transplant recipients who received ganciclover in controlled clinical trials, particularly in patients receiving concomitant administration of nephrotoxic agents such as cyclosporine and amphotericin B.

Data from four patients indicate that ganciclovir plasma levels are reduced approximately 50% following hemodialysis.

Carcinogenesis, mutagenesis, impairment of fertility: In mice, daily oral doses of 1,000 mg/kg may have caused an increased incidence of tumors in the preputial gland of males, nonglandular mucosa of the stomach of males and females, and ovary, vagina and liver of females. A slightly increased incidence of tumors occurred in the preputial gland (males), nonglandular mucosa of the stomach (males and females) and the liver (females) in mice given 20 mg/kg/day. Consider ganciclovir a potential carcinogen in humans.

Ganciclovir caused point mutations and chromosomal damage in mammalian cells in vitro and in vivo. Because of the mutagenic potential of ganciclovir, advise women of childbearing potential to use effective contraception during treatment. Similarly, advise male patients to practice barrier contraception during and for at least 90 days following treatment with ganciclovir.

Ganciclovir caused decreased mating behavior, decreased fertility and increased embryolethality in female mice at doses approximately equivalent to the recommended human dose. Animal data indicate that ganciclovir causes inhibition of spermatogenesis and subsequent infertility. These effects were reversible at lower doses and irreversible at higher doses. Although data in humans is lacking, IV ganciclovir at recommended doses probably causes temporary or permanent inhibition of spermatogenesis.

Elderly: Since elderly individuals frequently have reduced glomerular filtration, pay particular attention to assessing renal function before and during ganciclovir administration.

Pregnancy: Category C. Ganciclovir is teratogenic in rabbits and embryotoxic in mice in doses approximately equivalent to the recommended human dose. The adverse effects observed in mice were maternal/fetal toxicity and embryolethality. In rabbits, the effects were fetal growth retardation, embryolethality, teratogenicity and maternal toxicity. Teratogenic changes included cleft palate, anophthalmia/microphthalmia, aplastic organs (kidney and pancreas), hydrocephaly and brachygnathia.

Ganciclovir may be teratogenic or embryotoxic at the dose levels recommended for human use. There are no adequate and well-controlled studies in pregnant women. Use during pregnancy only if the potential benefit outweighs the potential risk to the fetus.

Lactation: It is not known if ganciclovir is excreted in breast milk. Carcinogenicity and teratogenicity occurred in animals treated with ganciclovir. Because of the potential for serious adverse reactions from ganciclovir in nursing infants, instruct mothers to discontinue nursing if they are receiving ganciclovir. The minimum interval before nursing can safely be resumed after the last dose is unknown.

Daily IV doses of 90 mg/kg administered to female mice prior to mating, during gestation and during lactation caused hypoplasia of the testes and seminal vesicles in the month-old male offspring, as well as pathologic changes in the nonglandular region of the stomach.

Children: The use of ganciclovir warrants extreme caution due to the probability of long-term carcinogenicity and reproductive toxicity. Administer to children only after careful evaluation and only if the potential benefits of treatment outweigh the risks.

There has been very limited clinical experience in treating CMV retinitis in patients under the age of 12 years. Two children (ages 9 and 5 years) showed improvement or stabilization of retinitis for 23 and 9 months, respectively. These children received induction treatment with 2.5 mg/kg 3 times daily followed by maintenance therapy with 6 to 6.5 mg/kg once per day, 5 to 7 days per week. When retinitis progressed during once-daily maintenance therapy, both children were treated with the 5 mg/kg twice-daily regimen. Two other children (ages 2.5 and 4 years) who received similar induction regimens showed only partial or no response to treatment. A 6-year-old with T-cell dysfunction showed stabilization of retinitis for 3 months while receiving continuous infusions of ganciclovir at doses of 2 to 5 mg/kg/24 hours. Continuous infusion treatment was discontinued due to granulocytopenia.

Adverse events reported in 120 immunocompromised children with serious CMV infections receiving ganciclovir were similar to those reported in adults. Granulocytopenia (17%) and thrombocytopenia (10%) were most commonly reported.

Precautions:

The maximum single dose administered was 6 mg/kg by IV infusion over 1 hour. Larger doses, or more rapid infusions, will probably result in increased toxicity.

Initially reconstituted ganciclovir solutions have a high pH (range 9 to 11). Despite further dilution in IV fluids, phlebitis or pain may occur at the site of IV infusion. Care must be taken to infuse solutions containing ganciclovir only into veins with adequate blood flow to permit rapid dilution and distribution.

Hydration: Administration of ganciclovir by IV infusion should be accompanied by adequate hydration, since ganciclovir is excreted by the kidneys, and normal clearance depends on adequate renal function.

Lab Tests: Perform neutrophil and platelet counts every 2 days during twice-daily dosing of ganciclovir and at least weekly thereafter. Monitor neutrophil counts daily in patients in whom ganciclovir or other nucleoside analogues have previously resulted in leukopenia, or in whom neutrophil counts are less than 1,000 cells/mm³ at the beginning of treatment. Because dosing must be modified in patients with renal impairment, monitor serum creatinine or Ccr at least once every 2 weeks.

Drug Interactions:

Cytotoxic drugs that inhibit replication of rapidly dividing cell populations such as bone marrow, spermatogonia and germinal layers of skin and GI mucosa may have additive toxicity when administered concomitantly with ganciclovir. Therefore, consider the concomitant use of drugs such as *dapsone, pentamidine, flucytosine, vincristine, vinblastine, adriamycin, amphotericin B, trimethoprim/sulfamethoxazole* combinations or other nucleoside analogues only if potential benefits are judged to outweigh the risks.

Imipenem-cilastatin: Generalized seizures occurred in six patients who received ganciclovir and imipenem-cilastatin. Do not use these drugs concomitantly unless the potential benefits outweigh the risks.

Probenecid and other drugs that inhibit renal tubular secretion or resorption may reduce renal clearance of ganciclovir.

Zidovudine: Patients with AIDS may be receiving, or may have received, treatment with zidovudine. Because both zidovudine and ganciclovir can cause granulocytopenia, it is recommended that these two drugs not be given concomitantly. Data from a small number of patients indicate that treatment with ganciclovir plus zidovudine at the recommended doses is not tolerated.

Adverse Reactions:

During clinical trials, ganciclovir was withdrawn or interrupted in approximately 32% of patients because of adverse reactions. In some instances, treatment was restarted and the reappearance of adverse reactions again necessitated withdrawal or interruption.

Most frequent: Hematopoietic system – Granulocytopenia (absolute neutrophil count less than 1,000 cells/mm³; 40%); thrombocytopenia (platelet count less than 50,000/mm³; 20%). In most cases, withdrawal of ganciclovir resulted in increased neutrophil or platelet counts. While granulocytopenia was generally reversible with discontinuation of treatment, patients may experience irreversible neutropenia or sepsis during neutropenic episodes. In an open label study of 522 immunocompromised patients with sight- or life-threatening CMV disease, five neutropenic patients died with severe bacterial or fungal infections.

Other – Anemia; fever; rash; abnormal liver function values (2%).

Adverse reactions that occurred in 1% or fewer patients:

Body as a whole – Chills; edema; infections; malaise.

Cardiovascular – Arrhythmia; hypertension; hypotension.

CNS – Abnormal thoughts or dreams; ataxia; coma; confusion; dizziness; headache; nervousness; paresthesia; psychosis; somnolence; tremor.

GI – Nausea; vomiting; anorexia; diarrhea; hemorrhage; abdominal pain.

Dermatologic – Alopecia; pruritus; urticaria.

GU – Hematuria; increased serum creatinine; increased blood urea nitrogen (BUN).

Injection site – Inflammation; pain; phlebitis.

Other – Dyspnea; eosinophilia; retinal detachment in CMV retinitis patients.

Laboratory abnormalities – Decrease in blood glucose.

Overdosage:

Overdosage has been reported in eleven patients. In three of these patients, no adverse effects were observed. The doses received were: 7 doses of 11 mg/kg over a 3-day period, 9 mg/kg twice daily for 3 days and 2 doses of 500 mg in a 21-month-old child.

Symptoms: Neutropenia in three patients: One had a history of bone marrow suppression prior to treatment and received ganciclovir 5 mg/kg twice daily for 14 days followed by 8 mg/kg given as single-daily doses for 4 days, and one patient received a single dose of 1,675 mg (approximately 24 mg/kg) and a 60 year old man with preexisting neutropenia received a single dose of 20 mg/kg. In all cases, the neutropenia was reversible (17 days and 1 day, respectively) following discontinuation of ganciclovir.

Toxic manifestations observed in animals given very high single doses of ganciclovir (500 mg/kg) included: Emesis; hypersalivation; anorexia; bloody diarrhea; inactivity; cytopenia; elevated liver function test results; elevated BUN; testicular atrophy; death.

Treatment: Hemodialysis and hydration may be of benefit in reducing drug plasma levels.

Patient Information:

Ganciclovir is not a cure for CMV retinitis. Immunocompromised patients may continue to experience progression of retinitis during or following treatment. Advise patients to have regular ophthalmologic examinations.

The major toxicities of ganciclovir are granulocytopenia and thrombocytopenia. Dose modifications may be required, including possible discontinuation. Emphasize the importance of close monitoring of blood counts while on therapy.

Patients with AIDS may be receiving zidovudine. Treatment with zidovudine or ganciclovir, and especially the combination, can result in severe granulocytopenia. Therefore, it is recommended that the two drugs not be given concomitantly.

Advise patients that ganciclovir has caused decreased sperm production in animals and may cause infertility in humans. Advise women of childbearing potential that ganciclovir causes birth defects in animals and should not be used during pregnancy; use effective contraception during ganciclovir treatment. Similarly, advise men to practice barrier contraception during, and for at least 90 days following, ganciclovir treatment.

Ganciclovir causes tumors in animals. Although there is no information from human studies, consider ganciclovir a potential carcinogen.

Administration and Dosage:

Do not administer ganciclovir by rapid or bolus IV injection. The toxicity of ganciclovir may be increased as a result of excessive plasma levels.

Administer IV. IM or SC injection of reconstituted ganciclovir may result in severe tissue irritation due to high pH (approximately 11).

Do not exceed the recommended dosage, frequency or infusion rates.

Induction Treatment: Initial dose for patients with normal renal function is 5 mg/kg (given IV at a constant rate over 1 hour) every 12 hours for 14 to 21 days.

Maintenance Treatment: Following induction treatment, 5 mg/kg given as an IV infusion over 1 hour once per day for 7 days, or 6 mg/kg once per day for 5 days each week. Patients who experience progression of retinitis while receiving maintenance therapy may be re-treated with the twice-daily regimen.

Perform frequent hematologic monitoring throughout treatment. Do not administer if the neutrophil count falls below 500 cells/mm³ or the platelet count falls below 25,000/mm³.

GANCICLOVIR DOSE IN RENAL IMPAIRMENT		
Ccr* (ml/1.73 m²/min)	Ganciclovir Dose (mg/kg)	Dosing Interval (hours)
≥ 80	5	12
50-79	2.5	12
25-49	2.5	24
< 25	1.25	24

* Ccr can be related to serum creatinine by the following formula:

$$\text{Males:} \quad \frac{\text{Weight (kg) x (140 - age)}}{72 \text{ x serum creatinine (mg/dl)}} \quad \text{x} \quad 1.73/\text{body surface [m}^2\text{]}$$

Females: 0.85 x above value

The optimal maintenance dose for patients with renal impairment is not known. Physicians may elect to reduce the dose to 50% of the induction dose and monitor the patient for disease progression.

Only limited data are available on ganciclovir elimination in patients undergoing hemodialysis. Do not exceed 1.25 mg/kg/24 hours. On days when hemodialysis is performed, administer shortly after the completion of the hemodialysis session, since hemodialysis reduces plasma levels by approximately 50%. Monitor neutrophil and platelet counts daily.

Patient Monitoring: Due to the frequency of granulocytopenia and thrombocytopenia in patients receiving ganciclovir (see Adverse Reactions), perform neutrophil and platelet counts every 2 days during twice-daily dosing, and at least weekly thereafter. In patients in whom ganciclovir or other nucleoside analogues have previously resulted in leukopenia, or in whom neutrophil counts are less than 1,000 cells/mm³ at the beginning of treatment, monitor neutrophil counts daily. Because dosing must be modified in renal impairment, monitor serum creatinine or Ccr at least once every 2 weeks.

Reduction of Dose: Perform frequent white blood cell counts. Severe neutropenia (ANC less than 500/mm³) or severe thrombocytopenia (platelets less than 25,000/mm³) requires a dose interruption until evidence of marrow recovery is observed (ANC greater than or equal to 750/mm³).

Method of Preparation: Each 10 ml vial contains ganciclovir sodium equivalent to 500 mg of the free base form of ganciclovir and 46 mg of sodium. Prepare the contents of the vial for administration in the following manner:

1. Reconstitute lyophilized ganciclovir by injecting 10 ml of Sterile Water for Injection into the vial.

   Do not use bacteriostatic water for injection containing parabens. It is incompatible with ganciclovir sterile powder and may cause precipitation.

2. Shake the vial to dissolve the drug.

3. If particulate matter or discoloration is observed, discard the vial.

4. Reconstituted solution in the vial is stable at room temperature for 12 hours.

   Do not refrigerate.

Admixture Preparation and Administration: Based on patient weight, remove the appropriate calculated dose volume from the vial (ganciclovir concentration 50 mg/ml) and add to an acceptable infusion fluid (typically 100 ml) for delivery over 1 hour. Infusion concentrations greater than 10 mg/ml are not recommended. The following infusion fluids are chemically and physically compatible with ganciclovir: 0.9% Sodium Chloride, 5% Dextrose, Ringer's Injection and Lactated Ringer's Injection.

Handling: Caution should be exercised. Avoid direct contact with the skin or mucous membranes. If contact occurs, wash thoroughly with soap and water; rinse eyes thoroughly with plain water.

Disposal: Because ganciclovir is a nucleoside analogue, consider procedures for proper handling and disposal of unused solution.

Storage: Powder – Store at room temperature 59° to 86°F (15° to 30°C). Avoid excessive heat above 104°F (40°C). *Infusion solution* – Because nonbacteriostatic infusion fluid must be used with ganciclovir, the infusion solution must be used within 24 hours of dilution to reduce the risk of bacterial contamination. Refrigerate the infusion solution. Freezing is not recommended.

Rx	**Cytovene** (Syntex)	**Powder:** 500 mg/vial ganciclovir (as sodium)	In 10 ml vials.

FOSCARNET SODIUM (Phosphonoformic acid)

> **Warning:**
>
> Renal impairment, the major toxicity of foscarnet, occurs to some degree in most patients. Consequently, continual assessment of a patient's risk and frequent monitoring of serum creatinine with dose adjustment for changes in renal function are imperative.
>
> Foscarnet causes alterations in plasma minerals and electrolytes that have led to seizures. Monitor patients frequently for such changes and their potential sequelae.

Actions:

Pharmacology: Foscarnet is an organic analog of inorganic pyrophosphate that inhibits replication of all known herpesviruses in vitro including cytomegalovirus (CMV), herpes simplex virus types 1 and 2 (HSV-1, HSV-2), human herpesvirus 6 (HHV-6), Epstein-Barr virus (EBV) and varicella-zoster virus (VZV).

Foscarnet exerts its antiviral activity by a selective inhibition at the pyrophosphate binding site on virus-specific DNA polymerases and reverse transcriptases at concentrations that do not affect cellular DNA polymerases. Foscarnet does not require activation (phosphorylation) by thymidine kinase or other kinases, and therefore is active in vitro against HSV mutants deficient in thymidine kinase. CMV strains resistant to ganciclovir may be sensitive to foscarnet.

The quantitative relationship between the in vitro susceptibility of human CMV to foscarnet and clinical response to therapy has not been clearly established in man and virus sensitivity testing has not been standardized. If no clinical response to foscarnet is observed, test viral isolates for sensitivity to foscarnet; naturally resistant mutants may emerge under selective pressure both in vitro and in vivo. The latent state of any of the human herpesviruses is not known to be sensitive to foscarnet and viral reactivation of CMV occurs after foscarnet therapy is terminated.

Pharmacokinetics: Foscarnet is 14% to 17% bound to plasma protein at plasma drug concentrations of 1 to 1000 mcM. Plasma foscarnet concentrations in two studies are summarized in the following table:

Foscarnet Plasma Concentrations			
Mean dose (Infusion time)	Day of sampling	Mean plasma concentration (mcM)	
		C_{max} (range)	C_{min} (range)
57 ± 6 mg/kg q 8 hr (1 hour)	1	573 (213 to 1305)[1]	78 (< 33 to 139)[3]
47 ± 12 mg/kg q 8 hr (1 hour)	14 or 15	579 (246 to 922)[2]	110 (< 33 to 148)[4]
55 ± 6 mg/kg q 8 hr (2 hours)	3	445 (306 to 720)[1]	88 (< 33 to 162)[3]
57 ± 7 mg/kg q 8 hr (2 hours)	14 or 15	517 (348 to 789)[2]	105 (43 to 205)[4]

[1] Observed 0.9 to 2.4 hr after start of infusion.
[2] Observed 0.8 to 2.6 hr after start of infusion.
[3] Observed 4 to 8.1 hr after start of infusion.
[4] Observed 6.3 to 8.7 hr after start of infusion.

Mean plasma clearances were 130 ± 44 and 178 ± 48 ml/min in two studies in which foscarnet was given by intermittent infusion and 152 ± 59 and 214 ± 25 ml/min/1.73 m² in two studies using continuous infusion. Approximately 80% to 90% of IV foscarnet is excreted unchanged in the urine of patients with normal renal function. Both tubular secretion and glomerular filtration account for urinary elimination of foscarnet. In one study, plasma clearance was less than creatinine clearance (Ccr), suggesting that foscarnet may also undergo tubular reabsorption. In three studies, decreases in plasma clearance of foscarnet were proportional to decreases in Ccr.

Two studies in patients with initially normal renal function who were treated with intermittent infusions showed average drug plasma half-lives of about 3 hours determined on days 1 or 3 of therapy. This may be an underestimate of the effective half-life due to the limited observation period. Plasma half-life increases with the severity of renal impairment. Half-lives of 2 to 8 hours occurred in patients having estimated or measured 24 hour Ccr of 44 to 90 ml/min. Careful monitoring of renal function and dose adjustment is imperative (see Warnings and Administration and Dosage).

Following continuous foscarnet infusion for 72 hours in six HIV-positive patients, plasma half-lives of 0.45 ± 0.32 and 3.3 ± 1.3 hours were determined. A terminal half-life of 18 ± 2.8 hours was estimated from foscarnet urinary excretion over 48 hours after stopping infusion. When foscarnet was given as a continuous infusion to 13 patients with HIV infection for 8 to 21 days, plasma half-lives of 1.4 ± 0.6 and 6.8 ± 5 hours were determined. A terminal half-life of 87.5 ± 41.8 hours was estimated from foscarnet urinary excretion over 6 days after the last infusion; however, renal function at the time of discontinuing the infusion was not known.

Measurements of urinary excretion are required to detect the longer terminal half-life assumed to represent release of foscarnet from bone. In animal studies (mice), 40% of an IV dose is deposited in bone in young animals and 7% in adults. Evidence indicates that foscarnet accumulates in human bone; however, the extent to which this occurs has not been determined. Mean volumes of distribution at steady state range from 0.3 to 0.6 L/kg.

Variable penetration into cerebrospinal fluid (CSF) has been observed. Intermittent infusion of 50 mg/kg every 8 hours for 28 days in 9 patients produced CSF levels of 150 to 260 mcM 3 hours after the end of infusion or 39% to 103% of the plasma levels. In another 4 patients, CSF concentrations were 35% to 69% of the plasma drug level after a dose of 230 mg/kg/day by continuous infusion for 2 to 13 days. However, the CSF:plasma ratio was only 13% in one patient receiving a continuous infusion at a rate of 274 mg/kg/day. Disease-related defects in the blood-brain barrier may be responsible for the variations seen.

Clinical trials: In most clinical studies, treatment for CMV retinitis was begun with an induction dosage regimen of 60 mg/kg every 8 hours for the first 2 to 3 weeks, followed by a once-daily maintenance regimen at doses ranging from 60 to 120 mg/kg.

A prospective, randomized, masked, controlled clinical trial was conducted in 24 patients with acquired immunodeficiency syndrome (AIDS) and CMV retinitis. Patients received induction treatment of 60 mg/kg every 8 hours for 3 weeks, followed by maintenance treatment with 90 mg/kg/day until retinitis progression (appearance of a new lesion or advancement of the border of a posterior lesion > 750 microns in diameter). The 13 patients randomized to treatment with foscarnet had a significant delay in progression of CMV retinitis compared to untreated controls. Median times to retinitis progression from study entry were 93 days (range, 21 to > 364) and 22 days (range, 7 to 42), respectively.

In another prospective clinical trial of CMV retinitis in AIDS patients, 33 were treated with 2 to 3 weeks of foscarnet induction (60 mg/kg 3 times a day) and then randomized to two maintenance dose groups, 90 and 120 mg/kg/day. Median times from study entry to retinitis progression were 96 days (range, 14 to > 176) and 140 days (range, 16 to > 233), respectively. This difference was not statistically significant.

Indications:

For the treatment of CMV retinitis in patients with AIDS. Safety and efficacy of foscarnet have not been established for: Congenital or neonatal CMV disease; treatment of other CMV infections (eg, pneumonitis, gastroenteritis); use in non-immunocompromised individuals.

Diagnosis of CMV retinitis is ophthalmologic and should be made by indirect ophthalmoscopy. The diagnosis of CMV retinitis may be supported by culture of CMV from urine, blood, throat, etc, but a negative CMV culture does not rule out CMV retinitis.

Contraindications:

Hypersensitivity to foscarnet.

Warnings:

Renal function impairment: The major toxicity of foscarnet is renal impairment, which occurs to some degree in most patients. Approximately 33% of 189 patients with AIDS and CMV retinitis who received IV foscarnet in clinical studies developed significant impairment of renal function, manifested by a rise in serum creatinine concentration to $\geq$ 2 mg/dl. Therefore, use foscarnet with caution in all patients, especially those with a history of renal function impairment. Patients vary in their sensitivity to foscarnet-induced nephrotoxicity, and initial renal function may not be predictive of the potential for drug-induced renal impairment.

Renal impairment is most likely to become clinically evident as assessed by increasing serum creatinine during the second week of induction therapy at 60 mg/kg 3 times a day. Renal impairment, however, may occur at any time in any patient during treatment; therefore, monitor renal function carefully (see Precautions).

Elevations in serum creatinine are usually, but not uniformly, reversible following discontinuation or dose adjustment. Recovery of renal function after foscarnet-induced impairment usually occurs within 1 week of drug discontinuation. However, of 35 patients who experienced grade II renal impairment (serum creatinine 2 to 3 times the upper limit of normal), two died with renal failure within 4 weeks of stopping foscarnet and three others died with renal insufficiency still present < 4 weeks after drug cessation.

Because of foscarnet's potential to cause renal impairment, dose adjustment for decreased baseline renal function and any change in renal function during treatment is necessary. In addition, it may be beneficial for adequate hydration to be established (eg, by inducing diuresis) prior to and during administration.

Mineral and electrolyte imbalances: Foscarnet has been associated with changes in serum electrolytes including hypocalcemia (15%), hypophosphatemia (8%) and hyperphosphatemia (6%), hypomagnesemia (15%) and hypokalemia (16%). Foscarnet is associated with a transient, dose-related decrease in ionized serum calcium, which may not be reflected in total serum calcium. This effect most likely is related to foscarnet's chelation of divalent metal ions such as calcium. Therefore, advise patients to report symptoms of low ionized calcium such as perioral tingling, numbness in the extremities and paresthesias. Be prepared to treat these as well as severe manifestations of electrolyte abnormalities, such as tetany and seizures. The rate of infusion may affect the transient decrease in ionized calcium; slowing the rate may decrease or prevent symptoms.

Transient changes in calcium or other electrolytes (including magnesium, potassium or phosphate) may also contribute to a patient's risk for cardiac disturbances and seizures (see Neurotoxicity and Seizures). Therefore, particular caution is advised in patients with altered calcium or other electrolyte levels before treatment, especially those with neurologic or cardiac abnormalities and those receiving other drugs known to influence minerals and electrolytes (see Precautions and Drug Interactions).

Neurotoxicity and seizures: Foscarnet was associated with seizures in 18/189 (10%) of AIDS patients in five controlled studies. Three patients were not taking foscarnet at the time of seizure. In most cases (15/18), the patients had an active CNS condition (eg, toxcplasmosis, HIV encephalopathy) or a history of CNS diseases. The rate of seizures did not increase with duration of treatment. Three cases were associated with overdoses of foscarnet (see Overdosage).

Statistically significant risk factors associated with seizures were low baseline absolute neutrophil count (ANC), impaired baseline renal function and low total serum calcium. Several cases of seizures were associated with death. However, occurrence of seizures did not always necessitate discontinuation of foscarnet. Ten of fifteen patients with seizures that occurred while receiving the drug continued or resumed foscarnet following treatment of their underlying disease, electrolyte disturbances or dose decreases. If factors predisposing a patient to seizures are present, carefully monitor electrolytes, including calcium and magnesium (see Precautions).

Other CMV infections: Safety and efficacy have not been established for the treatment of other CMV infections (eg, pneumonitis, gastroenteritis); congenital or neonatal CMV disease; non-immunocompromised individuals.

Mutagenesis: Foscarnet showed genotoxic effects in an in vitro transformation assay at concentrations > 0.5 mcg/ml and an increased frequency of chromosome aberrations in the sister chromatid exchange assay at 1000 mcg/ml. A high dose of foscarnet (350 mg/kg) caused an increase in micronucleated polychromatic erythrocytes in mice at doses that produced exposures comparable to that anticipated clinically.

Elderly: Since these individuals frequently have reduced glomerular filtration, pay particular attention to assessing renal function before and during administration (see Administration and Dosage).

Pregnancy: Category C. Daily SC doses up to 75 mg/kg administered to female rats prior to and during mating, during gestation and 21 days postpartum caused a slight increase (< 5%) in the number of skeletal anomalies compared with the control group. Daily SC doses up to 75 mg/kg (one-third the maximal daily human exposure) administered to rabbits and 150 mg/kg (one-eighth the maximal daily human exposure) administered to rats during gestation caused an increase in the frequency of skeletal anomalies/variations. These studies are inadequate to define the potential teratogenicity at levels to which women will be exposed. There are no adequate and well controlled studies in pregnant women. Use during pregnancy only if clearly needed.

Lactation: It is not known whether foscarnet is excreted in breast milk; however, in lactating rats administered 75 mg/kg, foscarnet was excreted in maternal milk at concentrations three times higher than peak maternal blood concentrations. Exercise caution if foscarnet is administered to a nursing woman.

Children: The safety and efficacy of foscarnet in children have not been studied. Foscarnet is deposited in teeth and bone, and deposition is greater in young and growing animals. Foscarnet adversely affects development of tooth enamel in mice and rats. The effects of this deposition on skeletal development have not been studied. Since deposition in human bone also occurs, it is likely that it does so to a greater degree in developing bone in children. Administer to children only after careful evaluation and only if the potential benefits for treatment outweigh the risks.

Precautions:

Toxicity/local irritation: The maximum single dose administered was 120 mg/kg by IV infusion over 2 hours. Larger doses, or more rapid infusions, will probably result in increased toxicity.

Care must be taken to infuse solutions containing foscarnet only into veins with adequate blood flow to permit rapid dilution and distribution, and to avoid local irritation (see Administration and Dosage). Local irritation and ulcerations of penile epithelium have been reported in male patients receiving foscarnet, possibly related to the presence of drug in the urine. One case of vulvovaginal ulcerations in a female receiving foscarnet has been reported. Adequate hydration with close attention to personal hygiene may minimize the occurrence of such events.

Hydration: Administration of foscarnet by IV infusion should be accompanied by adequate hydration. Diuresis both prior to and during treatment is recommended to minimize renal toxicity.

Anemia has been reported in 33% of patients. This anemia was usually manageable with transfusions and required discontinuation of foscarnet in less than 1% (1/189) of patients in the studies. Granulocytopenia has been reported in 17% of patients; however, only 1% (2/189) were terminated from these studies because of neutropenia.

Monitoring: The majority of patients will experience some decrease in renal function due to foscarnet administration. Therefore it is recommended that Ccr, either measured or estimated using the modified Cockcroft and Gault equation based on serum creatinine, be determined at baseline, 2 to 3 times per week during induction therapy and at least once every 1 to 2 weeks during maintenance therapy, with foscarnet dose adjusted accordingly (see Administration and Dosage). More frequent monitoring may be required for some patients. It is also recommended that a 24 hour Ccr be determined at baseline and periodically thereafter to ensure correct dosing. Discontinue foscarnet if Ccr drops to < 0.4 ml/min/kg.

Due to foscarnet's propensity to chelate divalent metal ions and alter levels of serum electrolytes, closely monitor patients for such changes. It is recommended that a schedule similar to that recommended for serum creatinine (see above) be used to monitor serum calcium, magnesium, potassium and phosphorus. Particular caution is advised in patients with decreased total serum calcium or other electrolyte levels before treatment, as well as in patients with neurologic or cardiac abnormalities, and in patients receiving other drugs known to influence serum calcium levels. Correct any clinically significant metabolic changes. Also, patients who experience mild (eg, perioral numbness or paresthesias) or severe symptoms (eg, seizures) of electrolyte abnormalities should have serum electrolyte and mineral levels assessed as close in time to the event as possible.

Careful monitoring and appropriate management of electrolytes, calcium, magnesium and creatinine are of particular importance in patients with conditions that may predispose them to seizures (see Warnings).

Drug Interactions:

Nephrotoxic drugs: The elimination of foscarnet may be impaired by drugs that inhibit renal tubular secretion. Because of foscarnet's tendency to cause renal impairment, avoid the use of foscarnet in combination with potentially nephrotoxic drugs such as aminoglycosides, amphotericin B and IV pentamidine unless the potential benefits outweigh the risks to the patient.

Pentamidine: Concomitant treatment of four patients with foscarnet and IV pentamidine may have caused hypocalcemia; one patient died with severe hypocalcemia. Toxicity associated with concomitant use of aerosolized pentamidine has not been reported.

Zidovudine: Foscarnet was used concomitantly with zidovudine in approximately one-third of patients in the US studies. Although the combination was generally well tolerated, additive effects on anemia may have occurred. However, no evidence of increased myelosuppression was seen.

Foscarnet decreases serum levels of ionized calcium. Exercise particular caution when other drugs known to influence serum calcium levels are used concurrently.

Adverse Reactions:

Most frequent: Fever (65%); nausea (47%); anemia (33%); diarrhea (30%); abnormal renal function including acute renal failure, decreased creatinine clearance and increased serum creatinine (27%); vomiting (26%); headache (26%); seizures (10%) (see Warnings and Precautions).

Adverse reactions categorized as "severe" were: Death (14%); abnormal renal function (14%); marrow suppression (10%); anemia (9%); seizures (7%). Although death was specifically attributed to foscarnet in only one case, other complications of foscarnet (ie, renal impairment, electrolyte abnormalities, seizures) may have contributed to patient deaths (see Warnings and Precautions).

The following list of adverse reactions has been compiled regardless of causal relationship to foscarnet. Evaluation of these reports was difficult because of the diverse manifestations of the underlying disease and because most patients received numerous concomitant medications.

Body as a whole: Fever, fatigue, rigors, asthenia, malaise, pain, infection, sepsis, death ($\geq$ 5%); back/chest pain, edema, influenza-like symptoms, bacterial/fungal infections, moniliasis, abscess (1% to 5%); hypothermia, leg edema, peripheral edema, syncope, ascites, substernal chest pain, abnormal crying, malignant hyperpyrexia, herpes simplex, viral infection, toxoplasmosis ($<$ 1%).

Central and peripheral nervous system: Headache, paresthesias, dizziness, involuntary muscle contractions, hypoesthesia, neuropathy, seizures including grand mal (see Warnings) ($\geq$ 5%); tremor, ataxia, dementia, stupor, generalized spasms, sensory disturbances, meningitis, aphasia, abnormal coordination, leg cramps, EEG abnormalities (see Warnings) (1% to 5%); vertigo, coma, encephalopathy, abnormal gait, hyperesthesia, hypertonia, visual field defects, dyskinesia, extrapyramidal disorders, hemiparesis, hyperkinesia, vocal cord paralysis, paralysis, paraplegia, speech disorders, tetany, hyporeflexia, hyperreflexia, neuralgia, neuritis, peripheral neuropathy, cerebral edema, nystagmus ($<$ 1%).

GI: Anorexia, nausea, diarrhea, vomiting, abdominal pain ($\geq$ 5%); constipation, dysphagia, dyspepsia, rectal hemorrhage, dry mouth, melena, flatulence, ulcerative stomatitis, pancreatitis (1% to 5%); enteritis, enterocolitis, glossitis, proctitis, stomatitis, tenesmus, increased amylase, pseudomembranous colitis, gastroenteritis, oral leukoplakia, oral hemorrhage, rectal disorders, colitis, duodenal ulcer, hematemesis, paralytic ileus, esophageal ulceration, ulcerative proctitis, tongue ulceration ($<$ 1%).

Hematologic: Anemia, granulocytopenia, leukopenia (see Precautions) ($\geq$ 5%); thrombocytopenia, platelet abnormalities, thrombosis, WBC abnormalities, lymphadenopathy (1% to 5%); pulmonary embolism, coagulation disorders, decreased coagulation factors, epistaxis, decreased prothrombin, hypochromic anemia, pancytopenia, hemolysis, leukocytosis, cervical lymphadenopathy, lymphopenia ($<$ 1%).

Metabolic/Nutritional: Mineral/electrolyte imbalances (see Warnings) including hypokalemia, hypocalcemia, hypomagnesemia, hypo- or hyperphosphatemia ($\geq$ 5%); hyponatremia, decreased weight, increased alkaline phosphatase, LDH and BUN, acidosis, cachexia, thirst, hypercalcemia (1% to 5%); dehydration, glycosuria, increased creatine phosphokinase, diabetes mellitus, abnormal glucose tolerance, hypervolemia, hypochloremia, periorbital edema, hypoproteinemia ($<$ 1%).

Psychiatric: Depression, confusion, anxiety ($\geq$ 5%); insomnia, somnolence, nervousness, amnesia, agitation, aggressive reaction, hallucination (1% to 5%); impaired concentration, emotional lability, psychosis, suicide attempt, delirium, personality disorders, sleep disorders ($<$ 1%).

Respiratory: Coughing, dyspnea (≥ 5%); pneumonia, sinusitis, pharyngitis, rhinitis, respiratory disorders or insufficiency, pulmonary infiltration, stridor, pneumothorax, hemoptysis, bronchospasm (1% to 5%); bronchitis, laryngitis, respiratory depression, abnormal chest x-ray, pleural effusion, lobar pneumonia, pulmonary hemorrhage, pneumonitis (< 1%).

Dermatologic: Rash, increased sweating (≥ 5%); pruritus, skin ulceration, seborrhea, erythematous rash, maculopapular rash, skin discoloration, facial edema (1% to 5%); acne, alopecia, dermatitis, anal pruritus, genital pruritus, aggravated psoriasis, psoriaform rash, skin disorders, dry skin, urticaria, verruca (< 1%).

Urinary: Alterations in renal function including serum creatinine, decreased Ccr and abnormal renal function (see Warnings) (≥ 5%); albuminuria, dysuria, polyuria, urethral disorder, urinary retention, urinary tract infections, acute renal failure, nocturia (1% to 5%); hematuria, glomerulonephritis, micturition disorders/frequency, toxic nephropathy, nephrosis, urinary incontinence, renal tubular disorders, pyelonephritis, urethral irritation, uremia (< 1%).

Special senses: Vision abnormalities (≥ 5%); taste perversions, eye abnormalities, eye pain, conjunctivitis (1% to 5%); diplopia, blindness, retinal detachment, mydriasis, photophobia, deafness, earache, tinnitus, otitis (< 1%).

Cardiovascular: Hypertension, palpitations, ECG abnormalities including sinus tachycardia, first degree AV block and non-specific ST-T segment changes, hypotension, flushing, cerebrovascular disorder (see Warnings) (1% to 5%); cardiomyopathy, cardiac failure/arrest, bradycardia, extrasystole, arrhythmias, atrial arrhythmias/fibrillation, phlebitis, superficial thrombophlebitis of arm, mesenteric vein thrombophlebitis (< 1%).

Application site: Injection site pain or inflammation (1% to 5%).

Hepatic/biliary: Abnormal A-G ratio, abnormal hepatic function, increased AST and ALT (1% to 5%); cholecystitis, cholelithiasis, hepatitis, cholestatic hepatitis, hepatosplenomegaly, jaundice (< 1%).

Musculoskeletal: Arthralgia, myalgia (1% to 5%); arthrosis, synovitis, torticollis (< 1%).

Neoplasms: Lymphoma-like disorder, sarcoma (1% to 5%); malignant lymphoma, skin hypertrophy (< 1%).

Endocrine: Antidiuretic hormone disorders, decreased gonadotropins, gynecomastia (< 1%).

Reproductive: Perineal pain in women, penile inflammation (< 1%).

Overdosage:

Overdosage has been reported in 10 patients. All 10 patients experienced adverse effects, and all but one made a complete recovery.

Symptoms: One patient died after receiving a total daily dose of 12.5 g for 3 days instead of the intended 10.9 g. The patient suffered a grand mal seizure and became comatose. Three days later the patient died with the cause of death listed as respiratory/cardiac arrest. The other nine patients received doses ranging from 1.14 times to 8 times their recommended doses with an average of 4 times their recommended doses. Overall, three patients had seizures, three patients had renal function impairment, four patients had paresthesias either in limbs or periorally, and five patients had documented electrolyte disturbances primarily involving calcium and phosphate.

Treatment: There is no specific antidote. Hemodialysis and hydration may be of benefit in reducing drug plasma levels, but these have not been evaluated in a clinical trial setting. Observe the patient for signs and symptoms of renal impairment and electrolyte imbalance. Institute medical treatment if clinically warranted.

Patient Information:

Foscarnet is not a cure for CMV retinitis. Immunocompromised patients may continue to experience progression of retinitis during or following treatment. Advise patients to have regular ophthalmologic examinations.

The major toxicities of foscarnet are renal impairment, electrolyte disturbances and seizures. Dose modifications may be required, including possible discontinuation. Emphasize the importance of close monitoring while on therapy.

Advise patients of the importance of perioral tingling, numbness in the extremities or paresthesias during or after infusion as possible symptoms of electrolyte abnormalities. Should such symptoms occur, stop the infusion, obtain appropriate laboratory samples for assessment of electrolyte concentrations and consult physician before resuming treatment. The rate of infusion must be no more than 1 mg/kg/min.

The potential for renal impairment may be minimized by accompanying administration with hydration adequate to establish and maintain diuresis during dosing.

Administration and Dosage:

Do not administer foscarnet by rapid or bolus IV injection. The toxicity of foscarnet may be increased as a result of excessive plasma levels.

Take care to avoid unintentional overdose by carefully controlling the rate of infusion. Therefore, an infusion pump must be used. In spite of the use of an infusion pump, overdoses have occurred.

Administer by controlled IV infusion, either by using a central venous line or by using a peripheral vein. The standard 24 mg/ml solution may be used without dilution when using a central venous catheter for infusion. When a peripheral vein catheter is used, dilute the 24 mg/ml solution to 12 mg/ml with 5% Dextrose in Water or with a normal saline solution prior to administration to avoid local irritation of peripheral veins. Since the dose is calculated on the basis of body weight, it may be desirable to remove and discard any unneeded quantity from the bottle before starting with the infusion to avoid overdosage. Use solutions thus prepared within 24 hours of first entry into a sealed bottle.

Do not exceed the recommended dosage, frequency or infusion rates. All doses must be individualized for patients' renal function.

Induction treatment: The recommended initial dose for patients with normal renal function is 60 mg/kg, adjusted for individual patients' renal function, given IV at a constant rate over a minimum of 1 hour every 8 hours for 2 to 3 weeks depending on clinical response. An infusion pump must be used to control the rate of infusion. Adequate hydration is recommended to establish diuresis, both prior to and during treatment to minimize renal toxicity (see Warnings), provided there are no clinical contraindications.

Maintenance treatment: 90 to 120 mg/kg/day (individualized for renal function) given as an IV infusion over 2 hours. Because the superiority of the 120 mg/kg/day has not been established in controlled trials, and given the likely relationship of higher plasma foscarnet levels to toxicity, it is recommended that most patients be started on maintenance treatment with a dose of 90 mg/kg/day. Escalation to 120 mg/kg/day may be considered should early reinduction be required because of retinitis progression. Some patients who show excellent tolerance to foscarnet may benefit from initiation of maintenance treatment at 120 mg/kg/day earlier in their treatment. An infusion pump must be used to control the rate of infusion with all doses. Again, hydration to establish diuresis both prior to and during treatment is recommended to minimize renal toxicity.

Patients who experience progression of retinitis while receiving maintenance therapy may be retreated with the induction and maintenance regimens given above.

Renal function abnormalities: Use with caution in patients with abnormal renal function because reduced plasma clearance of foscarnet will result in elevated plasma levels. In addition, foscarnet has the potential to further impair renal function (see Warnings). Foscarnet has not been specifically studied in patients with Ccr < 50 ml/min or serum creatinine > 2.8 mg/dl. Carefully monitor renal function at baseline and during induction and maintenance therapy with appropriate dose adjustments. If Ccr falls below the limits of the dosing nomograms (0.4 ml/min/kg) during therapy, discontinue foscarnet and monitor the patient daily until resolution of renal impairment is ensured.

Dose adjustment in renal impairment: Individualize foscarnet dosing according to the patient's renal function status. Refer to the table below for recommended doses and adjust the dose as indicated.

To use this dosing guide, actual 24 hour Ccr (ml/min) must be divided by body weight (kg) or the estimated Ccr in ml/min/kg can be calculated from serum creatinine (mg/dl) using the following formula (modified Cockcroft and Gault equation).

$$\text{Males:} \quad \frac{140 - \text{age}}{\text{serum creatinine} \times 72} = \text{Ccr}$$

Females: 0.85 x above value

Foscarnet Dosing Guide Based on Ccr	
Induction	
Ccr (ml/min/kg)	Equivalent to 60 mg/kg dose every 8 hours
≥ 1.6	60
1.5	57
1.4	53
1.3	49
1.2	46
1.1	42
1	39
0.9	35
0.8	32
0.7	28
0.6	25
0.5	21
0.4	18

Maintenance		
Ccr (ml/min/kg)	Equivalent to 90 mg/kg dose every 24 hours	Equivalent to 120 mg/kg dose every 24 hours
≥ 1.4	90	120
1.2-1.4	78	104
1-1.2	75	100
0.8-1	71	94
0.6-0.8	63	84
0.4-0.6	57	76

IV incompatibility: Other drugs and supplements can be administered to a patient receiving foscarnet. However, take care to ensure that foscarnet is only administered with normal saline or 5% Dextrose Solution and that no other drug or supplement is administered concurrently via the same catheter. Foscarnet is chemically incompatible with 30% dextrose, amphotericin B, and solutions containing calcium such as Ringer's Lactate and TPN. Physical incompatibility with other IV drugs includes: Acyclovir sodium, ganciclovir, trimetrexate, pentamidine, vancomycin, trimethoprim/ sulfamethoxazole, diazepam, midazolam, digoxin, phenytoin, leucovorin and prochlorperazine. Because of foscarnet's chelating properties, a precipitate can potentially occur when divalent cations are administered concurrently in the same catheter.

Storage: Store at room temperature 59° to 86°F (15° to 30°C). Avoid excessive heat above 104°F (40°C). Do not freeze. Use only if bottle and seal are intact and a vacuum is present. Do not use unless solution is clear and colorless.

Rx **Foscavir** (Astra)	**Injection:** 24 mg/ml	In 250 and 500 ml bottles.

Agents for Glaucoma

Glaucoma is a condition of the eye in which there is usually an elevation of the intraocular pressure (IOP) that leads to progressive cupping and atrophy of the optic nerve head, deterioration of the visual fields and ultimately to blindness. *Primary open-angle glaucoma* is the most common type of glaucoma. *Angle-closure glaucoma* and *congenital glaucoma* are treated primarily by surgical methods, although short-term drug therapy is used to decrease IOP prior to surgery.

Drugs used in the therapy of primary open-angle glaucoma include a variety of agents with different mechanisms of action. The therapeutic goal in treating glaucoma is reducing the IOP, a major risk factor in the pathogenesis of glaucomatous visual field loss. The higher the level of IOP, the greater the likelihood of glaucomatous visual field loss and optic nerve damage. IOP may be reduced by either 1) decreasing the rate of production of aqueous humor or 2) increasing the rate of outflow (drainage) of aqueous humor from the anterior chamber of the eye.

The five groups of agents used in the therapy of primary open-angle glaucoma are listed in Table 1, which summarizes their mechanism of decreasing IOP, effects on pupil size and ciliary muscle and duration of action.

SYMPATHOMIMETIC AGENTS

Sympathomimetic agents (adrenergic agonists) (eg, epinephrine [eg, *Epifrin*], dipivefrin [eg, *Propine*]) have both α and β activity. They lower IOP mainly by increasing nonpressure-dependent uveal-scleral outflow. Epinephrine, usually used as an adjunct to miotic therapy, is also used as primary therapy, especially in young patients who develop intolerable fluctuating myopia or in older patients with lens opacities. The combination of a miotic and epinephrine will have additive effects in lowering IOP.

Dipivefrin HCl is a prodrug which is metabolized to epinephrine in vivo. The IOP-lowering and intraocular effects are qualitatively and quantitatively similar to epinephrine; however, extraocularly, dipivefrin may be better tolerated and have a lower incidence of adverse effects because of its lower concentration.

Table 1: AGENTS FOR GLAUCOMA						
Drug	Strength	Duration (hrs)	Decrease Aqueous Production	Increase Aqueous Outflow	Effect on Pupil	Effect on Ciliary Muscle
Sympathomimetics						
Apraclonidine[1]	1%	3-5	NR	NR	NR	NR
Epinephrine	0.25%-2%	12	NR	++	mydriasis	NR
Dipivefrin	0.1%	12	NR	++	mydriasis	NR
Beta-Blockers						
Betaxolol	0.5%	12	+++	NR	NR	NR
Carteolol	1%	12	nd	nd	nd	nd
Levobunolol	0.5%	12-24	+++	NR	NR	NR
Metipranolol	0.3%	12-24	NR	+	NR	NR
Timolol	0.25%-0.5%	12-24	+++	+	NR	NR
Miotics, Direct-Acting						
Acetylcholine[2]	1%	10-20 min	NR	+++	miosis	accommodation
Carbachol[2]	0.75%-3%	8	NR	+++	miosis	accommodation
Pilocarpine	0.25%-10%	4-6	NR	+++	miosis	accommodation
Miotics, Cholinesterase Inhibitors						
Physostigmine	0.25%-0.5%	12-36	NR	+++	miosis	accommodation
Demecarium	0.125%-0.25%	days-wks	NR	+++	miosis	accommodation
Echothiophate	0.03%-0.25%	days-wks	NR	+++	miosis	accommodation
Isoflurophate	0.025%	days-wks	NR	+++	miosis	accommodation
Carbonic Anhydrase Inhibitors						
Dichlorphenamide	50 mg	6-12	+++	NR	NR	NR
Acetazolamide	125-250 mg	8-12	+++	NR	NR	NR
Methazolamide	25-50 mg	10-18	+++	NR	NR	NR

+++ = significant activity   ++ = moderate activity   + = some activity   NR = no activity reported
nd = no data available
[1] Used only to decrease IOP in surgery.
[2] Intraocular administration only for miosis during surgery.

BETA-ADRENERGIC BLOCKING AGENTS

Beta-adrenergic blocking agents (eg, betaxolol [*Betoptic*], levobunolol [*Betagan Liqui-film*], metipranolol [*OptiPranolol*] and timolol [*Timoptic*]) may be used alone or in conjunction with other agents. They may be more effective than either pilocarpine or epinephrine alone and have the advantage of not affecting either pupil size or accommodation. They lower IOP by decreasing the rate of aqueous production.

DIRECT-ACTING MIOTICS

Direct-acting miotics (eg, pilocarpine [eg, *Isopto Carpine*], carbachol [eg, *Isopto Carbachol*]) were considered the first step in glaucoma therapy. They have now yielded to the β-blockers. They are useful adjunctive agents that are additive to either the β-blockers or the sympathomimetics. Dosage and frequency of administration must be individualized. Recent information indicates pilocarpine 2%/carbachol 1.5% every 12 hours provides maximum effect. Increasing the concentration and dosage intervals may correct an inadequate response. Concentrations greater than pilocarpine 4% or carbachol 3% are occasionally required in patients with darkly pigmented irides.

CHOLINESTERASE INHIBITOR MIOTICS

Cholinesterase inhibitor miotics include both reversible/short-acting (eg, physostig-mine [eg, *Isopto Eserine*]) and irreversible/long-acting (eg, echothiophate [eg, *Phospholine Iodide*]) agents which enhance the effects of endogenous acetylcholine by inactivation of the enzyme acetylcholinesterase. These agents are more potent and longer acting than the direct-acting cholinergic agents. Side effects and systemic toxicity are more common and of greater significance. Using a direct-acting cholinergic and a cholinesterase inhibitor provides no improvement in response.

CARBONIC ANHYDRASE INHIBITORS

Carbonic anhydrase inhibitors (ie, acetazolamide [eg, *Diamox*], dichlorphenamide [*Daranide*], methazolamide [*Neptazane*]) are administered systemically. IOP is lowered by a direct action on the ciliary epithelium which decreases aqueous humor production. Carbonic anhydrase inhibitors are used as adjunctive therapy and do not replace topical therapy.

HYPEROSMOTIC AGENTS

Hyperosmotic agents (ie, mannitol [eg, *Osmitrol*], urea [*Ureaphil*], glycerin [*Osmoglyn*] and isosorbide [*Ismotic*]) are useful in lowering IOP in acute situations (see p. 201). These agents lower IOP by creating an osmotic gradient between the ocular fluids and plasma. These agents are not for chronic use.

Thom J. Zimmerman, MD, PhD
University of Louisville

For More Information

Becker B, Shaffer RN. Diagnosis and Therapy of the Glaucomas, ed. 4. St. Louis, MO: C.V. Mosby Co., 1987.

Chandler PA, Grant WM. Lectures on Glaucoma. Philadelphia, PA: Lea & Febiger, 1965.

Duane TD, ed. Clinical Ophthalmology. Philadelphia, PA: J.B. Lippincott Company, 1988.

Eskridge JB, Bartlett JD. The Glaucomas. In: Bartlett JD, Jaanus SD, eds. Clinical Ocular Pharmacology, ed. 2. Boston, MA: Butterworth, 1989.

APRACLONIDINE HYDROCHLORIDE

Actions:

Pharmacology: Apraclonidine HCl is a relatively selective α-adrenergic agonist that does not have significant membrane stabilizing (local anesthetic) activity. When instilled into the eyes, apraclonidine reduces intraocular pressure (IOP) and has minimal effect on cardiovascular parameters.

Optic nerve head damage and visual field loss may result from an acute elevation in IOP that can occur after argon or Nd:YAG laser surgical procedures. The higher the peak of IOP, the greater the likelihood of visual field loss and optic nerve damage, especially in patients with previously compromised optic nerves. The onset of action is usually within 1 hour and the maximum IOP reduction occurs 3 to 5 hours after application of a single dose. The mechanism of action is not completely established, although its predominant action may be related to a reduction of aqueous formation.

Controlled clinical studies of patients requiring argon laser trabeculoplasty, argon laser iridotomy or Nd:YAG posterior capsulotomy showed that apraclonidine controlled or prevented the postsurgical IOP rise typically observed in patients after undergoing those procedures. After surgery, the mean IOP was 1.2 to 4 mmHg below the corresponding presurgical baseline before apraclonidine. With placebo, postsurgical pressures were 2.5 to 8.4 mmHg higher than presurgical baselines. Overall, only 2% of patients treated with apraclonidine had severe IOP elevations (spike greater than or equal to 10 mmHg) during the first 3 hours after laser surgery, whereas 22% of placebo-treated patients responded with severe pressure spikes (Table 1). Of the patients that experienced a pressure spike after surgery, the peak IOP was above 30 mmHg in most patients (Table 2) and was above 50 mmHg in seven placebo-treated patients and one apraclonidine-treated patient.

Table 1: INCIDENCE OF IOP SPIKES $\geq$ 10 mmHg						
			Treatment			
			Apraclonidine		Placebo	
Study	Laser Procedure	P-Value	N[a]	(%)	N[a]	(%)
1	Trabeculoplasty	< 0.05	0/40	(0%)	6/35	(17%)
2	Trabeculoplasty	= 0.06	2/41	(5%)	8/42	(19%)
1	Iridotomy	< 0.05	0/11	(0%)	4/10	(40%)
2	Iridotomy	= 0.05	0/17	(0%)	4/19	(21%)
1	Nd:YAG Capsulotomy	< 0.05	3/80	(4%)	19/83	(23%)
2	Nd:YAG Capsulotomy	< 0.05	0/83	(0%)	22/81	(27%)

N[a] = Number Spikes/Number Eyes.

Table 2: MAGNITUDE OF POSTSURGICAL IOP IN TRABECULOPLASTY, IRIDOTOMY AND Nd:YAG CAPSULOTOMY PATIENTS WITH SEVERE PRESSURE SPIKES $\geq$ 10 mmHg					
		Maximum Postsurgical IOP (mmHg)			
Treatment	Total Spikes	20-29 mmHg	30-39 mmHg	40-49 mmHg	> 50 mmHg
Apraclonidine	8	1	4	2	1
Placebo	78	16	47	8	7

Indications:

To control or prevent postsurgical elevations in IOP that occur in patients after argon laser trabeculoplasty, argon laser iridotomy or Nd:YAG posterior capsulotomy.

Contraindications:

Patients receiving monoamine oxidase inhibitor therapy and patients with hypersensitivity to any component of the formulation or to *clonidine*.

Warnings:

Pregnancy: Category C. There are no adequate and well-controlled studies of apraclonidine in pregnant women. Use during pregnancy only when clearly needed and when the potential benefits outweigh the potential hazards to the fetus.

Lactation: It is not known if topically applied apraclonidine is excreted in breast milk. Consider discontinuing nursing for the day on which apraclonidine is used.

Children: Safety and efficacy in children have not been established.

Precautions:

Closely monitor patients who develop exaggerated reductions in IOP. Apraclonidine is a potent depressor of IOP.

Cardiovascular disease: Acute administration of two drops of apraclonidine has had minimal effect on heart rate or blood pressure; however, use caution in treating patients with severe cardiovascular disease, including hypertension.

Consider the possibility of a vasovagal attack occurring during laser surgery. Use caution in patients with a history of such episodes.

Corneal changes: Topical ocular administration of two drops of 0.5%, 1% and 1.5% apraclonidine to rabbits 3 times daily for 1 month resulted in sporadic and transient instances of minimal corneal cloudiness in the 1.5% group. No histopathological changes were noted. No adverse ocular effects were observed in monkeys treated with two drops of 1.5% solution 3 times daily for 3 months. No corneal changes were observed in 320 humans given at least one dose of 1% apraclonidine.

Adverse Reactions:

The following adverse effects were reported with the use of apraclonidine in laser surgery: Ocular injection (1.8%); upper lid elevation (1.3%); irregular heart rate (0.7%); ocular inflammation (0.45%); nasal decongestion (0.45%); conjunctival blanching (0.4%); mydriasis (0.4%).

The following adverse effects were observed in investigational studies with dosing once or twice daily for up to 28 days in nonlaser studies:

Ocular – Conjunctival blanching; upper lid elevation; mydriasis; burning; discomfort; foreign body sensation; dryness; itching; hypotony; blurred or dimmed vision; allergic response; conjunctival microhemorrhage.

GI – Abdominal pain; diarrhea; stomach discomfort; vomiting.

Cardiovascular – Bradycardia; vasovagal attack; palpitations; orthostatic episode.

CNS – Insomnia; dream disturbances; irritability; decreased libido.

Other – Taste abnormalities; dry mouth; nasal burning or dryness; headache; head cold sensation; chest heaviness or burning; clammy or sweaty palms; body heat sensation; shortness of breath; increased pharyngeal secretion; extremity pain or numbness; fatigue; paresthesias; pruritus not associated with rash.

Administration and Dosage:

Instill 1 drop in scheduled operative eye 1 hour before initiating anterior segment laser surgery. Instill second drop into same eye immediately upon completion of surgery. Use a separate container for each single-drop dose and discard after use.

Storage: Store at room temperature 59° to 86°F (15° to 30°C). Protect from light.

Rx **Iopidine** (Alcon)	**Solution:** 1% apraclonidine HCl, 0.01% benzalkonium chloride and NaCl	In 0.1 ml (24s).

EPINEPHRINE

Actions:

Epinephrine, a direct-acting sympathomimetic agent, acts on α and β receptors. Topical application, therefore, causes conjunctival decongestion (vasoconstriction), transient mydriasis (pupillary dilation) and reduction of intraocular pressure (IOP). It is believed IOP reduction is primarily due to increased aqueous outflow. The duration of decrease in IOP is 12 to 24 hours.

Systemic effects from ophthalmic instillation have occurred when conjunctival permeability has been increased by use of local anesthetics or tonometry.

Epinephrine is available as the hydrochloride and borate salts. These preparations are therapeutically equal when given in equivalent doses of epinephrine base. The borate salts may cause less local discomfort.

Indications:

Management of open-angle (chronic simple) glaucoma; may be used in combination with miotics, β-adrenergic blocking agents, hyperosmotic agents or carbonic anhydrase inhibitors.

Contraindications:

Hypersensitivity to epinephrine or any component of the formulation. Do not use in narrow- or shallow-angle (angle closure) glaucoma, aphakia or in patients with a narrow angle who do not have glaucoma.

Do not use while wearing soft contact lenses; discoloration of lenses may occur.

Do not use if nature of the glaucoma has not been clearly established.

Warnings:

For topical eye use only. Not for injection or intraocular use.

Since pupil dilation may precipitate an acute attack of narrow-angle glaucoma, evaluate anterior chamber angle by gonioscopy prior to beginning therapy.

Anesthesia: Discontinue use prior to general anesthesia with anesthetics that sensitize the myocardium to sympathomimetics (eg, cyclopropane, halothane).

Aphakic patients: Maculopathy with associated decrease in visual acuity may occur in the aphakic eye; if this occurs, promptly discontinue use.

Pregnancy: Category C. Safety for use during pregnancy has not been established. Use only when clearly needed and potential benefits outweigh the potential hazards to the fetus.

Lactation: It is not known whether this drug is excreted in breast milk. Safety for use in the nursing mother has not been established. Because many drugs are excreted in breast milk and because of the potential for serious adverse reactions in nursing infants, a decision should be made whether to discontinue nursing or the drug, taking into account the importance of the drug to the mother.

Children: Safety and efficacy for use in children have not been established.

Elderly: Use with caution.

Precautions:

Epinephrine is relatively uncomfortable upon instillation. Discomfort lessens as concentration of epinephrine decreases.

Use with caution in the presence or history of hypertension, diabetes, hyperthyroidism, heart disease, cerebral arteriosclerosis or bronchial asthma.

Potentially hazardous tasks: Epinephrine may cause temporary blurred or unstable vision after instillation. Observe caution while driving or operating machinery.

Sulfite Sensitivity: Some of these products contain sulfites which may cause allergic-type reactions (eg, hives, itching, wheezing, anaphylaxis) in certain susceptible persons. Although the overall prevalence of sulfite sensitivity in the general population is probably low, it is seen more frequently in asthmatics or in atopic nonasthmatic persons. Specific products containing sulfites are identified in the product listings.

Drug Interactions:

β-Blockers, topical: The use of epinephrine with topical β-blockers is controversial. Some reports indicate the initial effectiveness of the combination decreases over time.

Chymotrypsin: Epinephrine 1:100 (1%) will inactivate chymotrypsin in approximately 1 hour.

Cyclopropane or *halothane:* Discontinue use prior to general anesthesia with anesthetics which sensitize the myocardium to sympathomimetics.

Monoamine oxidase inhibitors: When administered simultaneously with or up to 21 days after administration of MAOIs, careful supervision and adjustment of dosages are required; exaggerated adrenergic effects may result.

Tricyclic antidepressants: The pressor response of adrenergic agents may be potentiated by concurrent use of tricyclic antidepressants.

Adverse Reactions:

Local: Transient symptoms of stinging and burning, eye pain/ache, browache, headache, allergic lid reaction and conjunctival hyperemia. Prolonged use may be associated with conjunctival or corneal pigmentation. Following prolonged administration, ocular irritation (hypersensitivity) and localized adrenochrome deposits may occur in the conjunctiva, cornea and lids. Reversible cystoid macular edema may result from use in aphakic patients.

Systemic effects: Headache, palpitations, tachycardia, extrasystoles, cardiac arrhythmias, hypertension, faintness, trembling, sweating and pallor.

Overdosage:

If ocular overdosage occurs, flush eye(s) with water or normal saline.

Patient Information:

To avoid contamination, do not touch tip of container to any surface. Replace cap after using.

Do not use if solution is brown or contains a precipitate.

Do not use while wearing soft contact lenses.

Transitory stinging and burning may occur upon initial instillation. Headache or browache may occur.

Patients should immediately report any decrease in visual acuity.

Discard product 3 months after dropper is first placed in the solution.

Administration and Dosage:

Instill 1 drop into affected eye(s) once or twice daily. Determine frequency of instillation by tonometry.

More frequent instillation than 1 drop 4 times daily does not usually elicit any further improvement in therapeutic response.

When used in conjunction with miotics, instill the miotic first.

Storage: Solutions are inherently unstable. Store at 36° to 75°F (2° to 24°C). Keep container tightly sealed. Protect solution from light; store in cool place. Do not freeze. Discard if solution becomes discolored or contains a precipitate.

EPINEPHRINE (as HCl)   C.I.*

Rx	Epinephrine HCl (Iolab)	Solution: 0.1%	In 1 ml Drop-perettes (12s).[1]	54
Rx	Epifrin (Allergan)	Solution: 0.25%	In 15 ml dropper bottles.[2]	48
Rx	Epifrin (Allergan)	Solution: 0.5%	In 15 ml dropper bottles.[3]	55
Rx	Epifrin (Allergan)	Solution: 1%	In 15 ml dropper bottles.[3]	59
Rx	Glaucon (Alcon)		In 10 ml Drop-Tainers.[4]	48
Rx	Epifrin (Allergan)	Solution: 2%	In 15 ml dropper bottles.[3]	67
Rx	Glaucon (Alcon)		In 10 ml Drop-Tainers.[4]	53

EPINEPHRINE (as Borate)   C.I.*

Rx	Epinal (Alcon)	Solution: 0.5%	In 7.5 ml.[5]	54
Rx	Eppy/N ½% (Sola/Barnes-Hind)		In 7.5 ml.[6]	44
Rx	Epinal (Alcon)	Solution: 1%	In 7.5 ml.[5]	58
Rx	Eppy/N 1% (Sola/Barnes-Hind)		In 7.5 ml.[7]	47
Rx	Eppy/N 2% (Sola/Barnes-Hind)	Solution: 2%	In 7.5 ml.[7]	35

* Cost Index based on cost per ml.
[1] With 0.5% chlorobutanol and sodium bisulfite.
[2] With benzalkonium chloride, sodium metabisulfite, EDTA and sodium chloride.
[3] With benzalkonium chloride, sodium metabisulfite and EDTA.
[4] With 0.01% benzalkonium chloride, sodium metabisulfite, EDTA and sodium chloride.
[5] With 0.01% benzalkonium chloride, ascorbic acid and acetylcysteine.
[6] With 0.01% benzalkonium chloride, erythorbic acid, povidone, polyoxyl 40 stearate and sodium chloride.
[7] With 0.01% benzalkonium chloride, erythorbic acid, povidone and polyoxyl 40 stearate.

DIPIVEFRIN HCl (Dipivalyl epinephrine)

Actions:

Pharmacology: Dipivefrin HCl is a prodrug of *epinephrine* formed by the diesterification of epinephrine and *pivalic acid*, enhancing its lipophilic character and, as a consequence, its penetration into the anterior chamber. Corneal penetration is approximately 17 times that of epinephrine.

Dipivefrin is converted to epinephrine within the eye by enzymatic hydrolysis. It appears to exert its action by decreasing aqueous production and enhancing outflow facility. Dipivefrin delivers the same therapeutic effects of epinephrine with fewer local and systemic side effects.

Pharmacokinetics: The onset of action with 1 drop occurs about 30 minutes after treatment, with maximum effect seen at about 1 hour.

Clinical Pharmacology: In patients with a history of epinephrine intolerance, only 3% of dipivefrin-treated patients exhibited intolerance, while 55% of those treated with epinephrine again developed an intolerance.

Response to dipivefrin twice daily is less than that of 2% epinephrine twice daily and comparable to 2% pilocarpine 4 times daily. Patients using dipivefrin twice daily in studies of 76 to 146 days experienced mean IOP reductions ranging from 20% to 24%.

Dipivefrin does not produce miosis or accommodative spasm that cholinergic agents produce. The blurred vision and night blindness often associated with miotic agents do not occur with dipivefrin. In patients with cataracts, the inability to see around lenticular opacities caused by constricted pupil is avoided.

Indications:

Initial therapy or as an adjunct with other antiglaucoma agents for the control of IOP in chronic open-angle glaucoma.

Contraindications:

Hypersensitivity to dipivefrin or any component of the formulation.

Narrow angles since any dilation of the pupil may predispose the patient to an attack of angle-closure glaucoma.

Warnings:

Pregnancy: Category B. Animal studies reveal no evidence of impaired fertility or fetal harm. There are no adequate and well-controlled studies in pregnant women. Safety for use in pregnancy has not been established. Use only when clearly needed.

Lactation: It is not known whether this drug is excreted in breast milk. Because safety for use has not been established, use caution in nursing mothers.

Children: Safety and efficacy for use in children have not been established.

Precautions:

Aphakic Patients: Macular edema occurs in up to 30% of aphakic patients treated with epinephrine. Discontinuation generally results in reversal of the maculopathy.

Adverse Reactions:

Cardiovascular: Tachycardia, arrhythmias and hypertension (reported with *epinephrine*).

Local: Burning and stinging (6%); conjunctival injection (6.5%). Infrequently, follicular conjunctivitis, mydriasis and allergic reactions occur. Epinephrine therapy can lead to adrenochrome deposits in the conjunctiva and cornea.

Dipivefrin 0.1% is less irritating than 1% epinephrine HCl. Only 1.8% of dipivefrin patients reported discomfort due to photophobia, glare or light sensitivity.

Patient Information:

Slight stinging or burning on initial instillation may occur.

Do not try to "catch up" on missed doses by applying more than one dose at a time.

Administration and Dosage:

Not for injection.

Initial glaucoma therapy: Instill 1 drop into the eye(s) every 12 hours.

Replacement therapy: When transferring patients to dipivefrin from antiglaucoma agents other than *epinephrine,* continue the previous medication the first day and add 1 drop of dipivefrin in affected eye(s) every 12 hours. The next day, discontinue the other antiglaucoma agent and continue with dipivefrin. Monitor with tonometry.

When transferring patients from conventional epinephrine therapy, discontinue the epinephrine and institute the dipivefrin regimen. Monitor with tonometry.

Concomitant therapy: When patients receiving other antiglaucoma agents require additional therapy, add 1 drop of dipivefrin every 12 hours. For difficult-to-control patients, the addition of dipivefrin to other agents such as *pilocarpine, carbachol, echothiophate iodide* or *acetazolamide* has been shown to be effective.

C.I.*

Rx	**Propine** (Allergan)	**Solution:** 0.1%	In 5, 10 and 15 ml Compliance Cap B.I.D.[1]	81

* Cost Index based on cost per ml.
[1] With 0.005% benzalkonium chloride, EDTA and sodium chloride.

BETA-ADRENERGIC BLOCKING AGENTS, General Monograph

Actions:

Pharmacology: Carteolol, levobunolol, metipranolol and timolol are noncardioselective $(\beta_1$ and $\beta_2)$ β-blockers; betaxolol is a cardioselective (β_1) β-blocker. Topical β-blockers do not have significant membrane-stabilizing (local anesthetic) actions or intrinsic sympathomimetic activity. Carteolol does have intrinsic sympathomimetic activity. They reduce elevated and normal intraocular pressure (IOP), with or without glaucoma.

The exact mechanism of ocular hypotensive action is not established, but it appears to be a reduction of aqueous production. However, some studies show a slight increase in outflow facility with timolol and metipranolol.

These agents reduce IOP with little or no effect on pupil size or accommodation. Blurred vision and night blindness often associated with miotics are not associated with these agents. In addition, in patients with cataracts, the inability to see around lenticular opacities when the pupil is constricted is avoided. These agents may be absorbed systemically (see Warnings).

Pharmacokinetics are summarized in the following table.

OPHTHALMIC β-ADRENERGIC BLOCKING AGENTS				
Drug	β-receptor selectivity	Onset (min)	Maximum Effect (hr)	Duration (hr)
Betaxolol	β_1	≤ 30	2	12
Carteolol	β_1 and β_2	nd	nd	12
Levobunolol	β_1 and β_2	≤ 60	2 to 6	12 to 24
Metipranolol	β_1 and β_2	≤ 30	≈ 2	12 to 24
Timolol	β_1 and β_2	≤ 30	1 to 2	12 to 24

nd = No data

Clinical Pharmacology: Ophthalmic betaxolol was compared to ophthalmic timolol and placebo in patients with reactive airway disease. Betaxolol had no significant effect on pulmonary function as measured by Forced Expiratory Volume (FEV$_1$), Forced Vital Capacity (FVC) and FEV$_1$/VC. Also, action of isoproterenol was not inhibited. Timolol significantly decreased these pulmonary functions. No evidence of cardiovascular β-blockade during exercise was observed with betaxolol. Mean arterial blood pressure was not affected by any treatment; however, ophthalmic timolol significantly decreased mean heart rate. Betaxolol reduced mean IOP 25% from baseline. In controlled studies, the magnitude and duration of the ocular hypotensive effects of betaxolol and timolol were clinically equivalent.

Clinical observation of glaucoma patients treated with betaxolol solution for up to 3 years shows that the IOP-lowering effect is well maintained.

Betaxolol has been successfully used in glaucoma patients who have undergone laser trabeculoplasty and have needed long-term hypotensive therapy. The drug is well tolerated in glaucoma patients with hard or soft contact lenses and in aphakic patients.

Carteolol – In clinical trials ranging from 1.5 to 3 months, carteolol produced a median percent IOP reduction of 22% to 25% when given twice daily.

Levobunolol – In controlled clinical studies of approximately 2 years' duration, IOP was controlled in approximately 80% of subjects treated with levobunolol 0.5% twice daily. The mean IOP decrease from baseline was 6.87 to 7.81 mmHg. No significant effects on pupil size, tear production or corneal sensitivity were observed. In a 3-month clinical study, one drop once a day of levobunolol 0.5% controlled the IOP of 72% of subjects achieving an overall mean decrease in IOP of 7 mmHg.

Metipranolol – The average IOP was reduced approximately 20% to 26% in controlled studies of patients with IOP greater than 24 mmHg at baseline. Clinical studies in patients with glaucoma treated for up to 2 years indicate that an IOP-lowering effect is maintained.

Timolol – In controlled studies of untreated IOP of greater than or equal to 22 mmHg, timolol 0.25% or 0.5% twice daily caused greater IOP reduction than 1%, 2%, 3% or 4% pilocarpine solution 4 times daily or 0.5%, 1% or 2% epinephrine HCl solution twice daily. In comparative studies, mean IOP reduction was 31% to 33% with timolol, 22% with pilocarpine and 28% with epinephrine.

In studies comparing timolol with pilocarpine, 61% of patients treated with timolol had IOP reduced to less than 22 mmHg compared to 32% with pilocarpine. For patients completing these studies, the mean reduction in pressure at the end of the study was 31% for patients treated with timolol and 22% with pilocarpine.

In studies comparing timolol with epinephrine, 69% of patients treated with timolol had IOP reduced to less than 22 mmHg compared to 42% with epinephrine. For patients completing these studies, the mean reduction in pressure at the end of the study was 33% for patients treated with timolol and 28% with epinephrine.

In ocular hypertension, effects of timolol and acetazolamide are additive. Timolol, which is generally well tolerated, produces fewer and less severe side effects than pilocarpine or epinephrine. Timolol has been well tolerated in patients wearing conventional (PMMA) hard contact lenses.

Indications:

Lowering IOP in patients with chronic open-angle glaucoma.

For specific approved indications, refer to individual drug monographs.

Contraindications:

Hypersensitivity to any component of the formulation.

Individuals with bronchial asthma, a history of bronchial asthma or severe chronic obstructive pulmonary disease; sinus bradycardia; second-degree and third-degree AV block; overt cardiac failure; cardiogenic shock.

Warnings:

Systemic absorption: All topical ocular agents may be absorbed systemically. The adverse reactions found with systemic β-blockers may occur with topical use. Severe respiratory and cardiac reactions, including death due to bronchospasm in asthmatics, and rarely, death associated with cardiac failure, have been reported with topical β-blockers. Detectable, perhaps significant serum timolol levels may be achieved in some patients. Exercise caution with all of these agents.

Cardiovascular: Timolol can decrease resting and maximal exercise heart rate even in normal subjects. Levobunolol and metipranolol may decrease heart rate and blood pressure, and betaxolol has minimal effect on pulmonary and cardiovascular parameters.

Cardiac failure – Sympathetic stimulation may be essential for circulation support in diminished myocardial contractility; its inhibition by β-receptor blockade may precipitate more severe failure.

In patients without a history of cardiac failure – Continued depression of myocardium with β-blockers may lead to cardiac failure. Discontinue at the first sign or symptom of cardiac failure.

Diminished pulmonary function: Non-allergic bronchospasm patients or patients with a history of chronic bronchitis, emphysema, etc, should receive β-blockers with caution. These drugs may block bronchodilation produced by catecholamine stimulation of β_2-receptors.

There have been reports of asthmatic attacks and pulmonary distress during betaxolol treatment. Although rechallenges with ophthalmic betaxolol have not adversely affected pulmonary function test results, the possibility of adverse pulmonary effects in patients unusually sensitive to β-blockers cannot be ruled out.

Major surgery: Withdrawing β-blockers before major surgery is controversial. Beta-receptor blockade impairs the heart's ability to respond to β-adrenergically mediated reflex stimuli. This may augment the risk of general anesthesia. Some patients on β-blockers have had protracted severe hypotension during anesthesia. Difficulty restarting and maintaining heartbeat has been reported. In elective surgery, gradual withdrawal of β-blockers may be appropriate.

If necessary, the effects of β-blocking agents may be reversed by β-agonists such as isoproterenol, dopamine, dobutamine or norepinephrine.

Diabetes mellitus: Administer with caution to patients subject to spontaneous hypoglycemia or to diabetic patients (especially labile diabetics) who are receiving insulin or oral hypoglycemic agents. These agents may mask signs and symptoms of acute hypoglycemia.

Thyroid: β-adrenergic blocking agents may mask clinical signs of hyperthyroidism (eg, tachycardia). Manage patients suspected of developing thyrotoxicosis carefully to avoid abrupt withdrawal of β-blockers which might precipitate a thyroid storm.

Cerebrovascular insufficiency: Because of the potential effects of β-blockers on blood pressure and pulse, use with caution in patients with cerebrovascular insufficiency. If signs or symptoms suggesting reduced cerebral blood flow develop, consider alternative therapy.

Carcinogenesis: In mice receiving oral metipranolol doses of 5, 50 and 100 mg/kg/day, females receiving the low dose had an increased number of pulmonary adenomas.

Pregnancy: Category C. There are no adequate and well-controlled studies in pregnant women. Use during pregnancy only if the potential benefits outweigh the potential hazards to the fetus.

Betaxolol – In oral studies with rabbits and rats, evidence of post-implantation loss was seen at dose levels above 12 mg/kg and 128 mg/kg, respectively. Betaxolol was not teratogenic, however, and there were no other adverse effects on reproduction at subtoxic dose levels.

Carteolol – Increased resorptions and decreased fetal weights occurred in rabbits and rats at maternally toxic oral doses $\approx$ 1052 and 5264 times the maximum human dose, respectively. A dose-related increase in wavy ribs was noted in the developing rat fetus when pregnant rats received oral daily doses $\approx$ 212 times the maximum human dose.

Levobunolol – Fetotoxicity was observed in rabbits at doses 200 and 700 times the glaucoma dose.

Metipranolol – Increased fetal resorption, fetal death and delayed development occurred in rabbits receiving 50 mg/kg orally during organogenesis.

Timolol – Doses 1000 times the maximum recommended human oral dose were maternotoxic in mice and resulted in increased fetal resorptions. Increased fetal resorptions were seen in rabbits at 100 times the maximum recommended human oral dose.

Lactation: It is not known whether betaxolol, levobunolol or metipranolol are excreted in breast milk. Systemic β-blockers and topical timolol maleate are excreted in milk. Carteolol is excreted in breast milk of animals. Exercise caution when administering to a nursing mother.

Because of the potential for serious adverse reactions from *timolol* in nursing infants, decide whether to discontinue nursing or the drug, taking into account the importance of the drug to the mother.

Children: Safety and efficacy for use in children have not been established.

Precautions:

Angle-closure glaucoma: The immediate objective is to reopen the angle, requiring constriction of the pupil with a miotic. These agents have little or no effect on the pupil. When they are used to reduce elevated IOP in angle-closure glaucoma, use with a miotic.

Muscle weakness: β-blockade may potentiate muscle weakness consistent with certain myasthenic symptoms (eg, diplopia, ptosis, generalized weakness). Timolol has increased muscle weakness in some patients with myasthenia gravis or myasthenic symptoms (rare).

Long-term therapy: Diminished responsiveness to betaxolol and timolol after prolonged therapy has been reported. However, in long-term studies (2 and 3 years), no significant differences in mean IOP were observed after initial stabilization.

Hypersensitivity: While taking β-blockers, patients with a history of severe anaphylactic reactions to a variety of allergens may be more reactive to repeated challenge, either accidental, diagnostic or therapeutic. Such patients may be unresponsive to the usual doses of epinephrine used to treat allergic reactions.

Sulfite Sensitivity: Some of these products contain sulfites which may cause allergic-type reactions (eg, hives, itching, wheezing, anaphylaxis) in certain susceptible persons. Although the overall prevalence of sulfite sensitivity in the general population is probably low, it is seen more frequently in asthmatics or in atopic nonasthmatic persons.

Drug Interactions:

Adrenergic psychotropic drugs: Exercise caution.

Beta-adrenergic blocking agents, oral: Use topical β-blockers with caution because of the potential for additive effects either on IOP or on systemic β-blockade.

Calcium Antagonists: Use caution in the coadministration of β-blockers and calcium antagonists because of possible AV conduction disturbances, left ventricular failure and hypotension. Avoid coadministration in patients with impaired cardiac function.

Calcium Antagonists and Digitalis: Concomitant use of β-blockers may have additive effects in prolonging AV conduction time.

Catecholamine-depleting drugs: Observe the patient when a β-blocker is administered with drugs such as reserpine because of possible additive effects and the production of hypotension or marked bradycardia, which may produce vertigo, syncope or postural hypotension.

Epinephrine, topical: Use with topical β-blockers is controversial. Some reports indicate the initial effectiveness of the combination decreases over time.

Quinidine, oral: One case of sinus bradycardia has been reported with the coadministration of ophthalmic timolol. The incidence was reaffirmed by a negative rechallenge with the β-blockers alone and positive rechallenge with the combination.

Verapamil: Use with ophthalmic timolol has caused bradycardia and asystole.

Other drugs that may interact with the systemic β-adrenergic blocking agents may also interact with the ophthalmic agents. These agents are listed below.

Antithyroid agents	Hydralazine	Phenothiazines
Calcium channel blockers	Insulin	Prazosin
Cimetidine	Lidocaine	Rifampin
Clonidine	Morphine	Salicylates
Contraceptives, oral	Neuromuscular blockers,	Smoking
Digoxin	nondepolarizing	Sympathomimetics
Disopyramide	NSAIDs	Theophylline
Haloperidol	Phenobarbital	Thyroid hormones

Adverse Reactions:

The following adverse reactions have occurred with ophthalmic use of the β_1 and β_2 (non-selective) adrenergic blocking agents:

Systemic:

CNS – Headache; depression.

Cardiovascular – Arrhythmia; syncope; heart block; cerebral vascular accident; cerebral ischemia; congestive heart failure; palpitation.

Digestive – Nausea.

Skin – Hypersensitivity, including localized and generalized rash.

Respiratory – Bronchospasm (predominantly in patients with preexisting bronchospastic disease); respiratory failure.

Endocrine – Masked symptoms of hypoglycemia in insulin-dependent diabetics (see Warnings).

Ophthalmic – Keratitis; blepharoptosis; visual disturbances including refractive changes (due to withdrawal of miotic therapy in some cases); diplopia; ptosis.

Betaxolol:

Ophthalmic – Brief discomfort (25%), occasional tearing, dryness of eyes, blurred vision, foreign body sensation, inflammation, discharge, ocular pain, decreased visual acuity and crusty lashes. *Rare:* Decreased corneal sensitivity, erythema, itching, edema, corneal punctate staining, keratitis, anisocoria and photophobia.

Systemic – Rare: Insomnia, dizziness, vertigo, headache, lethargy, depression, hives, toxic epidermal necrolysis, bradycardia, heart block, congestive heart failure, bronchospasm, thickened bronchial secretions, respiratory failure, asthma, dyspnea, alopecia, glossitis and increase in signs and symptoms of myasthenia gravis.

Carteolol:

Ophthalmic – Transient irritation, burning, tearing, conjunctival hyperemia and edema (≈ 25%). *Occasional:* Blurred/cloudy vision, photophobia, decreased night vision, ptosis, blepharoconjunctivitis, abnormal corneal staining and corneal sensitivity.

Systemic – Arrhythmia, palpitations, dyspnea, asthenia, headache, dizziness, insomnia, sinusitis and taste perversion.

Levobunolol:

Ophthalmic – Transient burning/stinging ($\leq$ 33%), blepharoconjunctivitis (5%), iridocyclitis (rare) and decreased corneal sensitivity.

Systemic – Bradycardia and hypotension. *Rare:* Headache, transient ataxia, dizziness, lethargy, urticaria and pruritus.

Metipranolol:

Ophthalmic – Transient local discomfort, conjunctivitis, eyelid dermatitis, blepharitis, blurred vision, tearing, browache, abnormal vision, photophobia and edema.

Systemic – Allergic reaction, headache, asthenia, hypertension, myocardial infarction, atrial fibrillation, angina, palpitations, bradycardia, nausea, rhinitis, dyspnea, epistaxis, bronchitis, coughing, dizziness, anxiety, depression, somnolence, nervousness, arthritis, myalgia and rash.

Timolol:

Ophthalmic – Ocular irritation including conjunctivitis, blepharitis, keratitis, blepharoptosis, decreased corneal sensitivity, visual disturbances including refractive changes (due, in some cases, to withdrawal of miotics), diplopia and ptosis.

CNS – Headache, asthenia, dizziness, depression, increased signs and symptoms of myasthenia gravis and paresthesias.

Cardiovascular – Chest pain, bradycardia, arrhythmia, hypotension, syncope, heart block, cerebral vascular accident, cerebral ischemia, heart failure, palpitations and cardiac arrest.

Respiratory – Bronchospasm (mainly in patients with preexisting bronchospastic disease), respiratory failure, dyspnea, nasal congestion and cough.

Other – Masked symptoms of hypoglycemia in insulin-dependent diabetics, nausea, diarrhea, hypersensitivity including localized and generalized rash, urticaria and alopecia.

Causal Relationship Unknown – Fatigue, hypertension, pulmonary edema, worsening of angina pectoris, dyspepsia, anorexia, dry mouth, behavioral changes including confusion, hallucinations, anxiety, disorientation, nervousness, somnolence and other psychic disturbances, aphakic cystoid macular edema, retroperitoneal fibrosis and impotence.

Oral β-adrenergic blocker-associated reactions should be considered potential effects with ophthalmic use. For example, severe respiratory and cardiac reactions, including death due to bronchospasm in asthmatic patients, and rarely, death in association with cardiac failure, have been reported.

Overdosage:

If ocular overdosage occurs, flush eye(s) with water or normal saline. If accidentally ingested, efforts to decrease further absorption may be appropriate (gastric lavage).

The most common signs and symptoms of overdosage from systemic β-blockers are bradycardia, hypotension, bronchospasm and acute cardiac failure. If these occur, discontinue therapy and initiate appropriate supportive therapy.

Patient Information:

Transient stinging/discomfort is relatively common. Notify physician if it becomes severe.

To avoid contamination, do not touch tip of container to any surface. Replace cap after using.

Do not use betaxolol with contact lenses in eyes.

Administration:

Monitoring: The IOP-lowering response to betaxolol and timolol may require a few weeks to stabilize. Determine the IOP during the first month of treatment. Thereafter, determine IOP on an individual basis.

Because of diurnal IOP variations in individual patients, satisfactory response to twice-a-day therapy is best determined by measuring IOP at different times during the day. IOP less than or equal to 22 mmHg may not be optimal to control glaucoma in each patient; therefore, individualize therapy.

Concomitant therapy: If IOP is not controlled with these agents, institute concomitant pilocarpine, other miotics, dipivefrin or systemic carbonic anhydrase inhibitors. The use of epinephrine in combination with topical β-blockers is controversial. Some reports indicate the initial effectiveness of the combination decreases over time (see Drug Interactions).

Cost Index:

In lieu of the cost index (a system based on the average wholesale prices for equivalent quantities of a drug), a comparison based on cost per drop of drug follows.

Assuming equivalence in terms of efficacy and patient compliance, cost becomes an important factor in drug selection. In order to determine the most cost effective β-blocker on a per-dose basis, the cost per drop for five ophthalmic β-blockers was compared. Retail prices in New Orleans, LA, Philadelphia, PA and San Francisco, CA were used. Relative cost was stable throughout the regions, although retail price and availability did vary. Patients, physicians and health-care agencies should find this information valuable when making cost-related choices between ophthalmic β-blockers (see table below).

	Comparison of Price per Drop in Three Cities[1]								
	Price in Cents Based on Bottle Size								
	New Orleans, LA			Philadelphia, PA			San Francisco, CA		
	5 ml	10 ml	15 ml	5 ml	10 ml	15 ml	5 ml	10 ml	15 ml
Optipranolol	6.3	4.6	—*	—*	—*	—*	8.1	5	—*
Timoptic	7	6.9	6.8	9.3	7.2	6.8	11.2	9.2	8.8
Betoptic	9.8	7.8	7.5	9.7	8.3	7.8	12.3	10.2	9
Betoptic-S	10.1	—*	7.8	10.1	—*	8.1	12.7	—*	9.4
Betagan	13.5	11.3	10.6	13.6	11.5	10.8	18.3	13	13.3

* Not available.
[1] Reprinted with permission from Ball SF, Schneider E. Cost of β-Adrenergic Receptor Blocking Agents for Ocular Hypertension. *Arch Ophthalmol* 1992;110:654-57.

Individual drug monographs are on the following pages.

BETAXOLOL HCl

For complete prescribing information see General Monograph p. 165.

Indications:

Treatment of ocular hypertension and chronic open-angle glaucoma. Betaxolol may be used alone or in combination with other antiglaucoma drugs.

Administration and Dosage:

Instill 1 to 2 drops twice daily.

Replacement therapy (single agent): Continue the agent being used and add 1 drop of betaxolol twice daily. The following day, discontinue the previous agent and continue betaxolol. Monitor with tonometry.

Replacement therapy (multiple agents): When transferring from several antiglaucoma agents, individualize dosage. Adjust one agent at a time at intervals of not less than 1 week. One approach is to continue the agents being used and add 1 drop of betaxolol twice daily. The next day, discontinue one of the other agents. Decrease or discontinue the remaining antiglaucoma agents according to patient response.

Storage: Store at room temperature 59° to 86°F (15° to 30°C). Shake suspension well before using.

Rx	**Betoptic S** (Alcon)	**Suspension:** 2.8 mg (equiv. to 2.5 mg base) per ml (0.25%)	In 2.5, 5, 10 and 15 ml Drop- Tainers.[1]
Rx	**Betoptic** (Alcon)	**Solution:** 5.6 mg (equiv. to 5 mg base) per ml (0.5%)	In 2.5, 5, 10 and 15 ml Drop- Tainers.[2]

CARTEOLOL HCl

For complete prescribing information see General Monograph p. 165.

Indications:

Lowering IOP in patients with chronic open-angle glaucoma or intraocular hypertension. It may be used alone or in combination with other IOP lowering drugs.

Administration and Dosage:

Usual dose: Instill 1 drop twice daily. If the patient's IOP is not at a satisfactory level on this regimen, concomitant therapy can be instituted.

Storage: Store at 59° to 77°F (15° to 25°C). Protect from light.

Rx	**Ocupress** (Otsuka America)	**Solution:** 1%	In 5 and 10 ml dropper bottles.[3]

[1] With 0.01% benzalkonium chloride, mannitol, poly sulfonic acid, carbomer 934P and EDTA.
[2] With 0.01% benzalkonium chloride, sodium chloride and EDTA.
[3] With 0.005% benzalkonium chloride.

LEVOBUNOLOL HCl

For complete prescribing information see General Monograph p. 165.

Indications:

Lowering IOP in patients with chronic open-angle glaucoma or ocular hypertension.

Administration and Dosage:

Instill 1 to 2 drops into the affected eye(s) once or twice daily.

Storage: Store at room temperature 59° to 86°F (15° to 30°C). Protect from light.

Rx	Betagan (Allergan)	Solution: 0.25%	In 5 and 10 ml Compliance Cap B.I.D.[1]
Rx	Betagan (Allergan)	Solution: 0.5%	In 2 ml standard cap and 5, 10 and 15 ml Compliance Cap Q.D. and B.I.D.[1]

METIPRANOLOL HCl

For complete prescribing information see General Monograph p. 165.

Indications:

Lowering IOP in patients with chronic open-angle glaucoma or ocular hypertension.

Administration and Dosage:

Usual dose: One drop twice daily. More frequent administration or a larger dose is not known to be of benefit. Concomitant therapy to lower IOP can be instituted.

Storage: Store at room temperature 59° to 86°F (15° to 30°C).

Rx	OptiPranolol (Bausch & Lomb)	Solution: 0.3%	In 2, 5 or 10 ml dropper bottles.[2]

[1] With 1.4% polyvinyl alcohol, 0.004% benzalkonium chloride, sodium metabisulfite, sodium chloride and EDTA.
[2] With 0.004% benzalkonium chloride, glycerol, povidone, sodium chloride and EDTA.

TIMOLOL MALEATE

For complete prescribing information see General Monograph p. 165.

Indications:

Lowering IOP in patients with chronic open-angle glaucoma; patients with aphakic glaucoma; some patients with secondary glaucoma; patients with elevated IOP who require lowering of the ocular pressure. In patients who respond inadequately to multiple antiglaucoma drug therapy, the addition of timolol may produce a further reduction of IOP.

Administration and Dosage:

Initial therapy: 1 drop of 0.25% twice daily. If clinical response is not adequate, change the dosage to 1 drop of 0.5% solution twice daily. If the IOP is maintained at satisfactory levels, change the dosage to 1 drop once daily. Since the pressure-lowering response may require a few weeks to stabilize, evaluation should include a determination of IOP after approximately 4 weeks of treatment.

Replacement therapy (single agent): When a patient is transferred from another topi-cal ophthalmic β-adrenergic blocking agent, discontinue that agent after proper dos-ing on one day and start treatment with timolol on the following day with 1 drop of 0.25% timolol twice daily. Increase the dose to 1 drop of 0.5% solution twice daily if clinical response is not adequate.

When changing from another antiglaucoma agent other than an ophthalmic β-block-ing agent, on day 1, continue with the agent being used and add 1 drop of 0.25% timolol twice daily. The next day, discontinue the previous agent completely and con-tinue with timolol. If a higher dosage is required, substitute 1 drop of 0.5% twice daily.

Replacement therapy (multiple agents): When transferring from several concomi-tantly administered agents, individualize dosage. If the agent is a β-blocker, discon-tinue before starting timolol. Adjust one agent at a time, at intervals of not less than 1 week. Continue the agents used and add 1 drop of 0.25% twice daily. The next day, discontinue one of the other agents. Decrease or discontinue remaining agents according to patient response. If higher dosage is required, use 1 drop of 0.5% twice daily.

Storage: Store at room temperature 59° to 86°F (15° to 30°C). Protect from light.

Rx	Timoptic (MSD)	Solution:	0.25%	In 2.5, 5, 10 and 15 ml Ocumeters.[1]
			0.5%	In 2.5, 5, 10 and 15 ml Ocumeters.[1]
Rx	Timoptic in Ocudose (MSD)	Solution:	0.25%	Preservative free. In UD 60s.
			0.5%	Preservative free. In UD 60s.

[1] With 0.01% benzalkonium chloride.

MIOTICS, DIRECT-ACTING, General Monograph

Actions:

The direct-acting miotics are parasympathomimetic drugs which duplicate the muscarinic effects of acetylcholine, but have no nicotinic effects. When applied topically, these drugs produce pupillary constriction, stimulate the ciliary muscles and increase aqueous humor outflow facility. Miosis, produced through contraction of the iris sphincter, causes increased tension on the scleral spur (reducing outflow resistance) and opening of the trabecular meshwork spaces facilitating outflow. With the increase in outflow facility, there is a decrease in intraocular pressure (IOP).

Pharmacokinetics: Onset, peak and duration of action of the oculohypotensive effect for the direct-acting topical miotics are summarized in the following table.

INTRAOCULAR PRESSURE REDUCTION			
Miotic	Onset (hours)	Peak (hours)	Duration (hours)
Carbachol	1	2 to 4	6 to 8
Pilocarpine Solution Gel Ocular System	 0.75 to 1 1 1	 1.25 3 to 12 1.5 to 2	 4 to 14 18 to 24 7 days

Miosis following topical application of pilocarpine occurs in 10 to 30 minutes, peaks in 20 minutes and lasts 4 to 8 hours.

Indications:

To decrease elevated IOP in glaucoma.

Acetylcholine is used only for intraocular administration to induce miosis during surgery.

For specific approved indications, refer to individual drug monographs.

Unlabeled Uses: Pilocarpine 5 mg has been used orally to successfully treat xerostomia (dry mouth) in patients with malfunctioning salivary glands.

Contraindications:

Hypersensitivity to any component of the formulation; where cholinergic effects such as constriction are undesirable (eg, acute iritis, some forms of secondary glaucoma, pupillary block glaucoma, acute inflammatory disease of the anterior chamber).

Warnings:

Use carbachol with caution in the presence of corneal abrasion to avoid excessive penetration.

Pregnancy: Category C (pilocarpine). Safety for use during pregnancy has not been established. Use only when clearly needed and potential benefits outweigh the potential hazards to the fetus.

Lactation: It is not known whether these drugs are excreted in breast milk. Because many drugs are excreted in breast milk, exercise caution when administering to a nursing woman.

Children: Safety and efficacy for use in children have not been established.

Precautions:

Systemic reactions rarely occur during the treatment of chronic glaucoma, but in treating acute angle-closure glaucoma, consider the possibility of such reactions because of the relatively high dosage required over a short period of time.

Caution is advised, although systemic effects are uncommon at usual doses in patients with acute cardiac failure, bronchial asthma, peptic ulcer, hyperthyroidism, GI spasm, urinary tract obstruction and Parkinson's disease.

Retinal detachment has been caused by miotics in susceptible individuals, in individuals with preexisting retinal disease or in those who are predisposed to retinal tears. Fundus examination is advised for all patients prior to initiation of therapy.

Miosis usually causes difficulty in dark adaptation. Advise patients to use caution while night driving or performing hazardous tasks in poor light.

Pilocarpine: Use with caution in patients with narrow angles; it may produce acute angle-closure.

Pilocarpine Ocular System (Ocusert): Carefully consider and evaluate patients with acute infectious conjunctivitis or keratitis prior to use.

Drug Interactions:

Nonsteroidal anti-inflammatory agents, topical: Although clinical studies with acetylcholine chloride and animal studies with acetylcholine chloride or carbachol revealed no interference, and there is no known pharmacological basis for an interaction, there have been reports that both of these drugs have been ineffective when used in patients treated with topical nonsteroidal anti-inflammatory agents.

Adverse Reactions:

Acetylcholine:

Ophthalmic – Corneal edema, corneal clouding and corneal decompensation.

Systemic – Bradycardia, hypotension, flushing, breathing difficulties and sweating.

Carbachol:

Ophthalmic – Transient stinging and burning, corneal clouding, persistent bullous keratopathy, postoperative iritis following cataract extraction with intraocular use. Retinal detachment, transient ciliary and conjunctival injection, ciliary spasm with resultant temporary decrease of visual acuity.

Systemic – Headache, salivation, GI cramps, vomiting, diarrhea, asthma, syncope, cardiac arrhythmia, flushing, sweating, epigastric distress, tightness in bladder.

Pilocarpine:

Ophthalmic – Transient stinging and burning, tearing, ciliary spasm, conjunctival vascular congestion, temporal, peri- or supra-orbital headache, superficial keratitis induced myopia (especially in younger individuals who have recently started administration), blurred vision, poor dark adaptation, conjunctival hyperemia, reduced visual acuity in poor illumination in older individuals and in individuals with lens opacity. A subtle corneal granularity has occurred with pilocarpine gel use. *Rare* – Retinal detachment. Lens opacity may occur with prolonged use of pilocarpine.

Systemic – Rare: Hypertension, tachycardia, bronchiolar spasm, pulmonary edema, salivation, sweating, nausea, vomiting, diarrhea.

Pilocarpine Ocular System (Ocusert): Conjunctival irritation, including mild erythema with or without a slight increase in mucus secretion with first use. These symptoms tend to lessen or disappear after the first week of therapy. Ciliary spasm may occur with pilocarpine usage but is not a contraindication to continued therapy unless the induced myopia is debilitating to the patient. Rarely, a sudden increase in pilocarpine effects has been reported during use.

Although withdrawal of the peripheral iris from the anterior chamber angle by miosis may reduce the tendency for narrow-angle closure, miotics can occasionally precipitate angle closure by increasing resistance to aqueous flow from posterior to anterior chamber. Miotic agents may also cause retinal detachment. Exercise care with all miotic therapy, especially in young myopic patients.

Irritation from pilocarpine has been infrequently encountered and may require cessation of therapy. True allergic reactions are uncommon, but require discontinuation of therapy. Corneal abrasion and visual impairment have been reported.

Overdosage:

Should accidental overdosage in the eye(s) occur, flush with water or normal saline.

Treatment includes usual supportive measures.

If accidentally ingested, induce emesis or perform gastric lavage. Observe patients for signs of toxicity (eg, salivation, lacrimation, sweating, nausea, vomiting and diarrhea). If these occur, therapy with anticholinergics (atropine) may be necessary. Bronchial constriction may be a problem in asthmatic patients.

Patient Information:

May sting on instillation, especially first few doses.

May cause headache, browache, alteration of distance vision and decreased night vision. Use caution while night driving or performing hazardous tasks in poor light.

To avoid contamination, do not touch tip of container to any surface. Replace cap after using. Keep bottle tightly closed when not in use.

Wash hands immediately after use.

Keep out of reach of children.

Discard solution after expiration date.

Individual drug monographs are on the following pages.

ACETYLCHOLINE CHLORIDE, INTRAOCULAR

For complete prescribing information see General Monograph p. 175.

Indications:

To produce complete miosis in seconds by irrigating the iris after delivery of the lens in cataract surgery. In penetrating keratoplasty, iridectomy and other anterior segment surgery where rapid, complete miosis may be required.

Administration and Dosage:

Open under aseptic conditions only.

Instill the solution into the anterior chamber before or after securing one or more sutures. The pupil is rapidly constricted and the peripheral iris drawn away from the angle of the anterior chamber if there are no mechanical hindrances. Any anatomical hindrance to miosis may require surgery to permit the desired effect of the drug.

In cataract surgery, use only after delivery of the lens.

Solution: 0.5 to 2 ml produces satisfactory miosis. Solution need not be flushed from the chamber after miosis occurs. Since acetylcholine has a short duration of action, pilocarpine may be applied topically before dressing to maintain miosis.

Preparation of solution: Aqueous solutions of acetylcholine are unstable. Prepare solution immediately before use. Do not use solution which is not clear and colorless. Discard any solution that has not been used.

Do not gas sterilize.

Storage: Store at room temperature 59° to 86°F (15° to 30°C). Do not freeze.

C.I.*

| Rx | Miochol (Iolab) | **Solution:** 1:100 acetyl-choline chloride when reconstituted | In 2 ml dual chamber univial (lower chamber 20 mg lyophilized acetylcholine chloride and 60 mg mannitol; upper chamber 2 ml Sterile Water for Injection). Also available in System Pak Plus with 15 ml (2s) *Iocare* balanced salt solution. | 320 |

CARBACHOL, INTRAOCULAR

For complete prescribing information see General Monograph p. 175.

Indications:

Intraocular use for miosis during surgery.

Administration and Dosage:

For single dose intraocular use only. Discard unused portion.

Open under aseptic conditions only.

Gently instill no more than 0.5 ml into the anterior chamber before or after securing sutures. Miosis is usually maximal 2 to 5 minutes after application.

Storage: Store at room temperature 59° to 86°F (15° to 30°C).

C.I.*

| Rx | Miostat (Alcon) | **Solution:** 0.01% | In 1.5 ml vials.[1] | 556 |

* Cost Index based on cost per ml.
[1] With 0.64% sodium chloride.

CARBACHOL, TOPICAL

For complete prescribing information see General Monograph p. 175.

Indications:

For lowering IOP in the treatment of glaucoma.

Administration and Dosage:

Instill 1 or 2 drops into eye(s) up to 3 times daily.

Storage: Store at 46° to 80°F (8° to 27°C).

				C.I.*
Rx	**Isopto Carbachol** (Alcon)	**Solution:** 0.75%	In 15 and 30 ml Drop-Tainers.[1]	33
		1.5%	In 15 and 30 ml Drop-Tainers.[1]	34
		2.25%	In 15 ml Drop-Tainers.[1]	36
		3%	In 15 and 30 ml Drop-Tainers.[1]	38

PILOCARPINE HCl

For complete prescribing information see General Monograph p. 175.

Indications:

To treat chronic simple glaucoma, especially open-angle glaucoma. Patients may be maintained on pilocarpine as long as IOP is controlled and there is no deterioration in the visual fields.

To treat chronic angle-closure glaucoma, especially after iridectomy.

To treat acute (angle-closure) glaucoma alone, or in combination with other miotics, β-adrenergic blocking agents, epinephrine, carbonic anhydrase inhibitors or hyperosmotic agents to decrease IOP prior to surgery.

To control pre- and post-operative intraocular tension.

To reverse mydriasis caused by mydriatic or cycloplegic agents.

Administration and Dosage:

Solution: 1 or 2 drops up to 6 times daily. The frequency of instillation and the concentration are determined by the response of the patient. Concentrations greater than 4% are occasionally more effective, especially in patients with dark pigmented eyes because pilocarpine is absorbed by melanin pigment; however, the incidence of adverse reactions is also increased.

During acute phases, the miotic must be instilled into the unaffected eye to prevent an attack of angle-closure glaucoma.

Storage – Store at 46° to 86°F (8° to 30°C). Protect from light.

---

* Cost Index based on cost per ml.
[1] With 0.005% benzalkonium chloride, 1% hydroxypropyl methylcellulose and sodium chloride.

Gel: Apply a 0.5 inch ribbon in the lower conjunctival sac of affected eye(s) once daily at bedtime. Under selected conditions, more frequent instillations may be indicated. If other glaucoma medication is also used at bedtime, the drops should be used at least 5 minutes before the gel.

> *Storage* – Refrigerate at 36° to 46°F (2° to 8°C) until dispensed to patient. Do not freeze. Patient may store at room temperature and should discard any unused portion after 8 weeks.

C.I.*

Rx	**Isopto Carpine** (Alcon)	**Solution:** 0.25%	In 15 ml Drop-Tainers.[1] 24
Rx	**Pilocarpine HCl** (Various, eg, Moore, Rugby, Schein)	**Solution:** 0.5%	In 15 and 30 ml. 7+
Rx	**Isopto Carpine** (Alcon)		In 15 and 30 ml Drop-Tainers.[1] 24
Rx	**Pilocar** (Iolab)		In 15 ml and twin-pack (2 x 15 ml).[2] 20
Rx	**Piloptic-½** (Optopics)		In 15 ml.[3] 5
Rx	**Pilostat** (Bausch & Lomb)		In 15 ml. 11
Rx	**Pilocarpine HCl** (Various, eg, Alcon, Fougera, Geneva, Goldline, Major, Moore, Rugby)	**Solution:** 1%	In 2, 15 and 30 ml and UD 1 ml. 7+
Rx	**Adsorbocarpine** (Alcon)		In 15 ml dropper bottles.[4] 24
Rx	**Akarpine** (Akorn)		In 15 ml dropper bottles.[5] 9
Rx	**Isopto Carpine** (Alcon)		In 15 and 30 ml Drop-Tainers.[1] 24
Rx	**Pilocar** (Iolab)		In 15 ml and twin-pack (2 x 15 ml) and 1 ml dropperettes.[2] 20
Rx	**Piloptic-1** (Optopics)		In 15 ml.[3] 6
Rx	**Pilostat** (Bausch & Lomb)		In 15 ml and twin-pack (2 x 15 ml). 11

* Cost Index based on cost per ml.
[1] With 0.5% hydroxypropyl methylcellulose, 0.01% benzalkonium chloride and sodium chloride.
[2] With hydroxypropyl methylcellulose, benzalkonium chloride and EDTA.
[3] With polyvinyl alcohol, benzalkonium chloride, EDTA and sodium chloride.
[4] With 0.004% benzalkonium chloride, EDTA, povidone, PEG, poloxamer 188 and hydroxyethyl cellulose.
[5] With hydroxypropyl methylcellulose, 0.01% benzalkonium chloride and EDTA.

PILOCARPINE HCl (Cont.)

C.I.*

Rx	Pilocarpine HCl (Various, eg, Alcon, Fougera, Geneva, Goldline, Major, Moore, Rugby, Schein, United Research)	Solution: 2%	In 2, 15 and 30 ml and UD 1 ml.	11+
Rx	Adsorbocarpine (Alcon)		In 15 ml dropper bottles.[1]	24
Rx	Akarpine (Akorn)		In 15 ml dropper bottles.[2]	11
Rx	Isopto Carpine (Alcon)		In 15 and 30 ml Drop-Tainers.[3]	24
Rx	Pilocar (Iolab)		In 15 ml and twin-pack (2 x 15 ml) and 1 ml dropperettes.[4]	20
Rx	Piloptic-2 (Optopics)		In 15 ml.[5]	7
Rx	Pilostat (Bausch & Lomb)		In 15 ml and twin-pack (2 x 15 ml).	15
Rx	Pilocarpine HCl (Various, eg, Goldline, Major, Schein)	Solution: 3%	In 15 ml.	11+
Rx	Isopto Carpine (Alcon)		In 15 and 30 ml Drop-Tainers.[3]	26
Rx	Pilocar (Iolab)		In 15 ml and twin-pack (2 x 15 ml).[4]	22
Rx	Piloptic-3 (Optopics)		In 15 ml.[6]	7
Rx	Pilostat (Bausch & Lomb)		In 15 ml.	17
Rx	Pilocarpine HCl (Various, eg, Alcon, Fougera, Geneva, Goldline, Major, Moore, Rugby, Schein)	Solution: 4%	In 2, 15 and 30 ml and UD 1 ml.	14+
Rx	Adsorbocarpine (Alcon)		In 15 ml dropper bottles.[1]	26
Rx	Akarpine (Akorn)		In 15 ml dropper bottles.[2]	14
Rx	Isopto Carpine (Alcon)		In 15 and 30 ml Drop-Tainers.[3]	26 ·
Rx	Pilocar (Iolab)		In 15 ml and twin-pack (2 x 15 ml) and 1 ml dropperettes.[4]	22
Rx	Piloptic-4 (Optopics)		In 15 ml.[6]	8
Rx	Pilostat (Bausch & Lomb)		In 15 ml and twin-pack (2 x 15 ml).	18
Rx	Isopto Carpine (Alcon)	Solution: 5%	In 15 ml Drop-Tainers.[3]	26

* Cost Index based on cost per g or ml.
[1] With 0.004% benzalkonium chloride, EDTA, povidone, PEG, poloxamer 188 and hydroxyethyl cellulose.
[2] With hydroxypropyl methylcellulose, 0.01% benzalkonium chloride and EDTA.
[3] With 0.5% hydroxypropyl methylcellulose and 0.01% benzalkonium chloride.
[4] With hydroxypropyl methylcellulose, benzalkonium chloride and EDTA.
[5] With polyvinyl alcohol, benzalkonium chloride and EDTA.
[6] With polyvinyl alcohol, benzalkonium chloride and EDTA.

PILOCARPINE HCl (Cont.)   C.I.*

Rx	**Pilocarpine HCl** (Various, eg, Moore, Rugby, Schein)	**Solution:** 6%	In 15 and 30 ml.	9+
Rx	**Isopto Carpine** (Alcon)		In 15 and 30 ml Drop-Tainers.[1]	28
Rx	**Pilocar** (Iolab)		In 15 ml and twin-pack (2 x 15 ml).[2]	22
Rx	**Piloptic-6** (Optopics)		In 15 ml.[3]	20
Rx	**Pilostat** (Bausch & Lomb)		In 15 ml.	26
Rx	**Pilocarpine HCl** (Alcon)	**Solution:** 8%	In 2 ml Drop-Tainers.	31
Rx	**Isopto Carpine** (Alcon)	**Solution:** 10%	In 15 ml Drop-Tainers.[1]	36
Rx	**Pilopine HS** (Alcon)	**Gel:** 4%	In 3.5 g.[4]	203

PILOCARPINE NITRATE

For complete prescribing information see General Monograph p. 175.

Indications:

To control IOP in glaucoma.

For emergency relief of mydriasis in an acutely glaucomatous situation.

To reverse mydriasis caused by cycloplegic agents.

Administration and Dosage:

Glaucoma: 1 to 2 drops 2 to 4 times daily. Patient response may vary.

Emergency miosis: 1 to 2 drops of higher concentrations.

Reversal of mydriasis: Dosage and strength required are dependent on the cycloplegic used.

Shake well before using. Do not freeze. Keep out of reach of children.

C.I.*

Rx	**Pilagan** (Allergan)	**Solution:** 1%	In 15 ml dropper bottles.[5]	21
		2%	In 15 ml dropper bottles.[5]	22
		4%	In 15 ml dropper bottles.[5]	22

* Cost Index based on cost per ml.
[1] With 0.5% hydroxypropyl methylcellulose and 0.01% benzalkonium chloride.
[2] With hydroxypropyl methylcellulose, benzalkonium chloride and EDTA.
[3] With polyvinyl alcohol, benzalkonium chloride and EDTA.
[4] With 0.008% benzalkonium chloride, carbopol 940 and EDTA.
[5] With 1.4% polyvinyl alcohol, 0.5% chlorobutanol, sodium chloride, menthol, camphor, phenol and eucalyptol.

PILOCARPINE OCULAR THERAPEUTIC SYSTEM

For complete prescribing information see General Monograph p. 175.

Actions:

An elliptical unit designed for continuous release of pilocarpine following placement in the cul-de-sac of the eye. Pilocarpine is released from the system as soon as it is placed in contact with the conjunctival surfaces.

Pharmacokinetics: Ocusert releases the drug at 3 times the rated value in the first hours and declines to the rated value in approximately 6 hours. A total of 0.3 to 0.7 mg pilocarpine is released during this initial 6-hour period (one drop of 2% pilocarpine solution contains 1 mg pilocarpine). During the remainder of the 7-day period, the release rate is within ± 20% of the rated value.

The ocular hypotensive effect is fully developed within 1½ to 2 hours after placement in the cul-de-sac. A satisfactory ocular hypotensive response is maintained around the clock. IOP reduction for an entire week is achieved with the system from either 3.4 mg or 6.7 mg pilocarpine (20 or 40 mcg/hour times 24 hours/day times 7 days, respectively), as compared with 28 mg administered as a 2% ophthalmic solution 4 times daily.

During the first several hours after insertion, induced myopia may occur. In contrast to the fluctuating and high levels of induced myopia typical of pilocarpine administration by eyedrop, the amount of induced myopia with *Ocusert* decreases after the first several hours to a low baseline level (approximately 0.5 diopters or less), which persists for the therapeutic life of the system. Pilocarpine-induced miosis approximately parallels the induced myopia.

Indications:

To control elevated IOP in pilocarpine-responsive patients.

Concurrent therapy: Ocusert has been used concomitantly with various ophthalmic medications. Its release rate is not influenced by other ophthalmic preparations.

Patient Information:

Patient package insert is available with the product.

Wash hands thoroughly with soap and water before touching or manipulating the system.

If a displaced system contacts unclean surfaces, rinse with cool tap water before replacing. Discard contaminated systems and replace with a fresh unit.

Check for the presence of the system before retiring at night and upon arising.

Administration and Dosage:

Damaged or deformed systems: Do not place or retain in the eye. Remove and replace systems believed to be associated with an unexpected increase in drug action.

Initiation of therapy: There is no direct correlation between the strength of *Ocusert* used and the strength of pilocarpine eyedrop solutions required to achieve a given level of pressure lowering. It has been estimated that *Ocusert* 20 mcg is roughly equal to 0.5% or 1% drops and 40 mcg is roughly equal to 2% or 3% drops. *Ocusert* reduces the amount of drug necessary to achieve adequate medical control; therefore, therapy may be started with the 20 mcg system, irrespective of the strength of pilocarpine solution the patient previously required. Depending on the patient's age, family history and disease status or progression, however, therapy may be started with the 40 mcg system. The patient should return during the first week of therapy for evaluation of IOP, and as often thereafter as deemed necessary.

If pressure is satisfactorily reduced with the 20 mcg system, the patient should continue its use, replacing each unit every 7 days. If IOP reduction greater than that achieved by the 20 mcg system is needed, transfer the patient to the 40 mcg system. If necessary, an epinephrine ophthalmic solution, β-blocker or carbonic anhydrase inhibitor may be used concurrently.

It is strongly recommended that the patient's ability to manage the placement and removal of the system be reviewed at the first patient visit after initiation of therapy.

Placement and removal of the system: The system is placed in and removed from the eye by the patient, according to patient instructions provided in the package.

Since pilocarpine-induced myopia may occur during the first several hours of therapy (average of 1.4 diopters), place the system into the conjunctival cul-de-sac at bedtime. By morning, the myopia is at a stable level (about 0.5 diopters or less).

In those patients in whom retention of the unit is a problem, superior cul-de-sac placement is often more desirable. The unit can be manipulated from the lower to the upper conjunctival cul-de-sac by gentle digital massage through the lid. If possible, move the unit before sleep to the upper conjunctival cul-de-sac for best retention. Should the unit slip out of the conjunctival cul-de-sac during sleep, its ocular hypotensive effect following loss continues for a period of time comparable to that following instillation of eyedrops.

Storage: Refrigerate at 36° to 46°F (2° to 8°C).

Rx	**Ocusert Pilo-20** (Alza)	**Ocular Therapeutic System:** Releases 20 mcg pilocarpine per hour for 1 week	In packages of 8 individual sterile systems.
Rx	**Ocusert Pilo-40** (Alza)	**Ocular Therapeutic System:** Releases 40 mcg pilocarpine per hour for 1 week	In packages of 8 individual sterile systems.

MIOTICS, CHOLINESTERASE INHIBITORS, General Monograph

Actions:

These indirect-acting agents inhibit the enzyme cholinesterase, potentiating the action of acetylcholine on the parasympathomimetic end organs. Topical application to the eye produces intense miosis and muscle contraction. Intraocular pressure (IOP) is reduced by a decreased resistance to aqueous outflow.

Pharmacokinetics: Cholinesterase inhibitors are subdivided into reversible and irreversible agents. Reversible agents (eg, physostigmine, demecarium) quickly combine with cholinesterase; the resulting complex is slowly hydrolyzed and the inhibited enzyme is regenerated. The demecarium-enzyme complex is hydrolyzed more slowly than the physostigmine complex; therefore, its duration of action is longer.

Irreversible agents (eg, echothiophate, isoflurophate) also bind to cholinesterase; however, the resulting covalent bond is not hydrolyzed. Therefore, cholinesterase is not regenerated. More cholinesterase must be synthesized or supplied from depots elsewhere in the body before ophthalmic action dependent on cholinesterase returns.

These effects are accompanied by increased capillary permeability of the ciliary body and iris, increased permeability of the blood-aqueous barrier and vasodilation. Myopia may be induced or, if present, may be augmented by the increased refractive power of the lens that results from the accommodative effect of the drug. Demecarium indirectly produces some of the muscarinic and nicotinic effects of acetylcholine as quantities of the latter accumulate.

CHOLINESTERASE-INHIBITING MIOTICS					
	Miosis		IOP Reduction		
Miotics	Onset (minutes)	Duration	Onset (hours)	Peak (hours)	Duration
Reversible Physostigmine Demecarium	20 to 30 15 to 60	12 to 36 hrs 3 to 10 days	— —	2 to 6 24	12 to 36 hrs 7 to 28 days
Irreversible Echothiophate Isoflurophate	10 to 30 5 to 10	1 to 4 weeks 1 to 4 weeks	4 to 8 —	24 24	7 to 28 days 1 week

Indications:

Therapy of open-angle glaucoma; conditions obstructing aqueous outflow (eg, synechial formation) that are amenable to miotic therapy; following iridectomy.

May be used in combination with adrenergic agents, β-blockers, carbonic anhydrase inhibitors or hyperosmotic agents.

Demecarium, echothiophate and *isoflurophate* are indicated in accommodative esotropia (convergent strabismus).

Physostigmine is indicated only for reduction of IOP in primary glaucoma.

Echothiophate iodide may be used in subacute or chronic angle-closure glaucoma after iridectomy or where surgery is refused or contraindicated and in certain nonuveitic secondary types of glaucoma, especially glaucoma following cataract surgery.

Contraindications:

Hypersensitivity to cholinesterase inhibitors or any component of the formulation.

Active uveal inflammation or any inflammatory disease of the iris or ciliary body; glaucoma associated with iridocyclitis.

Demecarium and *isoflurophate* are contraindicated in pregnancy.

Echothiophate is contraindicated in most cases of angle-closure glaucoma.

Warnings:

Myasthenia gravis: Because of possible additive adverse effects, administer demecarium, echothiophate and isoflurophate only with extreme caution to patients with myasthenia gravis who are receiving systemic anticholinesterase therapy. Conversely, exercise extreme caution in the use of anticholinesterase drugs for the treatment of myasthenia gravis patients who are already undergoing topical therapy with cholinesterase inhibitors.

Surgery: In patients receiving cholinesterase inhibitors such as demecarium and isoflurophate, administer succinylcholine with extreme caution before and during general anesthesia.

Pregnancy: Category X (Demecarium, isoflurophate). Because of the toxicity of cholinesterase inhibitors in general, these drugs are contraindicated in women who are or who may become pregnant. If this drug is used during pregnancy, or if the patient becomes pregnant while taking this drug, apprise the patient of the potential hazard to the fetus.

> *Category C* (physostigmine, echothiophate). Safety for use during pregnancy has not been established. Use only when clearly needed and when the potential benefits outweigh the potential hazards to the fetus.

Lactation: It is not known whether these drugs are excreted in human milk. Exercise caution when administering physostigmine to a nursing woman. Because of the potential for serious adverse reactions in nursing infants, decide whether to discontinue nursing or the drug, taking into account the importance of the drug to the mother.

Children: The occurrence of iris cysts is more frequent in children. Extreme caution should be exercised in children receiving demecarium and isoflurophate who may require general anesthesia. Safety and efficacy for use of physostigmine have not been established.

Precautions:

Use with caution in patients with chronic angle-closure (narrow-angle) glaucoma or in patients with narrow angles, because of the possibility of producing pupillary block and increasing angle blockage.

Use caution in patients with marked vagotonia, bronchial asthma, spastic GI disturbances, peptic ulcer, pronounced bradycardia and hypotension, recent MI, epilepsy, parkinsonism and other disorders that may respond adversely to vagotonic effects.

Ophthalmic ointments may retard corneal healing.

Miosis usually causes difficulty in dark adaptation. Use caution while driving at night or performing hazardous tasks in poor light.

Use in glaucoma only when shorter-acting miotics have proven inadequate. Gonioscopy is recommended prior to use of medication.

Concomitant ocular conditions: When an intraocular inflammatory process is present, breakdown of the blood-aqueous barrier from anticholinesterase therapy requires abstention from, or cautious use of, these drugs. Use with great caution, where there is a history of retinal detachment or quiescent uveitis.

After long-term use, blood vessel dilation and resultant greater permeability increase the possibility of hyphema during or prior to ophthalmic surgery. Discontinue 3 to 4 weeks before surgery.

Systemic effects: Repeated administration may cause depression of the concentration of cholinesterase in the serum and erythrocytes, with resultant systemic effects. Discontinue if salivation, urinary incontinence, diarrhea, profuse sweating, muscle weakness, respiratory difficulties, shock or cardiac irregularities occur.

Although systemic effects are infrequent, use digital compression of the nasolacrimal ducts for 1 to 2 minutes after instillation to minimize drainage into the nasopharyngeal area.

Sulfite Sensitivity: Some of these products contain sulfites which may cause allergic-type reactions (eg, hives, itching, wheezing, anaphylaxis) in certain susceptible persons. Although the overall prevalence of sulfite sensitivity in the general population is probably low, it is seen more frequently in asthmatics or in atopic nonasthmatic persons.

Drug Interactions:

Carbamate or *organophosphate insecticides* and *pesticides:* Warn persons on cholinesterase inhibitors who are exposed to these substances (gardeners, organophosphate plant or warehouse workers, farmers, etc) of systemic effects possible from absorption through the respiratory tract or skin. Advise use of respiratory masks, frequent washing and clothing changes.

Succinylcholine: Use extreme caution before or during general anesthesia of patients on cholinesterase inhibitors because of possible respiratory and cardiovascular collapse.

Systemic anticholinesterases: Additive effects are possible; coadminister topical cholinesterase inhibitors cautiously, regardless of which therapy is added (see Warnings).

Adverse Reactions:

Ocular: Stinging, burning, lacrimation, eczematoid dermatitis, allergic follicular conjunctivitis, accommodative spasm, lid muscle twitching, conjunctival and ciliary redness, browache from ciliary spasm (with initial therapy), headache, activation of latent iritis or uveitis and induced myopia with visual blurring may occur.

Iris cysts may form, enlarge and obscure vision (more frequent in children). The iris cyst usually shrinks upon discontinuance of the miotic, or following reduction in strength of the drops or frequency of instillation. Rarely, the cyst may rupture or break free into the aqueous humor. Frequent examination for this occurrence is advised.

Retinal detachment has been reported occasionally.

Prolonged use may cause conjunctival thickening and obstruction of nasolacrimal canals. Posterior synechiae to the lens may occur; dilation of the pupil once or twice yearly will prevent synechiae formation. Lens opacities have been reported. Routine slit-lamp examinations, including lens, should accompany prolonged use.

Paradoxical increase in IOP by pupillary block may follow instillation. Alleviate with pupil-dilating medication.

Systemic: Nausea, vomiting, abdominal cramps, diarrhea, urinary incontinence, faintness, sweating, salivation, difficulty in breathing or cardiac irregularities may occur.

Overdosage:

If systemic effects occur, give parenteral atropine sulfate (IV if necessary):

Adults – ≥ 0.4 to 0.6 mg.

Infants and children up to 12 years – 0.01 mg/kg repeated every 2 hours as needed until the desired effect is obtained, or adverse effects of atropine preclude further usage. The maximum single dose should not exceed 0.4 mg.

Children – 0.05 mg/kg IV initially, followed by maintenance with 0.02 to 0.05 mg/kg, titrated to signs of atropinization.

Much larger atropine doses for anticholinesterase intoxication in adults have been used. Initially, 2 to 6 mg followed by 2 mg every hour or more often, as long as muscarinic effects continue. Consider the greater possibility of atropinization with large doses, particularly in sensitive individuals.

Pralidoxime chloride has been useful in treating systemic effects due to cholinesterase inhibitors. However, use in addition to, not as a substitute for, atropine.

A short-acting barbiturate is indicated for convulsions not relieved by atropine. Promptly treat marked weakness or paralysis of respiratory muscles by maintaining a clear airway and by artificial respiration.

Patient Information:

Local irritation and headache may occur at initiation of therapy.

Notify physician if abdominal cramps, diarrhea or excessive salivation occurs.

Keep tube or bottle tightly closed. Keep out of reach of children.

To avoid contamination, do not touch tip of container to any surface. Replace cap after using.

Do not wash or allow the tip to touch the eyelid or other moist surface.

Drops: Apply continuous gentle pressure on the lacrimal duct with the index finger for several seconds immediately following instillation of the drops. This is to prevent drainage overflow of solution into the nasal and pharyngeal spaces, which might cause systemic absorption.

Wash hands immediately after administration.

Use caution while driving at night or performing hazardous tasks in poor light.

Individual drug monographs are on the following pages.

PHYSOSTIGMINE (ESERINE)

For complete prescribing information see General Monograph p. 185.

Administration and Dosage:

Ointment: Apply small quantity to lower fornix, up to 3 times daily.

    Storage: Keep tightly closed. Protect from heat.

Solution: Instill 2 drops into the eye(s), up to 4 times daily.

    Storage: Store at 46° to 80°F (8° to 27°C). Do not use if solution becomes cloudy or dark brown. Protect from heat. Keep tightly closed.

				C.I.*
Rx	**Eserine Sulfate** (Various, eg, Iolab)	**Ointment:** 0.25% (as sulfate)	In 3.5 g.	113+
Rx	**Isopto Eserine** (Alcon)	**Solution:** 0.25% (as salicylate)	In 15 ml Drop-Tainers.[1]	26
Rx	**Eserine Salicylate** (Alcon)	**Solution:** 0.5% (as salicylate)	In 2 ml Drop-Tainers.[2]	28
Rx	**Isopto Eserine** (Alcon)		In 15 ml Drop-Tainers.[1]	28

DEMECARIUM BROMIDE

For complete prescribing information see General Monograph p. 185.

Administration and Dosage:

Closely observe the patient during the initial period. If the response is not adequate within the first 24 hours, consider other measures. Keep frequency of use to a minimum in all patients, especially children, to reduce chance of iris cyst development.

Glaucoma: Initial – Place 1 or 2 drops into the eye. A decrease in IOP should occur within a few hours. During this period, keep patient under supervision and perform tonometric examinations at least hourly for 3 or 4 hours to be sure no immediate rise in pressure occurs.

    Usual dose – 1 or 2 drops twice a week to 1 or 2 drops twice a day. The 0.125% strength used twice daily usually results in smooth control of the physiologic diurnal variation in IOP.

Strabismus: Essentially equal visual acuity of both eyes is a prerequisite to successful treatment.

    Diagnosis – For initial evaluation, use as a diagnostic aid to determine if an accommodative factor exists. This is especially useful preoperatively in young children and in patients with normal hypermetropic refractive errors. Instill 1 drop daily for 2 weeks, then 1 drop every 2 days for 2 to 3 weeks. If the eyes become straighter, an accommodative factor is demonstrated. This technique may supplement or complement standard testing with atropine and trial with glasses for the accommodative factor.

    Therapy – In esotropia uncomplicated by amblyopia or anisometropia, instill not more than 1 drop at a time in both eyes every day for 2 to 3 weeks; too severe a

---

* Cost Index based on cost per g or ml.
[1] With 0.15% chlorobutanol, 0.5% hydroxypropyl methylcellulose, sodium bisulfite and sodium chloride.
[2] With sodium bisulfite and sodium chloride.

degree of miosis may interfere with vision. Then reduce dosage to 1 drop every other day for 3 to 4 weeks and re-evaluate the patient's status. Continue with a dosage of 1 drop every 2 days to 1 drop twice a week. The latter dosage may be maintained for several months. Evaluate the patient's condition every 4 to 12 weeks. If improvement continues, reduce to 1 drop once a week and eventually to a trial without medication. However, discontinue therapy after 4 months if control of the condition still requires 1 drop every 2 days.

Do not use more often than directed. Caution is necessary to avoid overdosage.

Individualize dosage to obtain maximal therapeutic effect.

Storage: Do not freeze. Protect from heat.

			C.I.*
Rx **Humorsol** (MSD)	**Solution:** 0.125%	In 5 ml Ocumeters.[1]	89
	0.25%	In 5 ml Ocumeters.[1]	95

ECHOTHIOPHATE IODIDE

For complete prescribing information see General Monograph p. 185.

Administration and Dosage:

Because of the prolonged duration of action of the irreversible cholinesterase inhibitors, administration of the drug is required only twice daily; some patients may achieve adequate control with once-daily or every other day administration. Because of the tendency to produce more severe adverse effects, including systemic reactions, use the lowest dose consistent with adequate control.

Tolerance may develop after prolonged use; a rest period restores response to the drug.

Glaucoma: Two doses per day are preferred to maintain as smooth a diurnal tension curve as possible, although 1 dose daily or every other day has been used with satisfactory results. It is unnecessary and undesirable to exceed a schedule of twice a day. Instill the daily dose or one of the two daily doses just before retiring to avoid inconvenience due to miosis.

Early chronic simple glaucoma – Instill a 0.03% solution just before retiring and in the morning in cases not controlled with pilocarpine. Control during the night and early morning hours may then be obtained. Change therapy if IOP fails to remain at an acceptable level.

Advanced chronic simple glaucoma and glaucoma secondary to cataract surgery – Instill a 0.03% solution twice daily, as above. When transferring a patient to echothiophate because of unsatisfactory control with other miotics, one of the higher strengths will usually be needed. In this case, a brief trial with the 0.03% solution will be advantageous because higher strengths will then be more easily tolerated.

Concomitant therapy: May be coadministered with epinephrine, a carbonic anhydrase inhibitor, or both.

Accommodative esotropia:

Diagnosis – Instill 1 drop of 0.125% solution once a day into both eyes on retiring, for 2 or 3 weeks. If the esotropia is accommodative, a favorable response may begin within a few hours.

---

* Cost Index based on cost per ml.
[1] With 1:5000 benzalkonium chloride and sodium chloride.

Treatment – Use the lowest concentration and frequency which gives satisfactory results. After initial period of treatment for diagnostic purposes, reduce schedule to 0.125% every other day or 0.06% every day. Dosages can often be gradually lowered as treatment progresses. The 0.03% strength has proven effective in some cases. The maximum recommended dose is 0.125% once daily, although more intensive therapy has been used for short periods.

Duration of treatment – In diagnosis, only a short period is required and little time will be lost in instituting other procedures if the esotropia proves to be unresponsive. In therapy, there is no definite limit if the drug is well tolerated. However, if the eyedrops, with or without eyeglasses, are gradually withdrawn after a year or two and deviation recurs, consider surgery.

Storage: Store at room temperature 59° to 86°F (15° to 30°C). After reconstitution, keep eye drops in refrigerator to obtain maximum useful life of 6 months. Use within a month if stored at room temperature.

C.I.*

Rx	**Phospholine Iodide** (Wyeth-Ayerst)	**Powder for Reconstitution:**	With 5 ml diluent.[1]	
		1.5 mg to make 0.03%		128
		3 mg to make 0.06%		134
		6.25 mg to make 0.125%		151
		12.5 mg to make 0.25%		170

ISOFLUROPHATE

For complete prescribing information see General Monograph p. 185.

Administration and Dosage:

Apply the required dose in the conjunctival sac, with the patient supine. Take care not to touch the cornea with the tip of the tube.

Whenever possible, apply before retiring to lessen blurring of vision. Wash hands immediately after administration.

Isoflurophate hydrolyzes in the presence of water to form hydrofluoric acid. To prevent absorption of moisture and loss of potency, keep ointment tube tightly closed.

Do not use more often than directed. Caution is necessary to avoid overdosage. Keep frequency of use to a minimum in all patients, especially children, to reduce the chance of iris cyst development. If tolerance develops, use another miotic. Isoflurophate therapy may be resumed later.

Glaucoma: Initial – Place 0.25 inch strip of ointment into the eye every 8 to 72 hours. A decrease in IOP should occur within a few hours. During this period, keep patient under supervision and perform tonometric examinations at least hourly for 3 or 4 hours to be sure that no immediate rise in pressure occurs.

Strabismus: Essentially equal visual acuity of both eyes is a prerequisite to successful treatment.

Diagnosis – For initial evaluation, use isoflurophate as a diagnostic aid to determine if an accommodative factor exists. This is especially useful preoperatively in young children and in patients with normal hypermetropic refractive errors. Not more than 0.25 inch strip of ointment is administered every night for 2 weeks. If the eyes become straighter, an accommodative factor is demonstrated. This technique may supplement or complement standard atropine testing and trial with glasses for the accommodative factor.

---

* Cost Index based on cost per ml.
[1] With potassium acetate, 0.55% chlorobutanol and 1.2% mannitol.

Therapy – In esotropia uncomplicated by amblyopia or anisometropia, use not more than 0.25 inch strip at a time in both eyes every night for 2 weeks, as too severe a degree of miosis may interfere with vision. Dosage is then reduced from 0.25 inch strip every other day to 0.25 inch strip once a week for 2 months, after which the patient's status should be re-evaluated. If benefit cannot be maintained with a dosage interval of at least 48 hours, discontinue therapy.

Frequency of administration and duration of maintenance therapy depend on how long the eyes remain straight without medication. Gradually increase intervals between administration to the greatest length compatible with good results. Therapy may need to be continued indefinitely. In a few instances, it has been possible to discontinue therapy entirely after several months.

Storage: Protect from moisture, freezing and excessive heat.

				C.I.*
Rx	**Floropryl** (MSD)	**Ointment:** 0.025% in a polyethylene mineral oil gel	In 3.5 g.	60

* Cost Index based on cost per g.

PILOCARPINE AND EPINEPHRINE COMBINATIONS

PILOCARPINE lowers IOP by a direct cholinergic action which improves outflow facility on chronic administration (p. 175).

EPINEPHRINE reduces IOP by increasing outflow facility (p. 160).

The combination of pilocarpine and epinephrine provides additive effects in lowering IOP; opposing actions on the pupil may prevent marked miosis or mydriasis. These fixed combinations do not permit the flexibility necessary to adjust the dosage of each agent.

Administration and Dosage:

Instill 1 or 2 drops into the eye(s) 1 to 4 times daily. Determine concentration and frequency of instillation by severity of the glaucoma and response of the patient.

Individuals with heavily pigmented irides may require larger doses.

Storage: Store at 46° to 86°F (8° to 30°C). Keep tightly closed. Do not use solution if it is brown or contains a precipitate. Protect from light and heat.

				C.I.*
Rx	E-Pilo-1 (Iolab)	Solution: 1% pilocarpine HCl and 1% epinephrine bitartrate	In 10 ml dropper bottles.[1]	39
Rx	P₁E₁ (Alcon)		In 15 ml Drop-Tainers.[2]	33
Rx	E-Pilo-2 (Iolab)	Solution: 2% pilocarpine HCl and 1% epinephrine bitartrate	In 10 ml dropper bottles.[1]	40
Rx	P₂E₁ (Alcon)		In 15 ml Drop-Tainers.[2]	33
Rx	E-Pilo-3 (Iolab)	Solution: 3% pilocarpine HCl and 1% epinephrine bitartrate	In 10 ml dropper bottles.[1]	41
Rx	P₃E₁ (Alcon)		In 15 ml Drop-Tainers.[2]	34
Rx	E-Pilo-4 (Iolab)	Solution: 4% pilocarpine HCl and 1% epinephrine bitartrate	In 10 ml dropper bottles.[1]	43
Rx	P₄E₁ (Alcon)		In 15 ml Drop-Tainers.[2]	36
Rx	E-Pilo-6 (Iolab)	Solution: 6% pilocarpine HCl and 1% epinephrine bitartrate	In 10 ml dropper bottles.[1]	45
Rx	P₆E₁ (Alcon)		In 15 ml Drop-Tainers.[2]	38

* Cost Index based on cost per ml.
[1] With benzalkonium chloride, EDTA, mannitol and sodium bisulfite.
[2] With 0.01% benzalkonium chloride, methylcellulose, EDTA, chlorobutanol, polyethylene glycol and sodium bisulfite.

PILOCARPINE AND PHYSOSTIGMINE COMBINATION

PILOCARPINE lowers IOP by a direct cholinergic action which improves outflow facility on chronic administration (p. 175).

PHYSOSTIGMINE is a reversible inhibitor of cholinesterase and has indirect cholinergic effects (p. 185).

Combinations of pilocarpine and physostigmine have been used on the theory that improved response may be obtained. Studies indicate that no additive pressure-lowering effects are achieved over either agent used alone. Such combinations are therefore not recommended.

Administration and Dosage:

Instill 1 or 2 drops into the eye(s) up to 4 times daily.

Storage: Store at 46° to 80°F (8° to 27°C).

C.I.*

Rx	**Isopto P-ES** (Alcon)	**Solution:** 2% pilocarpine HCl and 0.25% physostigmine salicylate	In 15 ml Drop-Tainers.[1] 33

* Cost Index based on cost per ml.
[1] With 0.5% hydroxypropyl methylcellulose and 0.15% chlorobutanol.

CARBONIC ANHYDRASE INHIBITORS, General Monograph

Actions:

Carbonic anhydrase inhibitors are nonbacteriostatic sulfonamides which act specifically on the enzyme, carbonic anhydrase. In the eye, this inhibitory action decreases the secretion of aqueous humor and results in a drop in intraocular pressure (IOP). Evidence suggests that bicarbonate ions are produced in the ciliary body under the influence of carbonic anhydrase and diffuse into the posterior chamber with sodium ions. The aqueous fluid contains more sodium and bicarbonate ions than does plasma and consequently is hypertonic. Water is attracted to the posterior chamber by osmosis. Systemic administration of carbonic anhydrase inhibitors has been shown to inactivate carbonic anhydrase in the ciliary body of the rabbit's eye and to reduce the high concentration of bicarbonate ions in ocular fluids. Carbonic anhydrase inhibitors in high doses cause some decrease in renal blood flow and glomerular filtration rate.

The diuretic effect is due to its action in the kidney on the reversible reaction involving hydration of carbon dioxide and dehydration of carbonic acid. The result is renal loss of bicarbonate ion, which carries out sodium, water and potassium. Alkalinization of the urine and promotion of diuresis are thus effected. Alteration in ammonia metabolism occurs due to increased reabsorption of ammonia by the renal tubules as a result of urinary alkalinization.

Pharmacokinetics of these agents are summarized in the table below:

Carbonic Anhydrase Inhibitor	INTRAOCULAR PRESSURE REDUCTION			Relative Inhibitor Potency
	Onset	Peak Effect	Duration	
Dichlorphenamide	0.5 to 1 hr	2 to 4 hr	6 to 12 hr	30
Acetazolamide				1
Tablets	1 to 1½ hr	2 to 4 hr	8 to 12 hr	
Sustained Release Capsules	2 hr	8 to 12 hr	18 to 24 hr	
Injection (IV)	2 min	15 to 30 min	4 to 5 hr	
Methazolamide	2 to 4 hr	6 to 8 hr	10 to 18 hr	†

† Quantitative data not available; reported to be more active than acetazolamide.

Indications:

Glaucoma: For adjunctive treatment of chronic simple (open-angle) glaucoma and secondary glaucoma; preoperatively in acute angle-closure glaucoma when delay of surgery is desired to lower IOP.

Acetazolamide (tablets, sustained release capsules and injection): For the prevention or amelioration of symptoms associated with acute mountain sickness in climbers attempting rapid ascent and in those who are susceptible to acute mountain sickness despite gradual ascent.

Acetazolamide (tablets and injection only): For adjunctive treatment of edema due to CHF, drug-induced edema and centrencephalic epilepsy (petit mal, unlocalized seizures).

Unlabeled Uses: Treatment of hyperkalemic and hypokalemic periodic paralysis.

Contraindications:

Hypersensitivity to these agents. *Cross-sensitivity* between antibacterial sulfona-mides and sulfonamide derivative diuretics, including acetazolamide and various thiazides, has been reported.

Depressed sodium or potassium serum levels, marked kidney and liver disease or dysfunction, hyperchloremic acidosis, suprarenal gland failure, cirrhosis, decreased sodium and potassium levels, adrenocortical insufficiency/failure.

Dichlorphenamide: Do not use in patients with severe pulmonary obstruction who are unable to increase alveolar ventilation since acidosis may be increased.

Severe or absolute glaucoma: Long-term use in chronic noncongestive angle-closure glaucoma, since organic closure of the angle may occur while worsening glaucoma is masked by lowered IOP.

Warnings:

Caution is advised for patients receiving concomitant high-dose aspirin and carbonic anhydrase inhibitors, as anorexia, tachypnea, lethargy, coma and death have been reported (see Drug Interactions).

Pregnancy: Category C (Acetazolamide, dichlorphenamide). Animal studies with some of these drugs have demonstrated teratogenic (skeletal anomalies) and embryocidal effects at high doses. While there is no evidence of increased fetal risk in humans, do not use during pregnancy, especially during the first trimester, unless the potential benefits outweigh the potential hazards.

Lactation: Safety for use in the nursing mother has not been established. It is not known whether these drugs are excreted in breast milk. Because many drugs are excreted in breast milk, exercise caution when administering to a nursing woman.

Children: Safety and efficacy for use in children have not been established.

Precautions:

Increasing the dose does not increase diuresis and may increase drowsiness or paresthesia. It often results in decreased diuresis. However, very large doses have been given with other diuretics to promote diuresis in complete refractory failure.

Electrolyte imbalance: Adequate and balanced electrolyte intake is essential in all patients whose clinical condition may cause an electrolyte imbalance.

> *Dichlorphenamide* – Hypokalemia may develop when severe cirrhosis is present, during concomitant use of steroids or ACTH and with interference with ade-quate oral electrolyte intake. Hypokalemia can sensitize or exaggerate the response of the heart to the toxic effects of digitalis (eg, increased ventricular irritability).

> *Methazolamide* – Potassium excretion is increased initially, upon administration, and in patients with cirrhosis or hepatic insufficiency, the drug could precipitate a hepatic coma. Use with caution in patients on steroid therapy because of the potentiality of a hypokalemic state.

Hypokalemia may be avoided or treated with potassium supplements or foods with a high potassium content.

Pulmonary: Use with caution in patients with severe degrees of respiratory acidosis. These drugs may precipitate or aggravate acidosis. Use with caution in patients with pulmonary obstruction or emphysema when alveolar ventilation may be impaired.

Monitor for hematologic reactions common to sulfonamides. Obtain baseline CBC and platelet counts before initiating therapy and at regular intervals during therapy. If significant changes occur, discontinue the drug and institute appropriate therapy. Periodic monitoring of serum electrolytes is also recommended.

Drug Interactions:

Cyclosporine: Acetazolamide may increase the pharmacologic effects of cyclosporine. Increased trough cyclosporine levels with possible nephrotoxicity and neurotoxicity may occur.

Digitalis: Carbonic anhydrase inhibitors may induce hypokalemia, which sensitizes the heart to the toxic effects of digitalis (see Precautions).

Lithium: Carbonic anhydrase inhibitors increase the renal clearance of lithium. Reduced serum levels affecting therapeutic response may occur.

Primidone: When given concurrently, oral acetazolamide may alter primidone metabolism. Primidone peak serum and urine levels may be delayed.

Quinidine: An increase in urine pH secondary to acetazolamide may result in an increased renal tubular reabsorption of quinidine and a decreased urinary excretion. A possible increase in pharmacologic and toxicologic effects of quinidine may occur.

Salicylates: Concurrent use of carbonic anhydrase inhibitors may result in carbonic anhydrase inhibitor accumulation and toxicity including CNS depression and metabolic acidosis. Salicylates displace the drugs from binding sites and inhibit renal clearance.

Adverse Reactions:

All sulfonamides:

> *Sulfonamide-type reactions:* Anaphylaxis, fever, rash (including erythema multiforme, Stevens-Johnson syndrome, toxic epidermal necrolysis), crystalluria, renal calculus, bone marrow depression, thrombocytopenia purpura, hemolytic anemia, leukopenia, pancytopenia and agranulocytosis. Precaution is advised for early detection of such reactions. If they occur, discontinue the drug and institute appropriate therapy.

> Fatalities have occurred, although rarely, due to Stevens-Johnson syndrome, toxic epidermal necrolysis, fulminant hepatic necrosis, agranulocytosis, aplastic anemia and other blood dyscrasias. Sensitization may recur when a sulfonamide is readministered irrespective of the route of administration. If signs of hypersensitivity or other serious reactions occur, discontinue use.

Acetazolamide:

> *Ophthalmic* – Transient myopia that subsides upon dosage reduction or discontinuance.

> *Systemic* – Adverse reactions, occurring most often early in therapy, include paresthesias (particularly "tingling" feeling in the extremities), hearing dysfunction or tinnitus, loss of appetite, taste alteration, GI disturbances (nausea, vomiting and diarrhea), polyuria, drowsiness, confusion, metabolic acidosis and electrolyte imbalance. Other adverse reactions include urticaria, melena, hematuria, glycosuria, hepatic insufficiency, flaccid paralysis, photosensitivity and convulsions.

Dichlorphenamide: Certain side effects characteristic of carbonic anhydrase inhibitors may occur, particularly with increasing doses. The most common effects include GI disturbances (anorexia, nausea and vomiting), drowsiness and paresthesias.

Methazolamide:

> *Systemic* – Anorexia, nausea, vomiting, malaise, fatigue, drowsiness, headache, vertigo, mental confusion, depression and paresthesias of fingers, toes, hands or feet and occasionally at the mucocutaneous junction of the lips, mouth and anus. Rarely, photosensitivity has been reported.
>
> Urinary citrate excretion and uric acid output are decreased, but urinary calculi have been reported only rarely. The effect on citrate excretion is less than that reported with acetazolamide.

Overdosage:

Acetazolamide: No data are available regarding acetazolamide overdosage in humans, as no cases of acute poisoning with this drug have been reported. Animal data suggest that acetazolamide is remarkably nontoxic. No specific antidote is known. Treatment should be symptomatic and supportive.

Electrolyte imbalance, development of an acidotic state and central nervous effects might be expected to occur. Monitor serum electrolyte levels (particularly potassium) and blood pH levels. Supportive measures are required to restore electrolyte and pH balance. The acidotic state can usually be corrected by the administration of bicarbonate.

Despite its high intraerythrocytic distribution and plasma protein binding properties, acetazolamide may be dialyzable. This may be particularly important in the management of acetazolamide overdosage when complicated by the presence of renal failure.

Dichlorphenamide: Symptoms of overdosage or toxicity may include drowsiness, anorexia, nausea, vomiting, dizziness, paresthesias, ataxia, tremor and tinnitus.

In the event of overdosage, induce emesis or perform gastric lavage. The electrolyte disturbance most likely to be encountered from overdosage is hyperchloremic acidosis that may respond to bicarbonate administration. Potassium supplementation may be required. Carefully observe patient and give supportive treatment.

Patient Information:

May cause drowsiness; observe caution while driving or performing other tasks requiring alertness.

Notify physician if sore throat, fever, unusual bleeding or bruising, tingling in the hands or feet, appetite loss, confusion, difficulty breathing, urinary incontinence or skin rash occurs.

Bioavailability:

Bioequivalence problems have been documented for carbonic anhydrase inhibitors marketed by different manufacturers. Brand interchange is not recommended unless comparative bioavailability data provide evidence of therapeutic equivalence.

Individual drug monographs are on the following pages.

ACETAZOLAMIDE

For more complete prescribing information see General Monograph p. 195.

Administration and Dosage:

Chronic simple (open-angle) glaucoma: Adults – 250 mg to 1 g/day, in divided doses for amounts over 250 mg. Dosage in excess of 1 g daily does not usually increase the effect.

Secondary glaucoma and preoperative treatment of acute congestive (closed-angle) glaucoma: Adults – 250 mg every 4 hours or 250 mg twice daily on short term therapy.

Acute cases: 500 mg followed by 125 or 250 mg every 4 hours.

Children – 5 to 10 mg/kg/dose, IM or IV, every 6 hours or 8 to 30 mg/kg/day, orally, in divided doses, every 6 to 8 hours.

Sustained release: 500 mg twice daily. Only indicated for use in glaucoma and acute mountain sickness.

Parenteral: IV therapy may be used for rapid relief of increased IOP. A complementary effect occurs when acetazolamide is used with miotics or mydriatics. Direct IV administration is preferred; IM use is painful because of the alkaline pH of the solution.

Preparation and storage of parenteral solution: Reconstitute each 500 mg vial with at least 5 ml of Sterile Water for Injection. Reconstituted solutions retain potency for 1 week if refrigerated. However, since this product contains no preservative, use within 24 hours of reconstitution.

If an *oral liquid dosage form* is required, acetazolamide tablets may be crushed and suspended in cherry syrup or a 2:1 simple syrup/cherry syrup mixture.

Storage: Store at room temperature 59° to 86°F (15° to 30°C).

				C.I.*
Rx	**Acetazolamide** (Various, eg, Moore, United Research)	**Tablets:** 125 mg	In 50s, 100s, 250s, 500s and 1000s.	16+
Rx	**Diamox** (Storz/Lederle)		(Diamox 125/D1 LL). White, scored. In 100s.[1]	18
Rx	**Acetazolamide** (Various, eg, Danbury, Major, Moore, Qualitest, Schein, United Research)	**Tablets:** 250 mg	In 50s, 100s, 250s, 500s, 1000s and UD 100s.	10+
Rx	**AK-Zol** (Akorn)		In 100s and 1000s.	9
Rx	**Dazamide** (Major)		In 100s, 1000s and UD 100s.	8
Rx	**Diamox** (Storz/Lederle)		(Diamox 250/D2 LL). White, scored. In 100s, 1000s and UD 100s.[1]	11

* Cost Index based on cost per 250 mg acetazolamide.
[1] With povidone.

ACETAZOLAMIDE (Cont.)   C.I.*

Rx	Diamox Sequels (Storz/Lederle)	Capsules, sustained release: 500 mg	(Diamox D3). Orange. In 30s and 100s.[1]	14
Rx	Diamox (Storz/Lederle)	Powder for Injection: 500 mg (as sodium) per vial.		1386

DICHLORPHENAMIDE

For more complete prescribing information see General Monograph p. 195.

Administration and Dosage:

Usually given with topical ocular hypotensive agents. In acute angle-closure glaucoma, dichlorphenamide may be used with miotics and osmotic agents to rapidly reduce intraocular tension. If quick relief does not occur, surgery may be mandatory.

Adults: Individualize dosage.

Initial dose – 100 to 200 mg, followed by 100 mg every 12 hours, until the desired response is obtained.

Maintenance dosage – 25 to 50 mg, 1 to 3 times daily.

C.I.*

Rx	Daranide (MSD)	Tablets: 50 mg	(MSD 49). Yellow, scored. In 100s.	15

METHAZOLAMIDE

For more complete prescribing information see General Monograph p. 195.

Administration and Dosage:

Glaucoma: 50 to 100 mg, 2 or 3 times daily. May be used with miotic and osmotic agents.

Storage: Store at room temperature 59° to 86°F (15° to 30°C).

C.I.*

Rx	Neptazane (Storz/Lederle)	Tablets: 25 mg	(N2/N). White. In 100s.	31
		50 mg	(N1/LL). White, scored. In 100s.	23

* Cost Index based on cost per 250 mg acetazolamide, 50 mg dichlorphenamide or 50 mg methazolamide.
[1] With ethylcellulose, glycerin, propylene glycol and parabens.

Hyperosmotic Agents

Hyperosmotic agents (also referred to as osmotic agents) can be administered topically, orally or intravenously to increase osmotic pressure of tears and plasma relative to that of the ocular structures. As a result of the osmotic gradient established, fluid moves from the eye to hyperosmotic tear fluid with topical instillation, or plasma of ocular blood vessels following oral or intravenous administration.

TOPICAL AGENTS

The clinical objective of topical osmotherapy is to enhance the rate of fluid movement from the edematous cornea. When these agents are applied to the eye, water is drawn from the cornea to the hyperosmolal tear film and eliminated through the usual tear flow mechanisms.

Sodium chloride, glycerol and glucose have proven useful for reducing corneal edema of various etiologies, including bullous keratopathy and Fuchs' endothelial dystrophy.

Hypertonic solutions of sodium chloride or glucose can be useful for prolonged treatment of corneal edema. Sodium chloride appears less effective when the corneal epithelium is traumatized due to its increased ability to penetrate the epithelial barrier. Both sodium chloride and glucose should be administered at regular intervals for maximum clinical effect. Since vision is usually worse upon arising, more frequent application during the first waking hours can be helpful.

Glycerol can reduce corneal edema within 1 to 2 minutes following topical instillation to the eye. Since application is painful, a topical anesthetic must be instilled prior to its use. The osmotic action of glycerol is transient since the molecules mix readily with water. Therefore, for diagnostic purposes, its primary clinical use is to facilitate ophthalmoscopy and gonioscopy with edematous corneas.

SYSTEMIC AGENTS

Hyperosmotic agents administered by oral and intravenous routes are useful for initial management of acute angle-closure glaucoma and prior to intraocular surgery to reduce intraocular pressure (IOP).

Following systemic administration, a relatively rapid increase in serum osmolarity can occur. Transfer of fluid from the eye to the circulation results in a decrease in IOP. Factors that determine the difference in osmotic pressure between the ocular fluids and plasma are as follows:

- Molecular weight and concentration

- Dose administered

- Rate of absorption

- Distribution in body water

- Ocular penetration

- Rate of excretion

- Nature of diuresis

The integrity of the ocular tissues can also influence the osmotic effect. Inflammation may enhance ocular penetration and decrease the osmotic gradient, resulting in a reduction in the pressure-lowering effect of these agents.

Systemic administration can result in a significant drop in IOP within 15 to 60 minutes, depending on the dosage given. The effect of systemic osmotherapy can last up to 8 hours. The primary use of these agents is to treat or prevent acute rises in IOP such as acute angle-closure glaucoma and postoperative spiking of IOP. Chronic administration is contraindicated.

SYSTEMIC HYPEROSMOTIC AGENTS			
Action	Glycerin (oral)	Isosorbide (oral)	Mannitol (IV)
Diuresis			
Onset (minutes)	10 to 30	< 30	30 to 60
Peak (hours)	1 to 1.5	1 to 1.5	1
Duration (hours)	4 to 6	5 to 6	6 to 9
Decrease in IOP			
Onset (minutes)	15 to 60	15 to 60	15 to 30
Peak (hours)	0.5 to 1.5	0.5 to 1.5	0.5 to 1
Half-Life	30 to 45 minutes	5 to 9.5 hours	15 to 100 minutes
Metabolized (%)	80	0	7 to 10
Ocular Penetration	moderate	good	poor
Distribution	E[1]	TBW[2]	E[1]

[1] E = extracellular
[2] TBW = total body water

Intravenous Administration

Mannitol (eg, *Osmitrol*) is currently the hyperosmotic of choice for intravenous use. It is not absorbed from the gastrointestinal tract and, therefore, is ineffective by the oral route. Intravenous administration can reduce IOP within 20 to 30 minutes. The effect can last for 4 to 8 hours. Mannitol exhibits minimal cellular penetration, is not metabolized and is excreted in the urine. It, therefore, can be used in diabetic patients, but should be administered with caution in patients with renal disease. Since mannitol is confined to the extracellular fluid, dehydration and a profound diuresis can result following administration.

Oral Administration

Glycerin and isosorbide *(Ismotic)* are both readily absorbed from the gastrointestinal tract and are effective when administered by the oral route.

Glycerin is metabolized in the body analogous to other carbohydrates and produces 4.32 kcal/g. Use caution when administering glycerin to diabetic patients since hyperglycemia and glycosuria can result. Although reduction in IOP is somewhat less than with mannitol, administration of the recommended dosage reduces pressure within 30 to 60 minutes. The osmotic effect can last for several hours.

Isosorbide is not metabolized, and about 95% is excreted unchanged in the urine. Therefore, it provides no calories and, unlike glycerin, can be administered to diabetic patients. Isosorbide reduces IOP within 30 to 60 minutes. The effect can last as long as 5 to 6 hours.

Although oral administration simplifies osmotherapy, both glycerin and isosorbide exhibit characteristics limiting their use. Neither agent can be administered to patients who are nauseated or vomiting. Since both agents have a sweet taste, they may induce nausea or vomiting. In addition, the increase in serum osmolarity can cause dehydration, headache, confusion and disorientation.

Siret D. Jaanus, PhD
Southern California College of Optometry

For More Information

Bartlett JD, Jaanus SD, eds. Clinical Ocular Pharmacology, ed. 2. Boston, MA: Butterworth, 1989.

Becker B, et al. Hyperosmotic agents. In: Leopold IE, ed. Symposium in Ocular Therapy. St. Louis, MO: C.V. Mosby Co., 1968.

Becker B, et al. Isosorbide: An oral hyperosmotic agent. *Arch Ophthalmol* 1967;78:147-50.

Galin MA, et al. Ophthalmological use of osmotic therapy. *Am J Ophthalmol* 1966;62:629-34.

Kolker AE. Hyperosmotic agents in glaucoma. *Invest Ophthalmol* 1970;9:418-23.

Lambert DW. Topical hyperosmotic agents and secretory stimulants. *Int Ophthalmol Clin* 1980;20:163-69.

Luxenberg MN, Green K. Reduction of corneal edema with topical hypertonic agents. *Am J Ophthalmol* 1970;9:418-23.

McCurdy DK, et al. Oral glycerol: The mechanism of intraocular hypotension. *Am J Ophthalmol* 1966;61: 1244-49.

GLUCOSE, TOPICAL

Indications:

For topical osmotherapy in the treatment of corneal edema.

Contraindications:

Hypersensitivity to any component of the formulation.

Precautions:

If irritation develops, discontinue use.

Administration and Dosage:

May be used 2 to 6 times daily.

Depress lower lid with index finger while looking upward. Introduce a small amount of ointment behind depressed eyelid into conjunctival sac. Close and open eyes twice. Wipe off excess ointment. If eyelids are sticky, clean them before each application with a pledget of cotton and lukewarm boiled water.

Storage: Store at room temperature 59° to 86°F (15° to 30°C). Keep tightly closed. Protect from heat.

				C.I.*
Rx	**Glucose-40** (Iolab)	**Ointment:** 40% in white petrolatum and anhydrous lanolin with parabens	In 3.5 g.	264

GLYCERIN, TOPICAL

Actions:

Glycerin ophthalmic solution is used only for topical application to the cornea. By virtue of its osmotic action, it promptly reduces edema and causes clearing of corneal haze. The action is transient, and it is, therefore, used primarily for diagnostic purposes.

Indications:

To clear an edematous cornea in order to facilitate ophthalmoscopic and gonioscopic examination in acute glaucoma, bullous keratitis and Fuchs' endothelial dystrophy.

Contraindications:

Hypersensitivity to any component of the formulation.

Warnings:

Pregnancy: Category C. Safety for use during pregnancy has not been established. Use only when clearly needed and when the potential benefits outweigh the potential hazards to the fetus.

Lactation: It is not known whether glycerin is excreted in breast milk. Safety for use in the nursing mother has not been established.

Children: Safety and efficacy for use in children have not been established.

---

* Cost Index based on cost per g.

Precautions:

Because glycerin is an irritant and may cause pain, instill a local anesthetic before use.

Adverse Reactions:

Some pain or irritation may occur upon instillation.

Administration and Dosage:

Instill 1 or 2 drops prior to examination. In gonioscopy of an edematous cornea, additional glycerin may be used as a lubricant.

Storage: Keep bottle tightly closed. Store at room temperature 59° to 86°F (15° to 30°C). Discard product 6 months after dropper is first placed in the drug solution.

			C.I.*
Rx **Ophthalgan** (Wyeth-Ayerst)	**Solution:** Glycerin with 0.55% chlorobutanol	In 7.5 ml.	65

SODIUM CHLORIDE, HYPERTONIC (TOPICAL)

Actions:

A hypertonic solution exerts an osmotic gradient greater than that present in the body tissues and fluids, so that water is drawn from the body tissues and fluids across semi-permeable membranes. Applied topically to the eye, a hypertonicity agent creates an osmotic gradient which draws water out of the cornea.

Indications:

For temporary relief of corneal edema.

Contraindications:

Hypersensitivity to any component of the formulation.

Adverse Reactions:

May cause temporary burning and irritation upon instillation.

Patient Information:

To avoid contamination, do not touch tip of container to any surface. Replace cap after using.

Do not use this product except under the advice and supervision of a physician. If you experience eye pain, changes in vision, continued redness or irritation of the eye or if condition worsens or persists, discontinue use and consult a physician.

Product may cause temporary burning and irritation upon being instilled into the eye.

If solution changes color or becomes cloudy, do not use.

* Cost Index based on cost per ml.

Administration and Dosage:

Solution: Instill 1 or 2 drops in affected eye(s) every 3 or 4 hours, or as directed.

Ointment: Apply once a day or more often, as directed.

Storage: Store at 46° to 86°F (8° to 30°C). Keep tightly closed. Protect from light.

				C.I.*
otc	**AK-NaCl** (Akorn)	**Ointment:** 5%	In 3.5 g.[1]	197
otc	**Muro 128** (Bausch & Lomb)		In 3.5 g single and twin packs.[1]	264
otc	**Adsorbonac** (Alcon)	**Solution:** 2%	In 15 ml.[2]	68
otc	**Muro 128** (Bausch & Lomb)		In 15 ml dropper bottles.[3]	59
otc	**Adsorbonac** (Alcon)	**Solution:** 5%	In 15 ml.[2]	73
otc	**AK-NaCl** (Akorn)		In 15 ml.[4]	46
otc	**Muro 128** (Bausch & Lomb)		In 15 and 30 ml.[3]	79
otc	**Muroptic-5** (Optopics)		In 15 ml.[5]	46

* Cost Index based on cost per g or ml.
[1] With mineral oil, white petrolatum and anhydrous lanolin.
[2] With povidone, hydroxyethyl cellulose, PEG-90M, poloxamer 188, 0.004% thimerosal and EDTA.
[3] With hydroxypropyl methylcellulose, 0.023% methylparaben, 0.01% propylparaben and propylene glycol.
[4] With hydroxypropyl methylcellulose, propylene glycol, 0.023% methylparaben and 0.01% propylparaben.
[5] With benzalkonium chloride, EDTA, polyvinyl alcohol and propylene glycol.

GLYCERIN (GLYCEROL), ORAL

Actions:

An oral osmotic agent for reducing IOP. It adds to the tonicity of the blood until metabolized and eliminated by the kidneys.

Indications:

For the short-term reduction of IOP. May be used prior to and after intraocular surgery. May be used to interrupt an attack of acute glaucoma.

Contraindications:

Well-established anuria; severe dehydration; frank or impending acute pulmonary edema; severe cardiac decompensation.

Hypersensitivity to any components of the formulation.

Warnings:

For oral use only. Not for injection.

Use cautiously in hypervolemia, confused mental states, congestive heart disease, as well as in certain diabetic patients and dehydrated individuals.

Pregnancy: Category C. Safety for use during pregnancy has not been established. Use only when clearly needed and when the potential benefits outweigh the potential hazards to the fetus.

Precautions:

When administered prior to surgery, ensure that the patient's bladder is emptied. Prolonged use may cause excessive weight gain. Administer with caution to patients with cardiac, renal or hepatic disease. Altered hydration may lead to pulmonary edema and congestive heart failure.

Adverse Reactions:

Nausea, vomiting, headache, confusion and disorientation may occur. Severe dehydration, cardiac arrhythmias and hyperosmolar nonketotic coma, which can result in death, have been reported.

Administration and Dosage:

2 to 3 ml/kg of body weight (approximately 4 to 6 oz per individual), given 1 to 1½ hours prior to surgery.

C.I.*

Rx **Osmōglyn** (Alcon)	**Solution:** 50% (0.6 g glycerin/ml)	Lime flavor. In 220 ml.[1]	355

* Cost Index based on cost per 30 ml glycerin.
[1] With 0.05% potassium sorbate.

ISOSORBIDE, ORAL

Actions:

Isosorbide is rapidly absorbed after oral administration. It is essentially non-metabolized, and in the circulation, it contributes to the tonicity of the blood until it is eliminated by the kidneys unchanged. In the blood, isosorbide acts as an osmotic agent to promote redistribution of water toward the circulation with ultimate elimination in the urine. The physical action is similar to that of other osmotic agents.

Indications:

For the short-term reduction of IOP. May be used prior to and after intraocular surgery.

May be used to interrupt an acute attack of glaucoma. Use where less risk of nausea and vomiting than that posed by other oral hyperosmotic agents is needed.

Contraindications:

Well-established anuria; severe dehydration; frank or impending acute pulmonary edema; severe cardiac decompensation.

Hypersensitivity to any component of the formuation.

Warnings:

For oral use only. Not for injection.

With repeated doses, maintain adequate fluid and electrolyte balance.

If urinary output continues to decrease, closely review the patient's clinical status. Accumulation may result in overexpansion of the extracellular fluid.

Pregnancy: Category B. Reproduction studies in animals have shown no evidence of harm to the fetus. There is no adequate information on whether this drug affects fertility in humans or has a teratogenic potential or other adverse fetal effects. Use during pregnancy only if clearly needed.

Precautions:

Use repetitive doses with caution, particularly in patients with diseases associated with salt retention. Ensure the patient's bladder has been emptied prior to surgery.

Adverse Reactions:

Nausea, vomiting, headache, confusion and disorientation may occur. Gastric discomfort, thirst, hiccoughs, hypernatremia, hyperosmolarity, rash, irritability, syncope, lethargy, dizziness, vertigo and lightheadedness have also been reported.

Administration and Dosage:

Initial dose: 1.5 g/kg (equivalent to 1.5 ml/lb).

Dose range: 1 to 3 g/kg 2 to 4 times daily as indicated.

Palatability may be improved if the medication is poured over cracked ice and sipped.

Storage: Store at room temperature 59 ° to 86° F (15° to 30° C).

Rx	Ismotic (Alcon)	Solution: 45% (100 g/220 ml)	With 4.6 mEq sodium and 0.9 mEq potassium per 220 ml. With potassium sorbate, 0.3% alcohol, saccharin and sorbitol. Vanilla-mint flavor. In 220 ml.

MANNITOL, INTRAVENOUS

Actions:

Mannitol is a nonelectrolyte osmotic diuretic that is pharmacologically inert.

IV mannitol is confined to the extracellular space. Only small amounts are metabolized. Mannitol is readily diffused through the glomeruli. Approximately 80% of a 100 g dose will appear in the urine in 3 hours, with lesser amounts thereafter. Even at peak concentrations, mannitol will exhibit less than 10% of tubular reabsorption, and is not secreted by tubular cells. Mannitol will hinder tubular reabsorption of water and enhance excretion of sodium and chloride by elevating the osmolarity of the glomerular filtrate.

This increase in extracellular osmolarity effected by the IV administration of mannitol will induce the movement of intracellular water to the extracellular and vascular spaces. This action underlies the role of mannitol in reducing intracranial pressure, intracranial edema and elevated intraocular pressure (IOP).

Indications:

To reduce elevated IOP when the pressure cannot be lowered by other means.

To promote diuresis in the prevention or treatment of the oliguric phase of acute renal failure before irreversible renal failure becomes established.

To reduce intracranial pressure and treatment of cerebral edema.

To promote urinary excretion of toxic substances.

To measure glomerular filtration rate.

Contraindications:

Hypersensitivity to any component of the formulation.

Well-established anuria due to severe renal disease; severe pulmonary congestion or frank pulmonary edema; active intracranial bleeding except during craniotomy; severe dehydration; progressive renal damage or dysfunction after instituting mannitol therapy, including increasing oliguria and azotemia; progressive heart failure or pulmonary congestion after mannitol therapy.

Warnings:

Impaired renal function: Use a test dose; try a second test dose if there is an inadequate response. Do not attempt more than two test doses. (See Administration and Dosage.)

If urine output continues to decline during infusion, closely review the patient's clinical status and suspend mannitol infusion, if necessary. Accumulation of mannitol may result in overexpansion of the extracellular fluid, which may intensify existing or latent congestive heart failure and pulmonary edema.

Fluid and electrolyte imbalance: By sustaining diuresis, mannitol may obscure and intensify inadequate hydration or hypovolemia. Excessive loss of water and electrolytes may lead to serious imbalances. Loss of water in excess of electrolytes can cause hypernatremia. Shift of sodium-free intracellular fluid into the extracellular compartment following mannitol infusion may lower serum sodium concentration and aggravate preexisting hyponatremia.

Osmotic nephrosis, a reversible vacuolization of the tubules of unknown clinical significance, may proceed to severe irreversible nephrosis. Closely monitor renal function during mannitol infusion.

Neurosurgical patients: Mannitol injection may increase cerebral blood flow and the risk of postoperative bleeding.

Pregnancy: Category C. Safety for use during pregnancy has not been established. Use only when clearly needed and potential benefits outweight the potential hazards to the fetus.

Lactation: It is not known whether this drug is excreted in breast milk. Exercise caution when administering to a nursing woman.

Children: Safety and efficacy for use in children under 12 have not been established.

Precautions:

Carefully evaluate the patient's cardiovascular status before rapid administration of mannitol, since sudden expansion of the extracellular fluid may lead to fulminating congestive heart failure.

Do not give electrolyte-free mannitol solutions with blood. If blood is given simultaneously, add at least 20 mEq of sodium chloride to each liter of mannitol solution to avoid pseudoagglutination.

The obligatory diuretic response following rapid infusion of 15%, 20% or 25% mannitol may further aggravate preexisting hemoconcentration.

Patient monitoring of sodium and potassium blood levels, degree of hemoconcentration or hemodilution, and renal, cardiac and pulmonary function are paramount in avoiding excessive fluid and electrolyte shifts. The routine features of physical examination and clinical chemistries suffice in achieving an adequate degree of appropriate patient monitoring.

Adverse Reactions:

Isolated cases reported during or following mannitol infusion include:

Cardiovascular: Thrombophlebitis; hypotension; hypertension; tachycardia; angina-like chest pains.

GI: Nausea; vomiting; diarrhea.

GU: Marked diuresis; urinary retention.

Other: Rhinitis; local pain; skin necrosis; chills; urticaria; fever; dehydration; dizziness.

If unrecognized, fluid and electrolyte shift can produce pulmonary congestion, acidosis, electrolyte loss, dryness of mouth, thirst, edema, headache, blurred vision, convulsions and congestive cardiac failure.

These are not truly adverse reactions to the drug and can be prevented by: Evaluation of renal failure with a test-dose response to mannitol when indicated; evaluation of hypervolemia and hypovolemia; sodium and potassium levels; hemodilution or hemoconcentration; and evaluation of renal, cardiac and pulmonary function at the onset of therapy (see Warnings and Precautions).

Overdosage:

Symptoms: Larger than recommended doses may result in increased electrolyte excretion, particularly sodium, chloride and potassium. Sodium depletion can result in orthostatic tachycardia or hypotension and decreased central venous pressure.

Chloride metabolism closely follows that of sodium. Potassium deficit can impair neuromuscular function and cause intestinal dilation and ileus. If urine flow is inadequate, pulmonary edema or water intoxication may occur.

Administration and Dosage:

Administer by IV infusion only. Individualize total dosage, concentration and rate of administration. The adult dose ranges from 50 to 200 g/24 hours; in most instances, an adequate response will be achieved with 100 g/24 hours. Adjust the administration rate to maintain a urine flow of at least 30 to 50 ml/hour.

Test dose: For patients with marked oliguria or inadequate renal function, give 0.2 g/kg (about 75 ml of a 20% solution, 100 ml of a 15% solution or 50 to 60 ml of a 25% solution) infused over 3 to 5 minutes to produce a urine flow of at least 30 to 50 ml/hour. If urine flow does not increase, administer a second test dose. If response is inadequate, reevaluate the patient.

Reduction of IOP: 1.5 to 2 g/kg as a 20% solution (7.5 to 10 ml/kg) or as a 15% solution (10 to 13 ml/kg) over a period as short as 30 minutes. When used preoperatively, administer 1 to 1½ hours before surgery to achieve maximal effect.

Preparation of solution: When exposed to low temperatures, mannitol solution may crystallize. Concentrations greater than 15% have a greater tendency to crystallize. If crystals are observed, redissolve by warming the solution up to 70°C, with agitation. Heat solution by using a dry-heat cabinet with overwrap intact. Do not use a water-bath. Cool to body temperature or less before reinspecting for crystals. Administer IV using sterile, filter-type administration set.

The use of supplemental additive medication is not recommended.

Storage: Store at room temperature 59° to 86° F (15° to 30° C). Avoid excessive heat. Do not freeze. Brief exposure up to 104°F (40°C) does not adversely affect the product.

Rx	**Mannitol** (Abbott)	**Injection:** 5%	In 1000 ml.
Rx	**Osmitrol** (Baxter)		In 1000 ml.
Rx	**Mannitol** (Various, eg, Abbott, McGaw, Inc.)	**Injection:** 10%	In 1000 ml.
Rx	**Osmitrol** (Baxter)		In 500 and 1000 ml.
Rx	**Mannitol** (Abbott)	**Injection:** 15%	In 150 and 500 ml.
Rx	**Osmitrol** (Baxter)		In 500 ml.
Rx	**Mannitol** (Various, eg, Abbott, McGaw, Inc.)	**Injection:** 20%	In 250 and 500 ml.
Rx	**Osmitrol** (Baxter)		In 250 and 500 ml.
Rx	**Mannitol** (Various, eg, Abbott, American Regent, Astra, LyphoMed, Pasadena Research)	**Injection:** 25%	In 50 ml vials and syringes.

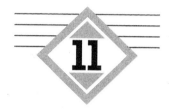

Surgical Adjuncts

Irrigating solutions, viscoelastic agents, botulinum toxin type A, absorbable gelatin film and proteolytic enzymes are adjuncts to a variety of ophthalmologic procedures and surgeries.

INTRAOCULAR IRRIGATING SOLUTIONS

Irrigating solutions are aqueous solutions used to cleanse and to maintain moisture of ocular tissue. Ideally these solutions are isotonic. The optimum pH is 7.4. A pH less than 7 or greater than 8 has caused cellular stress and death when the tissues have been exposed for a prolonged period of time.

The commercially available intraocular irrigating solutions (eg, *BSS* and *BSS Plus*) are used during ocular surgery to protect the lens and corneal endothelium. Unlike physiological saline and lactated Ringer's solution, these balanced salt solutions provide the ions magnesium and calcium as cellular nutrients. These nutrients are required for intercellular and intracellular function during prolonged ocular surgery. In addition to magnesium and calcium, bicarbonate, glucose and glutathione are in these perfusion media *(BSS Plus)*. These components help to maintain a deturgesced or thin cornea by avoiding corneal swelling.

For information on extraocular irrigating solutions see Nonsurgical Adjuncts.

VISCOELASTIC AGENTS

Viscoelastic agents sodium hyaluronate and hydroxymethylcellulose are used in many ophthalmic surgical procedures, including intraocular lens implantation and keratoplasty. In surgical procedures in the anterior segment of the eye, instillation maintains a deep anterior chamber, allowing for more efficient manipulation with less trauma to the corneal endothelium and surrounding tissues. The viscoelasticity of these agents helps push back the vitreous face and prevent formation of a post-operative flat chamber.

Viscoelastic agents are tissue protective substances and do not interfere with normal wound healing. They are nonantigenic and do not contain proteins that may cause inflammation or foreign body reactions.

BOTULINUM TOXIN TYPE A

Botulinum toxin is a form of purified botulinum toxin type A, produced from a culture of the Hall strain of *Clostridium botulinum.* Botulinum toxin type A blocks neuromuscular conduction by binding to receptor sites on motor nerve terminals, entering the nerve terminals and inhibiting the release of acetylcholine. When injected IM at therapeutic doses, the drug produces a localized chemical denervation muscle paralysis. When the muscle is chemically denervated, it atrophies and may develop extra-junctional acetylcholine receptors. There is evidence that the nerve can sprout and reinnervate the muscle, with the weakness thus being reversible. The paralytic effect on muscles injected with botulinum toxin type A is useful in reducing the excessive, abnormal contractions associated with blepharospasm.

ABSORBABLE GELATIN FILM

In the dry state, absorbable gelatin film has the appearance and texture of cellophane. When moistened, it assumes a rubbery consistency and can be cut to desired size and shape and fitted to rounded or irregular surfaces.

It is used in many surgical procedures including glaucoma filtration operations (ie, iridencleisis and trephination), extraocular muscle surgery and diathermy or scleral "buckling" operations for retinal detachment to aid in preventing formation of adhesions between contiguous ocular structures.

Absence of undue tissue reaction incident to implantation and absorption of gelatin film, with consequent decreased likelihood of developing adhesions, has been found to be of particular value in dural and ocular implants.

SURGICAL ENZYMES

Alpha-chymotrypsin is a proteolytic surgical enzyme used to dissolve zonules of the lens during intracapsular cataract surgery. Destruction of the equatorial pericapsular membrane of the lens occurs in 5 minutes. Zonular fibers are lysed within 10 to 15 minutes of application; complete lysis of the entire zonular membrane may take up to 30 minutes.

Many chemicals and natural body fluids are capable of inactivating alpha-chymotrypsin. Examples of products that may cause zonulysis to fail include: Serum, blood, detergents, alkalis, acids, antiseptics and epinephrine 1:100. These products may be used to inactivate alpha-chymotrypsin after zonulysis is complete. Pilocarpine (eg, *Isopto Carpine*), tetracaine (eg, *Pontocaine HCl*), acetylcholine (*Miochol*) and epinephrine 1:1000 will not inactivate this surgical enzyme.

Two other enzymes have been used during ocular surgery: Hyaluronidase and urokinase. *Hyaluronidase* is added to local anesthetic solutions to increase drug absorption and dispersion. This enzyme hydrolyzes hyaluronic acid in the connective tissue, which increases tissue permeability.

Urokinase has been used to irrigate hyphemas and to treat acute retinal artery and vein occlusions. The conversion of plasminogen to the proteolytic enzyme plasmin by urokinase causes degradation of plasma proteins, fibrinogen and fibrin clots.

J. James Rowsey, MD
University of South Florida

For More Information

Duane TD, ed. Clinical Ophthalmology. Philadelphia, PA: J.B. Lippincott Company, 1988.

Ellis PP. Ocular Therapeutics and Pharmacology, ed. 7. St. Louis, MO: C.V. Mosby, 1985.

Goodman LS, Gilman A. The Pharmacological Basis of Therapeutics, ed. 7. New York, NY: MacMillan, 1985.

Havener WH. Ocular Pharmacology, ed. 5. St. Louis, MO: C.V. Mosby, 1983.

Whikehart DR. Irrigating Solutions. In: Bartlett JD, Jaanus SD, eds. Clinical Ocular Pharmacology, ed. 2. Boston, MO: Butterworth, 1989:285-99.

INTRAOCULAR IRRIGATING SOLUTIONS

Actions:

Sterile irrigating solution is a sterile physiological balanced salt solution (BSS), each ml containing sodium chloride 0.64%, potassium chloride 0.075%, calcium chloride dihydrate 0.048%, magnesium chloride hexahydrate 0.03%, sodium acetate trihydrate 0.39%, sodium citrate dihydrate 0.17%, sodium hydroxide and/or hydrochloric acid (to adjust pH), and water. This solution is isotonic to ocular tissue and contains electrolytes required for normal cellular metabolic functions.

Indications:

For irrigation during various surgical procedures of the eyes. May also be used for the ears, nose and throat.

Warnings:

Not for injection or IV infusion.

Use aseptic technique only.

Precautions:

Preservative-free solutions: Do not use for more than one patient.

Do not use solution if it is cloudy or if seal assembly or packaging is damaged.

Do not use reconstituted solution if it is discolored or contains a precipitate.

Corneal clouding and edema have been reported following ocular surgery in which BSS solution was used as an irrigating solution. Take appropriate measures to minimize trauma to the cornea and other ocular tissues.

Addition of any medication to BSS solution may result in damage to intraocular tissue.

Diabetics: Studies suggest that intraocular irrigating solutions which are iso-osmotic with normal aqueous fluids should be used with caution in diabetic patients undergoing vitrectomy since intraoperative lens changes have been observed.

Adverse Reactions:

When the corneal endothelium is abnormal, irrigation or any other trauma may result in bullous keratopathy. Postoperative inflammatory reactions as well as incidents of corneal edema and corneal decompensation have been reported. Their relationship to the use of BSS solution has not been established.

Overdosage:

BSS solution has no pharmacological action and thus has no potential for overdosage. However, as with any intraocular surgical procedure, the duration of intraocular manipulation should be kept to a minimum.

Administration and Dosage:

Use BSS solution according to the established practices for each surgical procedure. Follow the manufacturer directions for the particular administration set to be used.

Storage: Store at 46° to 86°F (8° to 30°C). Avoid excessive heat. Do not freeze. Discard prepared solution after 6 hours.

Rx	**Balanced Salt Solution** (Various, eg, Abbott, Bausch & Lomb)	**Solution:** 0.64% NaCl, 0.075% KCl, 0.03% magnesium chloride, 0.048% calcium chloride, 0.39% sodium acetate, 0.17% sodium citrate and sodium hydroxide and/or hydrochloric acid	In 15, 30, 300 and 500 ml.
Rx	**AMO Endosol** (Allergan)		Preservative free. In 18 and 500 ml.
Rx	**BSS** (Alcon)		In 15, 30, 250 and 500 ml Drop-Tainers.
Rx	**Iocare Balanced Salt Solution** (Iolab)		Preservative free. In 15 and 500 ml.
Rx	**AMO Endosol Extra** (Allergan)	**Solution:** Mix aseptically just prior to use. **Part I:** 7.14 mg NaCl, 0.38 mg KCl, 0.154 mg calcium chloride dihydrate, 0.2 mg magnesium chloride hexahydrate, 0.92 mg dextrose and hydrochloric acid and/or sodium hydroxide/ml	Preservative free. In 515 ml.
		Part II: 1081 mg sodium bicarbonate, 216 dibasic sodium phosphate (anhydrous) and 95 mg glutathione disulfide (oxidized glutathione)/vial	Preservative free. In 60 ml.
Rx	**BSS Plus** (Alcon)	**Solution:** Mix aseptically just prior to use. **Part I:** 7.44 mg NaCl, 0.395 mg KCl, 0.433 mg dibasic sodium phosphate, 2.19 mg sodium bicarbonate and hydrochloric acid and/or sodium hydroxide/ml	Preservative free. In 500 ml.
		Part II: 3.85 mg calcium chloride dihydrate, 5 mg magnesium chloride hexahydrate, 23 mg dextrose and 4.6 mg glutathione disulfide/ml	Preservative free. In 20 ml.

SODIUM HYALURONATE

Actions:

Sodium hyaluronate and sodium chondroitin sulfate are widely distributed in extra-cellular matrix of connective tissues. They are found in synovial fluid, skin, umbilical cord and vitreous and aqueous humor of the eye. The cornea is the ocular tissue having the greatest concentration of sodium chondroitin sulfate, while the vitreous and aqueous humor contain the greatest concentration of sodium hyaluronate.

This preparation is a specific fraction of sodium hyaluronate developed for use in anterior segment and vitreous procedures as a viscoelastic agent. It has high molec-ular weight, is nonantigenic, does not cause inflammatory or foreign body reactions and has a high viscosity.

The 1% solution is transparent and remains in the anterior chamber for less than 6 days. It protects corneal endothelial cells and other ocular structures. It does not interfere with epithelialization and normal wound healing.

Indications:

For use as a surgical aid in cataract extraction (intra- and extracapsular), intraocular lens implantation (IOL), corneal transplant, glaucoma filtration and retinal attach-ment surgery.

To maintain a deep anterior chamber in surgical procedures in the anterior segment of the eye, allowing for efficient manipulation with less trauma to the corneal endothelium and other surrounding tissues.

To push back the vitreous face and prevent formation of a postoperative flat chamber.

As a surgical aid in posterior segment surgery to gently separate, maneuver and hold tissues.

To create a clear field of vision, facilitating intra- and postoperative inspection of the retina and photocoagulation.

Unlabeled use: Sodium hyaluronate has been used in the treatment of refractory dry eye syndrome.

Precautions:

For intraocular use. Use only if solution is clear.

Postoperative intraocular pressure (IOP) may be elevated as a result of preexisting glaucoma, compromised outflow and by operative procedures and sequelae, includ-ing enzymatic zonulysis, absence of an iridectomy, trauma to filtration structures and by blood and lenticular remnants in the anterior chamber. Since the exact role of these factors is difficult to predict in any individual case, the following precautions are recommended:

Do not overfill the anterior chamber (except in glaucoma surgery) (see Adminis-tration and Dosage).

Carefully monitor IOP, especially during the immediate postoperative period. Treat significant increases appropriately.

In posterior segment surgery in aphakic diabetics, exercise special care to avoid using large amounts of the drug.

Remove some of the preparation by irrigation or aspiration at the close of surgery (except in glaucoma surgery) (see Administration and Dosage).

Avoid trapping air bubbles behind the drug.

Hypersensitivity: Because this preparation is extracted from avian tissues and contains minute amounts of protein, potential risk of hypersensitivity may exist.

Drug Interactions:

Reports have been received indicating that the drug may become cloudy or form a slight precipitate after instillation. The clinical significance is not known since the majority do not indicate any harmful effects on ocular tissues. Be aware of this phenomenon and remove cloudy or precipitated material by irrigation and/or aspiration.

In vitro studies suggest that this phenomenon may be related to interactions with certain concomitantly administered ophthalmic medications.

Adverse Reactions:

Although well tolerated, a transient, postoperative increase in IOP has been reported.

Causal relationship not established: Postoperative inflammatory reactions (iritis, hypopyon); corneal edema; corneal decompensation.

Administration and Dosage:

Cataract surgery – IOL implantation: A sufficient amount is slowly introduced (using a cannula or needle) into the anterior chamber.

Inject either before or after delivery of the lens. Injection before lens delivery protects the corneal endothelium from possible damage arising from removal of the cataractous lens. May be used to coat surgical instruments and the IOL prior to insertion.

Additional amounts can be injected during surgery to replace any of the drug lost.

Glaucoma filtration surgery: In conjunction with the performance of the trabeculectomy, inject slowly and carefully through a corneal paracentesis to reconstitute the anterior chamber. Further injection can be continued to allow it to extrude into the subconjunctival filtration site through and around the sutured outer scleral flap.

Corneal transplant surgery: After removal of the corneal button, fill the anterior chamber with the drug. Then, suture the donor graft in place. An additional amount may be injected to replace the lost amount as a result of surgical manipulation.

Sodium hyaluronate has also been used in the anterior chamber of the donor eye prior to trepanation to protect the corneal endothelial cells of the graft.

Retinal attachment surgery: Slowly introduce into the vitreous cavity. By directing the injection, sodium hyaluronate can be used to separate membranes away from the retina for safe excision and release of traction. It also serves to maneuver tissues into the desired position (eg, to gently push back a detached retina or unroll a retinal flap) and aids in holding the retina against the sclera for reattachment.

Storage: Store *Amvisc* and *Amvisc Plus* at 36° to 46°F (2° to 8°C). Store *AMO Vitrax* at room temperature 59° to 86°F (15° to 30°C). Do not freeze. Protect from light. Allow the drug to attain room temperature before use (≈ 30 minutes).

Rx	Amvisc (Iolab)	Injection: 12 mg per ml[1]	In 0.5 or 0.8 ml disp. syringe.
Rx	Amvisc Plus (Iolab)	Injection: 16 mg per ml[1]	In 0.5 or 0.8 ml disp. syringe.
Rx	AMO Vitrax (Allergan)	Injection: 30 mg per ml[2]	In 0.65 ml disp. syringe.

[1] With 9 mg NaCl per ml.
[2] With 3.2 mg NaCl, 0.75 mg KCl, 0.48 mg calcium chloride, 0.3 mg magnesium chloride, 3.9 mg sodium acetate and 1.7 mg sodium citrate per ml.

CHONDROITIN SULFATE and SODIUM HYALURONATE

For complete prescribing information see Sodium Hyaluronate p. 218.

Indications:

A surgical aid in anterior segment procedures including cataract extraction and intraocular lens implantation.

Administration and Dosage:

Carefully introduce (using a 27-gauge cannula) into the anterior chamber. May inject prior to or following delivery of the crystalline lens. Instillation prior to lens delivery provides additional protection to corneal endothelium, protecting it from possible damage arising from surgical instrumentation. May also be used to coat intraocular lens and tips of surgical instruments prior to implantation surgery. May inject additional solution during anterior segment surgery to fully maintain the chamber or to replace solution lost during surgery. At the end of surgery, remove solution by thoroughly irrigating with a balanced salt solution. Alternatively, the solution may be left in the eye when used as directed.

Storage: Store at 36° to 46°F (2° to 8°C). Do not freeze.

Rx	**Viscoat** (Alcon)	**Solution:** 40 mg sodium chondroitin, 30 mg sodium hyaluronate, 0.45 mg sodium dihydrogen phosphate hydrate, 2 mg disodium hydrogen phosphate and 4.3 mg NaCl per ml	In 0.5 ml disp. syringe.

HYDROXYPROPYL METHYLCELLULOSE

Actions:

Hydroxymethylcellulose is a nonpyrogenic viscoelastic solution with a high molecular weight (greater than 80,000 daltons). It maintains a deep chamber during anterior segment surgery and allows for more efficient manipulation with less trauma to the corneal endothelium and other ocular tissues. The viscoelasticity helps the vitreous face to be pushed back, preventing formation of a postoperative flat chamber. It is also used as a demulcent agent.

Indications:

2% Solution: An ophthalmic surgical aid in anterior segment surgical procedures including cataract extraction and intraocular lens implantation.

2.5% Solution: For professional use in gonioscopic examinations.

Precautions:

Transient increased intraocular pressure (IOP) may occur following surgery because of preexisting glaucoma or due to the surgery itself. If the postoperative IOP increases above expected values, appropriate therapy should be administered.

Adverse Reactions:

Although well tolerated, a transient, postoperative increase in IOP has been reported.

Causal relationship not established: Postoperative inflammatory reactions (iritis, hypopyon); corneal edema; corneal decompensation.

Administration and Dosage:

Anterior segment surgery: Carefully introduce into the anterior chamber using a 20-gauge or smaller cannula. The 2% solution may be used prior to or following delivery of the crystalline lens. Injection of 2% solution prior to lens delivery will provide additional protection to the corneal endothelium and other ocular tissues.

The 2% solution may also be used to coat an intraocular lens and tips of surgical instruments prior to implantation surgery. May inject during anterior segment surgery to fully maintain the chamber, or to replace fluid lost during the surgical procedure. Remove solution from the anterior chamber at the end of surgery.

Gonioscopic examinations: Fill gonioscopic prism with solution, as necessary.

Stability: If this solution dries on optical surfaces, let them stand in cool water before cleansing. If solution changes color or becomes cloudy, do not use. Not for use with hot laser treatment. Solution clouding will occur.

To avoid contamination, do not touch tip of container to any surface. Replace cap after using. Keep container tightly closed.

Storage: Store at room temperature 59° to 86°F (15° to 30°C). Avoid excessive heat (140°F). Protect from light.

				C.I.*
Rx	**Occucoat** (Storz)	**Solution:** 2% in a balanced salt solution	In 1 ml syringe with cannula.	NA
otc	**Gonak** (Akorn)	**Solution:** 2.5%	In 15 ml dropper bottles.[1]	71
otc	**Goniosol** (Iolab)		In 15 ml.[1]	55

HYDROXYETHYL CELLULOSE

Indications:

For use in bonding gonioscopic prisms to the eye.

Storage: Store at room temperature 59° to 86°F (15° to 30° C).

Rx	**Gonioscopic** (Alcon)	**Solution:** Hydroxyethyl cellulose	In 15 ml.[2]	88

* Cost Index based on cost per ml.
[1] With 0.01% benzalkonium chloride and EDTA.
[2] With 0.004% thimerosal and 0.1% EDTA.

GELATIN FILM, ABSORBABLE

Actions:

Absorbable gelatin film is approximately 0.075 mm in thickness. In the dry state, absorbable gelatin film has the appearance and texture of cellophane. When moistened, it assumes a rubbery consistency and can be cut to desired size and shape and fitted to rounded or irregular surfaces.

Rate of absorption of gelatin ophthalmic film after implantation ranges from 1 to 6 months depending on size of the implant and site of implantation. Pleural and muscle implants have been reported to be completely absorbed in 8 to 14 days, whereas dural and ocular implants usually required at least 2 to 5 months of absorption. Absence of undue tissue reaction incident to implantation and absorption of gelatin film, with consequent decreased likelihood of developing adhesions, has been found to be of particular value in dural and ocular implants.

Indications:

For use in various ocular surgical procedures including: glaucoma filtration operations (ie, iridencleisis and trephination); extraocular muscle surgery and diathermy or scleral "buckling" operations for retinal detachment; as an aid in preventing formation of adhesions between contiguous ocular structures.

Precautions:

Infections: The rate of absorption of gelatin ophthalmic film is likely to be increased in the presence of purulent exudation. It is recommended that absorbable gelatin film not be implanted in grossly contaminated or infected surgical wounds.

Administration and Dosage:

To prepare for use, immerse absorbable gelatin film in sterile saline solution and allow to soak until it becomes pliable. It may then be cut to desired size and shape without difficulty.

For use as a seton in iridencleisis: Place a small piece of sterile ophthalmic gelatin film (approximately 4 x 10 mm) over the prolapsed iris pillar parallel to the limbus. Then close Tenon's capsule and the conjunctiva with continuous absorbable sutures spaced to insure tight closure.

In diathermy or scleral "buckling" operations: Place gelatin sterile ophthalmic film over the sclera, the muscle and the conjunctiva, then suture over the underlying gelatin film.

In extraocular muscle surgery: Place sterile ophthalmic gelatin film over and beneath the muscle before Tenon's capsule and the conjunctiva are closed in layers.

Storage: Store at room temperature 59° to 86°F (15° to 30°C). Once the envelopes have been opened, contents are subject to contamination. To insure sterility, it is recommended that absorbable gelatin film be used immediately after withdrawal from the envelope.

| Rx | Gelfilm (Upjohn) | Absorbable film: 0.075 mm | In 25 x 50 mm sterile envelopes (6s). |

MIOTICS, DIRECT-ACTING

For complete prescribing information see General Monograph p. 175.

Actions:

The direct-acting miotics are parasympathomimetic drugs that duplicate the muscarinic effects of acetylcholine, but have no nicotinic effects. When applied topically, these drugs produce pupillary constriction, stimulate the ciliary muscle and increase aqueous humor outflow facility.

ACETYLCHOLINE CHLORIDE, INTRAOCULAR

Indications:

To produce complete miosis in seconds by irrigating the iris after delivery of the lens in cataract surgery, in penetrating keratoplasty, iridectomy and other anterior segment surgery where rapid, complete miosis may be required.

Administration and Dosage:

Solution: Instill into the anterior chamber before or after securing one or more sutures. Instillation should be gentle and parallel to the iris face and tangential to the pupil border. In most cases, 0.5 to 2 ml produces satisfactory miosis. The pupil is rapidly constricted and the peripheral iris drawn away from the angle of the anterior chamber if there are no mechanical hindrances. Any anatomical hindrance to miosis may require surgery to permit the desired effect of the drug. In cataract surgery, use only after delivery of the lens.

Solution need not be flushed from the chamber after miosis occurs. Since acetylcholine has a short duration of action, pilocarpine may be applied topically before dressing to maintain miosis.

Preparation: Aqueous solutions of acetylcholine are unstable. Prepare immediately before use. Do not use solution that is not clear and colorless. Discard any solution that has not been used. Do not gas sterilize.

Storage: Store at room temperature 59° to 86°F (15° to 30°C). Do not freeze.

C.I.*

Rx	Miochol (Iolab)	Solution: 1:100 acetyl-choline chloride when reconstituted	In 2 ml sterile univial (lower chamber 20 mg lyophilized acetylcholine chloride and 60 mg mannitol; upper chamber 2 ml Sterile Water for Injection), one pack *Iocare Steri-Tags* sterile labels. Also available in System Pak Plus with 15 ml (2s) *Iocare* balanced salt solution.	305

CARBACHOL, INTRAOCULAR

Indications:

Intraocular use for miosis during surgery.

Administration and Dosage:

For single dose intraocular use only. Discard unused portion.

Gently instill no more than 0.5 ml into the anterior chamber before or after securing sutures. Miosis is usually maximal 2 to 5 minutes after application.

Storage: Store at room temperature 59° to 86°F (15° to 30°C).

C.I.*

Rx	Miostat (Alcon)	Solution: 0.01%	In 1.5 ml vials.[1]	465

* Cost Index based on cost per ml.
[1] In a balanced salt solution.

CHYMOTRYPSIN

Actions:

Chymotrypsin is a proteolytic enzyme. The principal proteolytic effect is exerted by the splitting of peptide bonds of amino acids in the zonular fibers attached to the lens and ocular tissues.

Destruction of the equatorial pericapsular membrane of the lens occurs in 5 minutes. Zonular fibers are lysed within 10 to 15 minutes of application; complete lysis of the entire zonular membrane may take up to 30 minutes.

Indications:

For enzymatic zonulysis prior to or during intracapsular lens extraction.

Contraindications:

Hypersensitivity to chymotrypsin or any component of the formulation; significant anterior displacement of the lens iris diaphragm with impending vitreous loss; other conditions in which loss of vitreous is a significant problem (eg, intracapsular extraction of congenital cataracts); high vitreous pressure; gaping incisional wound; congenital cataracts; patients under 20 years of age because of probable lens-vitreous adhesion not responsive to alpha-chymotrypsin lysis.

Warnings:

Do not use the reconstituted solution if cloudy or if it contains a precipitate.

Do not autoclave the powder or the reconstituted solution. Excessive heat, alcohol and other chemicals used for sterilization inactivate the enzyme. Syringes and instruments must be free of alcohol and disinfectants, which may inactivate the enzyme.

The enzyme solution should be freshly prepared. Discard any unused portion including the diluent.

The solution contains no preservative. Do not use for more than one patient.

Precautions:

Chymotrypsin may produce an acute rise in intraocular pressure (IOP) following surgery, especially in patients with poor facility of outflow.

The enzyme will not lyse the synechiae that may exist between the lens and other eye structures.

Children: Use is contraindicated in patients under 20 years of age.

Drug Interactions:

Serum, blood, detergents, alkalis, acids and *antiseptics* (eg, alcohol) will inactivate chymotrypsin.

Isoflurophate and *chloramphenicol* inhibit chymotrypsin.

Epinephrine 1:100 will inactivate chymotrypsin in approximately 1 hour.

Adverse Reactions:

Transient increases in IOP; moderate uveitis; corneal edema; striation. Delayed healing of incisions has been reported, but not confirmed.

Administration and Dosage:

Instruments and syringes must be free of alcohol and other chemicals. Do not auto-clave the powder or reconstituted solution. Do not use solution if it is cloudy or contains a precipitate. (See Warnings.)

Irrigate the posterior chamber with 1 to 2 ml of 1:5,000 solution. Wait 2 to 4 minutes, then irrigate anterior chamber with suitable irrigating solution, if desired.

If zonules are still intact, irrigate the posterior chamber with an additional 0.5 to 2 ml. Wait an additional 2 to 4 minutes, then irrigate with suitable irrigating solution, if desired. Extract lens.

Storage – Refrigerate at 36° to 46°F (2° to 8°C). Do not freeze. Shake gently before using.

C.I.*

Rx	Catarase 1:5,000 (Iolab)	For Ophthalmic Solution: 300 units with 2 ml NaCl diluent per dual chamber univial	359

* Cost Index based on cost per 150 units.

BOTULINUM TOXIN TYPE A

Actions:

Pharmacology: Botulinum toxin is a sterile, lyophilized form of purified botulinum toxin type A, produced from a culture of the Hall strain of *Clostridium botulinum* grown in a medium containing N-Z amine and yeast extract. Botulinum toxin type A blocks neuromuscular conduction by binding to receptor sites on motor nerve terminals, entering the nerve terminals and inhibiting the release of acetylcholine. When injected IM at therapeutic doses, the drug produces a localized chemical denervation muscle paralysis. When the muscle is chemically denervated, it atrophies and may develop extrajunctional acetylcholine receptors. There is evidence that the nerve can sprout and reinnervate the muscle, with the weakness thus being reversible.

The paralytic effect on muscles injected with botulinum toxin type A is useful in reducing the excessive, abnormal contractions associated with blepharospasm. When used for the treatment of strabismus, the drug may affect muscle pairs by inducing an atrophic lengthening of the injected muscle and a corresponding shortening of the muscle's antagonist. Following peri-ocular injection, distant muscles show electrophysiologic changes, but no clinical weakness or other clinical change for a period of several weeks or months, parallel to the duration of local clinical paralysis.

Clinical trials: In one study, botulinum toxin was evaluated in 27 patients with essential blepharospasm; 26 had previously undergone drug treatment utilizing benztropine mesylate, clonazepam or baclofen without adequate clinical results. Three of these patients then underwent muscle stripping surgery still without an adequate outcome. Upon using botulinum toxin, 25 of the 27 patients reported improvement within 48 hours. One of the other patients was later controlled with a higher dosage. The remaining patient reported only mild improvement but remained functionally impaired.

In another study, 12 patients with blepharospasm were evaluated in a double-blind, placebo-controlled study. All patients receiving botulinum toxin (n = 8) were improved compared with no improvements in the placebo group (n = 4). The mean dystonia score improved by 72%, the self-assessment score rating improved by 61% and a videotape evaluation rating improved by 39%. The effects of the treatment lasted a mean of 12.5 weeks. Patients with blepharospasm (n = 1684) evaluated in an open trial also showed clinical improvement lasting an average of 12.5 weeks prior to the need for retreatment.

Patients with strabismus (n = 677) treated with one or more injections of botulinum toxin type A were evaluated in an open trial; 55% were improved to an alignment of 10 prism diopters or less when evaluated at 6 months or more following injection. These results are consistent with results from additional open label trials.

Indications:

Treatment of strabismus and blepharospasm associated with dystonia, including benign essential blepharospasm or VII nerve disorders in patients 12 years of age or older.

The efficacy of botulinum toxin type A in deviations over 50 prism diopters, in restrictive strabismus, in Duane's syndrome with lateral rectus weakness and in secondary strabismus caused by prior surgical over-recession of the antagonist is doubtful, or multiple injections over time may be required. Botulinum toxin type A is ineffective in chronic paralytic strabismus except to reduce antagonist contracture in conjunction with surgical repair.

Contraindications:

Hypersensitivity to any component of the formulation.

Warnings:

Do not exceed the recommended dosage and frequency of administration. There have been no reported instances of systemic toxicity resulting from accidental injection or oral ingestion of botulinum toxin type A. Should accidental injection or oral ingestion occur, medically supervise the person for several days on an outpatient basis for signs or symptoms of systemic weakness or muscle paralysis. The entire contents of a vial is below the estimated dose for systemic toxicity in humans weighing 6 kg or greater.

Hypersensitivity: As with all biologic products, have epinephrine and other precautions available should an anaphylactic reaction occur.

Pregnancy: Category C. It is not known whether botulinum toxin type A can cause fetal harm when administered to a pregnant woman or can affect reproduction capacity. Administer to pregnant women only if clearly needed.

Lactation: It is not known whether this drug is excreted in breast milk. Exercise caution when botulinum toxin type A is administered to a nursing woman.

Children: Safety and efficacy in children under 12 have not been established.

Precautions:

Safe and effective use of botulinum toxin type A depends upon proper storage of the product, selection of the correct dose and proper reconstitution and administration techniques. Physicians administering botulinum toxin type A must understand the relevant neuromuscular and orbital anatomy, any alterations to the anatomy due to prior surgical procedures and standard electromyographic techniques.

Retrobulbar hemorrhages: During the administration of botulinum toxin type A for the treatment of strabismus, retrobulbar hemorrhages sufficient to compromise retinal circulation have occurred from needle penetrations into the orbit. Have appropriate instruments to decompress the orbit accessible. Ocular (globe) penetrations by needles have also occurred. Have an ophthalmoscope available to diagnose this condition.

Reduced blinking from botulinum toxin type A injection of the orbicularis muscle can lead to corneal exposure, persistent epithelial defect and corneal ulceration, especially in patients with VII nerve disorders. One case of corneal perforation in an aphakic eye requiring corneal grafting has occurred because of this effect. Carefully test corneal sensation in eyes previously operated upon, avoid injection into the lower lid area to avoid ectropion and vigorously treat any epithelial defect. This may require protective drops, ointment, therapeutic soft contact lenses or closure of the eye by patching or other means.

Presence of antibodies to botulinum toxin type A may reduce the effectiveness of therapy. In clinical studies, reduction in effectiveness due to antibody production has occurred in one patient with blepharospasm receiving 3 doses over a 6-week period totaling 92 U, and in several patients with torticollis who received multiple doses experimentally, totaling over 300 U in 1 month. For this reason, keep the dose of botulinum toxin type A for strabismus and blepharospasm as low as possible, in any case below 200 U in a 1-month period.

Drug Interactions:

Aminoglycosides: The effect of botulinum toxin may be potentiated by aminoglycoside antibiotics or any other drug that interferes with neuromuscular transmission. Exercise caution when botulinum toxin type A is used in patients taking any of these drugs.

Adverse Reactions:

Local: Diffuse skin rash (n = 7) and local swelling of the eyelid skin (n = 2) lasting for several days following eyelid injection have occurred.

Strabismus: Inducing paralysis in one or more extraocular muscles may produce spatial disorientation, double vision or past-pointing. Covering the affected eye may alleviate these symptoms. Extraocular muscles adjacent to the injection site are often affected, causing ptosis or vertical deviation, especially with higher doses. Side effects in 2058 adults who received 3650 injections for horizontal strabismus included: ptosis (15.7%); vertical deviation (16.9%). The incidence of ptosis was much less after inferior rectus injection (0.9%) and much greater after superior rectus injection (37.7%).

Side effects persisting for longer than 6 months in an enlarged series of 5587 injections of horizontal muscles in 3104 patients included: ptosis lasting over 180 days (0.3%); vertical deviation greater than 2 prism diopters lasting over 180 days (2.1%).

In these patients, the injection procedure itself caused 9 scleral perforations. A vitreous hemorrhage occurred and later cleared in one case. No retinal detachment or visual loss occurred in any case; 16 retrobulbar hemorrhages occurred. No eye lost vision from retrobulbar hemorrhage. Decompression of the orbit after 5 minutes was done to restore retinal circulation in one case. Five eyes had pupillary change consistent with ciliary ganglion damage (Adies pupil).

Blepharospasm: In 1684 patients who received 4258 treatments (involving multiple injections) for blepharospasm, the incidence rates per treated eye were: ptosis (11%); irritation/tearing, including dry eye, lagophthalmos and photophobia (10%); ectropion, keratitis, diplopia and entropion occurred rarely (less than 1%).

Ecchymosis occurs easily in the soft eyelid tissues. This can be prevented by applying pressure at the injection site immediately after the injection. In two cases of VII nerve disorder (one case of an aphakic eye), reduced blinking from botulinum toxin type A injection of the orbicularis muscle led to serious corneal exposure, persistent epithelial defect and corneal ulceration. Perforation requiring corneal grafting occurred in one case, an aphakic eye (see Precautions).

Two patients previously incapacitated by blepharospasm experienced cardiac collapse attributed to overexertion within 3 weeks following botulinum toxin type A therapy. Caution sedentary patients to resume activity slowly and carefully following the administration of botulinum toxin type A.

Overdosage:

In the event of overdosage or injection into the wrong muscle, additional information may be obtained by contacting Allergan Pharmaceuticals at (800) 347-5063 from 8 am to 4 pm Pacific Time, or at (714) 724-5954 for a recorded message at other times.

Patient Information:

Patients with blepharospasm may have been extremely sedentary for a long time. Caution sedentary patients to resume activity slowly and carefully following administration.

Administration and Dosage:

Dilution Technique: To reconstitute lyophilized botulinum toxin type A, use sterile normal saline without a preservative; 0.9% Sodium Chloride Injection is the recommended diluent. Draw up the proper amount of diluent in the appropriate size syringe. Since botulinum toxin type A is denatured by bubbling or similar violent agitation, inject the diluent into the vial gently. Discard the vial if a vacuum does not pull the diluent into the vial. Record the date and time of reconstitution on the space on the label. Administer within 4 hours after reconstitution.

During this time period, store reconstituted botulinum toxin type A in a refrigerator (see Storage). The use of one vial for more than one patient is not recommended because the product and diluent do not contain a preservative.

DILUTION OF BOTULINUM TOXIN TYPE A	
Diluent Added (0.9% Sodium Chloride Injection)	Resulting dose
1 ml	10 U
2 ml	5 U
4 ml	2.5 U
8 ml	1.25 U

These dilutions are calculated for an injection volume of 0.1 ml. A decrease or increase in the botulinum toxin type A dose is also possible by administering a smaller or larger injection volume – from 0.05 ml (50% decrease in dose) to 0.15 ml (50% increase in dose).

Strabismus: Botulinum toxin type A is intended for injection into extraocular muscles utilizing the electrical activity recorded from the tip of the injection needle as a guide to placement within the target muscle. Do not attempt injection without surgical exposure or electromyographic guidance. Physicians should be familiar with electromyographic technique.

To prepare the eye for injection, give several drops of a local anesthetic and an ocular decongestant several minutes prior to injection.

Draw into a sterile 1 ml tuberculin syringe an amount of the properly diluted toxin (see Dilution Table) slightly greater than the intended dose. Expel air bubbles in the syringe barrel and attach the syringe to the electromyographic injection needle, preferably a 1½ inch, 27-gauge needle. Expel injection volume in excess of the intended dose through the needle into an appropriate waste container to assure patency of the needle and to confirm that there is no syringe-needle leakage. Use a new, sterile needle and syringe to enter the vial on each occasion for dilution or removal of botulinum toxin type A.

The initial doses of the diluted botulinum toxin type A (see Dilution Table) typically create paralysis of injected muscles beginning 1 to 2 days after injection and increasing in intensity during the first week. The paralysis lasts for 2 to 6 weeks and gradually resolves over a similar time period. Overcorrections lasting over 6 months have been rare. About one half of patients will require subsequent doses because of inadequate paralytic response of the muscle to the initial dose, mechanical factors such as large deviations or restrictions, or the lack of binocular motor fusion to stabilize the alignment.

The volume of botulinum toxin type A injected for treatment of strabismus should be between 0.05 to 0.15 ml per muscle.

   I. Initial doses in units (U). Use low doses for treatment of small deviations. Use larger doses only for large deviations.

     A. *For vertical muscles, and for horizontal strabismus of less than 20 prism diopters:* 1.25 to 2.5 U in any one muscle.

     B. *For horizontal strabismus of 20 prism diopters to 50 prism diopters:* 2.5 to 5 U in any one muscle.

     C. *For persistent VI nerve palsy of 1 month or longer duration:* 1.25 to 2.5 U in the medial rectus muscle.

   II. Subsequent doses for residual or recurrent strabismus.

     A. Re-examine patients 7 to 14 days after each injection to assess the effect of that dose.

     B. Patients experiencing adequate paralysis of the target muscle who require subsequent injections should receive a dose comparable to the initial dose.

     C. Subsequent doses for patients experiencing incomplete paralysis of the target muscle may be increased up to twice the size of the previously administered dose.

     D. Do not administer subsequent injections until the effects of the previous dose have dissipated as evidenced by substantial function in the injected and adjacent muscles.

     E. The maximum recommended dose as a single injection for any one muscle is 25 U.

Blepharospasm: Diluted botulinum toxin type A (see Dilution Table) is injected using a sterile 27- to 30-gauge needle without electromyographic guidance.

   Initial – 1.25 to 2.5 U (0.05 to 0.1 ml volume at each site) injected into the medial and lateral pre-tarsal orbicularis oculi of the upper lid and into the lateral pre-tarsal orbicularis oculi of the lower lid.

   In general, the initial effect of the injections is seen within 3 days and reaches a peak at 1 to 2 weeks post-treatment. Each treatment lasts approximately 3 months, following which the procedure can be repeated indefinitely. At repeat treatment sessions, the dose may be increased up to two-fold if the response from the initial treatment is considered insufficient (usually defined as an effect that does not last longer than 2 months). However, there appears to be little benefit obtainable from injecting more than 5 U per site. Some tolerance may be found when botulinum toxin type A is used in treating blepharospasm if treatments are given any more frequently than every 3 months, and it is rare for the effect to be permanent.

   The cumulative dose of botulinum toxin type A in a 30-day period should not exceed 200 U.

Storage: Store the lyophilized product in a freezer at or below 23°F (-5°C). Administer within 4 hours after the vial is removed from the freezer and reconstituted. During these 4 hours, store reconstituted botulinum toxin type A in a refrigerator 36° to 46°F (2° to 8°C). Reconstituted botulinum toxin type A should be clear, colorless and free of particulate matter.

Rx **Oculinum** (Allergan)	**Powder for Injection (lyophilized):** 100 units of lyophilized *Clostridium botulinum* Toxin type A[1]	Preservative free. In vials with 0.5 mg albumin (human) and 0.9 mg NaCl.

[1] One unit corresponds to the calculated median lethal intraperitoneal dose (LD/50) in mice of the reconstituted drug injected.

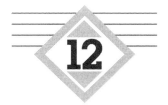

Nonsurgical Adjuncts

Dapiprazole HCl, extraocular irrigating solutions, lid scrubs and vitamins and minerals are adjuncts to a variety of ophthalmologic procedures and conditions.

DAPIPRAZOLE HCl

Dapiprazole is classified pharmacologically as an alpha-adrenergic antagonist. This drug demonstrates rapid reversal of mydriasis produced by phenylephrine and, to a lesser extent, tropicamide. The miosis produced by dapiprazole 0.5% begins 10 minutes following instillation and results in a significant reduction in pupil size. About half the pupils of treated eyes will achieve their premydriatic diameter within two hours of dilation with phenylephrine 2.5% and tropicamide 1%. In patients with brown irides, the rate of pupillary constriction may be slightly slower than in individuals with blue or green irides. The most siginificant side effect is conjunctival hyperemia associated with the alpha-receptor blockade of the conjunctival vasculature. The conjunctival injection lasts about 20 minutes in more than 80% of patients, and burning or stinging on instillation of the drug is reported in about half the patients.

EXTRAOCULAR IRRIGATING SOLUTIONS

Extraocular irrigating solutions are sterile isotonic solutions for general ophthalmic use. Office uses include irrigating procedures following tonometry, gonioscopy, foreign body removal or use of fluorescein. They are also used to soothe and cleanse the eye, and in conjunction with hard contact lenses. Because these solutions have a short contact time with the eye, they do not need to provide nutrients to cells. Unlike intraocular irrigants, irrigants for extraocular use contain preservatives that prevent bacterial contamination. However, the preservatives are exceedingly toxic to the corneal endothelium, and intraocular use of extraocular irrigating fluids is contraindicated.

LID SCRUBS

The mainstay of therapy for blepharitis is generally careful eyelid hygiene. This is easily accomplished at home by the patient. Although baby shampoo is frequently used for this purpose, commercially available eyelid cleansers are now available and are known to be effective with potentially less ocular stinging, burning and toxicity. Commercial lid scrub products are designed to aid in the removal of oils, debris or desquamated skin associated with the inflamed eyelid. The lid scrubs can also be used for hygienic eyelid cleansing in contact lens wearers. These products are designed to be used full strength on eyelid tissues but must be instilled directly into the eyes. Some of the commercial products are packaged with gauze or cotton pads, which provide an abrasive action to augment the cleansing properties of the detergent solution.

VITAMINS AND MINERALS

Deficiencies of vitamin A and zinc have sometimes been associated with certain adverse ocular effects. Beyond replacement of documented deficiencies, however, treatment or prevention of ophthalmic diseases using vitamins and minerals is not clearly established. Recently, various investigators have explored the use of vitamins A, C and E, as well as zinc, as preventative measures for degenerative ophthalmic changes often associated with the aging process. The primary mechanisms of action offered to explain the effectiveness of such therapy include antioxidation and free radical scavenging. Several products are now commercially available for the prevention and treatment of macular degeneration, but considerably more data will be required before the efficacy of these products becomes well established.

Jimmy D. Bartlett OD, DOS
University of Alabama at Birmingham

For More Information

Doughty MJ, Lyle WM. A review of the clinical pharmacokinetics of pilocarpine, moxisylyte (thymoxamine), dapiprazole in the reversal of diagnostic pupillary dilation. *Optom Vis Sci* 1992;69:358-68.

Allison RW, et al. Reversal of mydriasis by dapiprazole. *Ann Ophthalmol* 1990;92:131-38.

Bartlett JD, Classe JG. Dapiprazole: Will it affect the standard of care for pupillary dilation? *Optom Clin* 1992;2(3): 65-75.

Whikehart DR. Irrigating solutions. In: Bartlett JD, Jaanus SD, eds. Clinical Ocular Pharmacology. Boston, MA: Butterworth, 1989.

Polack FM, Goodman DF. Experience with a new detergent lid scrub in the management of chronic blepharitis. *Arch Ophthalmol* 1988;106:719-20.

Sperduto RD, et al. Do we have a nutritional treatment for age-related cataract or macular degeneration? *Arch Ophthalmol* 1990;108:1403-05.

DAPIPRAZOLE HCl

Actions:

Dapiprazole acts through blocking the alpha-adrenergic receptors in smooth muscle and produces miosis through an effect on the dilator muscle of the iris.

Dapiprazole does not have any significant activity on ciliary muscle contraction, and, therefore, does not induce a significant change in the anterior chamber depth or the thickness of the lens.

Dapiprazole has demonstrated safe and rapid reversal of mydriasis produced by phenylephrine and, to a lesser degree, tropicamide. In patients with decreased accommodative amplitude due to treatment with tropicamide, the miotic effect of dapiprazole may partially increase the accommodative amplitude.

Eye color affects the rate of pupillary constriction. In individuals with brown irides, the rate of pupillary constriction may be slightly slower than in individuals with blue or green irides. Eye color does not appear to affect the final pupil size.

Dapiprazole does not significantly alter IOP in normotensive eyes or in eyes with elevated IOP.

Indications:

For the treatment of iatrogenically induced mydriasis produced by adrenergic (phenylephrine) or parasympatholytic (tropicamide) agents.

Not indicated for the reduction of IOP or in the treatment of open-angle glaucoma.

Contraindications:

Hypersensitivity to any component of the formulation.

When constriction is undesirable, such as in acute iritis.

Warnings:

For topical use only. Not for injection.

Do not use in the same patient more frequently than once a week.

Precautions:

May cause difficulty in dark adaptation and may reduce field of vision. Patients should exercise caution in night driving or when performing other activities in poor illumination.

Pregnancy: Category B. There are no adequate and well-controlled studies in pregnant women. Use during pregnancy only when clearly needed and when potential benefits outweigh the potential hazards to the fetus.

Lactation: It is not known whether this drug is excreted in breast milk. Because many drugs are excreted in breast milk, caution should be exercised when dapiprazole is administered to a nursing woman.

Children: Safety and efficacy for use in children have not been established.

Adverse Reactions:

The most frequent reaction to dapiprazole was conjunctival injection lasting 20 minutes in over 80% of patients. Burning on instillation was reported in approximately half of all patients. Reactions occurring in 10% to 40% of patients include ptosis, lid erythema, lid edema, chemosis, itching, punctate keratitis, corneal edema, browache, photophobia and headache. Other reactions reported less frequently include dryness of the eye, tearing and blurring of vision.

Patient Information:

May cause difficulty in dark adaptation and may reduce field of vision. Exercise caution when driving at night or performing other activities in poor illumination.

To avoid contamination, do not touch tip of container to any surface.

Do not use in the same patient more frequently than once a week.

Discard any solution that is not clear and colorless.

Dosage and Administration:

Instill 2 drops into the conjunctiva of each eye followed 5 minutes later by an additional 2 drops. This should be administered after the ophthalmic examination to reverse the diagnostic mydriasis.

Shake well before using.

Storage: Store at room temperature 59° to 86°F (15° to 30°C) for 21 days.

Rx	Rêv-Eyes (Storz/Lederle)	Powder, lyophilized: 25 mg (0.5% solution when reconstituted)	In vials with 5 ml diluent and dropper.[1]

[1] With 0.4% hydroxypropyl methylcellulose, 2% mannitol, 0.01% benzalkonium chloride, 0.01% EDTA and sodium chloride.

EXTRAOCULAR IRRIGATING SOLUTIONS

Indications:

For irrigating the eye to help relieve irritation by removing loose foreign material, air pollutants (smog or pollen) or chlorinated water.

Contraindications:

Hypersensitivity to any component of the formulation.

Warnings:

Not for injection or intraocular surgery.

Not to be used as a saline solution for rinsing and soaking contact lenses.

Patient Information:

If you experience eye pain, changes in vision, continued redness or irritation of the eye, or if the condition worsens or persists, consult a doctor.

Obtain immediate medical treatment for all open wounds in or near the eyes.

If solution changes color or becomes cloudy, do not use.

Do not use with a wetting solution for contact lenses or with other eye care products containing polyvinyl alcohol.

Do not use these products with contact lenses.

To avoid contamination, do not touch tip of the container to any surface. Replace cap after using.

Keep out of the reach of children.

Administration and Dosage:

Solution: Flush the affected eye(s) as needed, controlling the rate of flow of solution by pressure on the bottle.

Eyecup: Fill the sterile eyecup halfway with eye wash. Apply the cup tightly to the affected eye and tilt the head backward. Open eyes wide, rotate eye and blink several times to insure that the solution completely floods the eye. Discard the wash. Rinse the cup with clean water and repeat the procedure with the other eye.

Rinse the eyecup before and after every use. Avoid contamination of the rim or inside surfaces of the cup. Cap the bottle tightly after use.

Storage: Store at 46° to 86°F (8° to 30°C).

				C.I.*
otc	**AK-Rinse** (Akorn)	Solution: NaCl, KCl, calcium chloride, magnesium chloride, sodium acetate and sodium citrate with 0.013% benzalkonium chloride	In 30 and 120 ml.	8
otc	**Blinx** (Sola/Barnes-Hind)	Solution: NaCl, KCl and sodium phosphate with 0.005% benzalkonium chloride and 0.02% EDTA	In 120 ml.	10
otc	**Collyrium for Fresh Eyes Eye Wash** (Wyeth-Ayerst)	Solution: Boric acid, sodium borate and 0.002% thimerosal	In 120 ml.	4

* Cost Index based on cost per ml.

EXTRAOCULAR IRRIGATING SOLUTIONS (Cont.)   C.I.*

otc	**Dacriose** (Iolab)	**Solution:** NaCl, KCl, sodium phosphate and sodium hydroxide with benzalkonium chloride and EDTA	In 15, 30 and 120 ml. **20**
otc	**Eye Irrigating Solution** (Rugby)	**Solution:** NaCl and sodium phosphate mono- and dibasic with benzalkonium chloride and EDTA	In 118 ml. **10**
otc	**Eye-Stream** (Alcon)	**Solution:** 0.64% NaCl, 0.075% KCl, 0.03% magnesium chloride, 0.048% calcium chloride, 0.39% sodium acetate and 0.17% sodium citrate with 0.013% benzalkonium chloride	In 30 and 120 ml. **14**
otc	**Eye Wash** (Bausch & Lomb)	**Solution:** Boric acid, sodium borate and NaCl with 0.025% EDTA and 0.1% sorbic acid	In 118 ml with eye cup. **12**
otc	**Eye Wash** (Goldline)	**Solution:** Boric acid, KCl, EDTA, anhydrous sodium carbonate and 0.01% benzalko- nium chloride	In 118 ml. **NA**
otc	**Eye Wash** (Lavoptik)	**Solution:** 0.49% NaCl, 0.4% sodium biphos- phate and 0.45% sodium phosphate with 0.005% benzalkonium chloride	In 180 ml with eyecup. **1**
otc	**Eye Irrigating Wash** (Hauck)	**Solution:** 1.2% boric acid, 0.38% KCl and 0.014% sodium carbonate anhydrous with 0.05% EDTA and 0.01% benzalkonium chloride	In 120 ml. **2**
otc	**Optigene** (Pfeiffer)	**Solution:** NaCl and sodium phosphate mono- and dibasic with EDTA and benzalkonium chloride	In 118 ml. **NA**
otc	**Star-Optic Eye Wash** (Stellar)	**Solution:** NaCl and sodium phosphate mono- and dibasic with EDTA and benzalkonium chloride	In 118 ml with eye cup. **NA**

* Cost Index based on cost per ml.

LID SCRUBS

Indications:

To aid in the removal of oils, debris or desquamated skin associated with blepharitis.

For hygenic eyelid cleansing for contact lens wearers.

Precautions:

For external use only. Do not instill directly into eye.

Do not dilute.

Administration and Dosage:

Close eye(s) and gently scrub on eyelid(s) and lashes using lateral side-to-side strokes. Rinse thoroughly. Repeat twice daily or as directed.

otc	I-Scrub (Spectra)	**Solution:** PEG-200 glyceryl monotallowate, disodium laureth sulfosuccinate, cocoamido propyl amine oxide, PEG-78 glyceryl monococoate, benzyl alcohol and EDTA	In 240 ml.
otc	OcuClenz (Storz/ Lederle)	**Solution:** Disodium oleamido PEG-2 sulfosuccinate, cocoamphodiacetate, poloxamer 185, poloxamer 188, methylparaben, propylparaben, citric acid and EDTA	In 120 ml.
otc	Lid Wipes-SPF (Akorn)	**Solution:** PEG-200 glyceryl monotallowate, PEG-80 glyceryl monococate, laureth-23, cocoamido propylamine oxide, NaCl, glycerin, sodium dihydrogen phosphate and sodium hydroxide	In UD 30s (Pads).
otc	OCuSOFT (Cynacon/ OCuSOFT)	**Solution:** PEG-80 sorbitan laurate, sodium trideceth sulfate, PEG-150 distearate, cocamido propyl hydroxysultaine, lauroamphocarboxyglycinate, sodium laureth-13 carboxylate, PEG-15 tallow polyamine, quaternium-15	In UD 30s (Pads) and 120 ml.

MISCELLANEOUS PREPARATIONS

otc **Schirmer Tear Test** (Various, eg, Alcon, Iolab)   In strips.

    Strips: Sterile test strips.

    Use: Test I – To diagnose dry eye syndrome, to evaluate lacrimal gland function in contact lens wearers, to check tear production prior to eyelid surgery, and prior to corneal transplantation and cataract surgery.

        Test II – To assess the adequacy of reflex lacrimation.

    Administration: Strips are placed at the junction of the middle and temporal one-third of the eyelid margin. Do not touch the cornea which can produce increased reflex lacrimation and pain.

---

otc **Sno Strips** (Akorn)   In strips
                                                                 (100s).

    Strips: Sterile tear flow test strips

    Use: Test performed on eye before any topical medication (especially anesthetic) is administered or other procedures are carried out (eg, manipulation of eyelids).

    Administration: Apply to lower temporal lid margin of eye. Distance between notch and shoulder of strip is 10 mm which should be wetted in ≈ 3 minutes. Repeat if in excess of 5 minutes; > 10 minutes indicates reduced tear secretion.

Rx **Succus Cineraria Maritima** (Walker Pharm.)   In 7 ml.

    Solution: An aqueous and glycerin solution of senecio compositae, hamamelis water and boric acid

    Use: The manufacturer claims usefulness for the treatment of "optic opacity caused by cataract." Not intended for use in glaucoma.

    Administration: Instill 2 drops, morning and night, into affected eye(s).

VITAMINS AND MINERALS

Actions:

Certain vitamin and mineral deficiencies have been associated with adverse ocular effects, most notably vitamin A and zinc. Beyond replacement of documented deficiency, treatment or prevention of ophthalmic diseases with vitamins and minerals is not well established.

However, investigators are beginning to explore this area. Some claims are being made for vitamins A, C and E as well as zinc as preventatives for degenerative ophthalmic changes often associated with aging. The principal mechanisms of action are offered as antioxidation and free radical scavenging.

Much more data are required before actual recommendations can be made. However, products are available, labeled with such claims.

Administration and Dosage:

Take with meals.

Adults: 1 to 2 tablets or packets 1 or 2 times daily or as directed by a physician.

Storage: Store at room temperature 59° to 86°F (15° to 30°C).

otc	Icaps Plus (La Haye Labs.)	**Tablets:** 5000 IU vitamin A[1], 250 mg C[2], 10 mg B_2, 50 IU E[3], 20 mg Zn[4], 1 mg Cu[5], 5 mg Mn[6], 20 mcg Se[7] and 25 mg L-cysteine	Golden. Oval. Film coated. In 60s and 120s.
otc	OcuCaps (Akorn)	**Caplets:** 5000 IU vitamin A[1], 400 mg C[2], 200 IU E[3], 40 mg Zn[8], 5 mg L-glutathione, 3 mg sodium pyruvate, 2 mg Cu[9], 40 mcg Se[7]	In 60s.
otc	**OCUSOFT VMS** (Cynacon/ OCuSOFT)	**Tablets:** 40 mg Zn, 2 mg Cu, 40 mcg Se, 5000 IU vitamin A, 30 IU E and 60 mg C	In 60s.
otc	Ocuvite (Storz/Lederle)	**Tablets:** 40 mg elemental Zn[4], 2 mg elemental Cu[10], 40 mcg elemental Se[11], 5000 IU vitamin A[1], 30 IU E[3] and 60 mg C[2]	(LL/04). Two-tone peach. Eye shaped. Film coated. In 60s.
otc	**Ophthalmic Nutrients** (Health Maintenance Programs)	**Yellow Capsules:** 1000 mg vitamin C[2], 100 mg glutathione, 20 mg B_3, 20 mg B_2, 10 mg B_5, 2 mg B_6, 1.5 mg B_1, 125 IU D_3, 100 mcg B_{12}, 250 mg calcium[12], 30 mg Zn[4], 5 mg Mn[13], 1 mg Cu[10] and 25 mcg Se[11] **Red Capsules:** 15 mg beta carotene and 100 IU vitamin E[3]	Blister packs of 2 yellow and 1 red capsule. In 60s.

[1] As Beta-carotene.
[2] As ascorbic acid.
[3] As dl-alpha tocopheryl acetate.
[4] As zinc oxide.

[5] As copper amino acid chelate.
[6] As manganese amino acid chelate.
[7] As selenomethionine.
[8] As zinc ascorbate.

[9] As copper ascorbate.
[10] As cupric oxide.
[11] As sodium selenate.
[12] As calcium carbonate.
[13] As manganese sulfate.

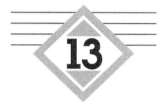

Contact Lens Care

Approximately 24 million Americans wear contact lenses. Contact lenses can offer patients a natural appearance, increased visual performance and convenience. They can successfully correct most refractive errors such as myopia, hyperopia and astigmatism. Bifocal contact lenses are available for the presbyopic patient. Tinted contact lenses can enhance or completely change the color of a patient's eyes. Research and development by major ophthalmic corporations have produced a variety of new lens materials and designs. With new contact lens products and patient education, contact lens use should continue to grow.

The number of contact lens care products has also increased dramatically. The sale of contact lens solutions has increased faster than any other category of goods sold in pharmacies. Over $400 million per year is spent on contact lens care products. Patients may become confused because there are over 150 products sold for contact lens care.

COMPLIANCE

Successful contact lens wear includes good vision, lens comfort and normal ocular health. Successful wear is dependent upon patient compliance in caring for their contact lenses. Several recent studies indicate that between 40% and 74% of soft contact lens patients are not following the care regimen prescribed by their doctor. In another study, it was found that 50% of the patients harbored potentially pathogenic microorganisms in their care systems. Noncompliance among contact lens wearers can have many consequences. Inadequate cleaning can lead to lens discoloration and lens surface buildup of protein, lipids, minerals and other environmental contaminants, which can contribute to giant papillary conjunctivitis, superficial punctate keratitis and corneal abrasion. Irregular contact lens disinfection can cause severe ocular infection.

Doctors, pharmacists and opticians must have a thorough understanding of all contact lens materials and care systems. With this knowledge, they can educate the patient, increase compliance and therefore decrease lens-related complications.

Compliance has been defined by the Food and Drug Administration (FDA) as the use of an approved contact lens care regimen in a manner both in agreement with the manufacturer's instructions and consistent with good general hygiene. Compliance must meet four criteria:

1. The patient should always wash his or her hands before lens manipulation;
2. The patient should use an FDA approved care system in an appropriate manner;
3. The patient should wear lenses only on a daily wear schedule unless the lenses are approved by the FDA for extended wear;
4. All solutions should be free of bacterial contamination.

CONTACT LENS GUIDELINES

- Proper contact lens care will increase success and decrease complications.
- Cleaning does not disinfect lenses.
- Disinfecting does not clean lenses.
- Enzyme solutions are not a substitute for disinfection.
- Wash and rinse hands thoroughly before handling contact lenses.
- Do not insert contact lenses if eyes are red or irritated. If eyes become painful or vision worsens while wearing lenses, remove lenses and consult an eye-care practitioner immediately.
- Do not wear contact lenses while sleeping unless they have been prescribed for extended wear.
- For soft lens care, use only products designed for soft lenses.
- For rigid lens care, use only products designed for rigid lenses.
- Do not change or substitute products from a different manufacturer without consulting a doctor.
- Do not use non-sterile, home-prepared saline solutions unless recommended by your eye care practitioner.
- Always follow label directions or doctor's recommendations.
- Do not store lenses in tap water.
- After removal, lenses must be cleaned, rinsed and disinfected before wearing again.
- Lenses that are stored longer than 12 hours may again require cleaning, rinsing and disinfection; consult package insert or eye-care practitioner.
- Never use saliva to wet contact lenses.
- Keep lens care products out of the reach of children.
- Do not instill topical medications while contact lenses are being worn unless directed by a doctor.
- Do not get cosmetic lotions, creams or sprays in your eyes or on lenses. It is best to put on lenses before putting on make up and remove them before removing make up. Water-base cosmetics are less likely to damage lenses than oil-base products.
- Schedule and keep follow-up appointments with your eye-care practitioner (approximately every 6 to 12 months or as recommended).
- Contact lenses wear out with time and should be replaced regularly. Throw away disposable lenses after the recommended wearing period.
- Check with your eye-care practitioner regarding wearing lenses during sports activities.

CONTACT LENS MATERIALS

Three types of contact lenses are manufactured: Hard, rigid gas permeable and soft.

Hard Contact Lenses

Hard contact lenses are made from polymethylmethacrylate (PMMA). PMMA does not transmit the oxygen needed for normal corneal integrity. Hard contact lenses have caused chronic corneal edema, corneal distortion, edematous corneal formations, spectacle blur, polymegathism and corneal abrasions. Because of these ocular complications, hard lenses are seldom the lens of choice for a new contact lens patient. Less than 1% of the contact lens population wear hard contact lenses.

Rigid Gas Permeable Lenses

Approximately 20% of contact lens patients wear rigid gas permeable (RGP) lenses. These lenses are oxygen permeable. Therefore, the RGP patient does not have the severe physiological complications of the hard lens patient. Most doctors prescribe daily wear RGP lenses. Several lens polymers with a high degree of oxygen permeability have been approved by the FDA for extended wear. RGP lenses provide the patient with good vision, durability and easy care.

Soft Contact Lenses

The majority of soft contact lenses are made of hydroxyethylmethacrylate (HEMA), a plastic compound that had been used for making artificial blood vessels and organs. The first soft lens was marketed in the US in 1971. Today, most soft lenses manufactured from HEMA contain 30% to 55% water.

Daily wear soft contact lenses are designed to be worn all day (12 to 14 hours), but must be removed nightly to be cleaned and disinfected. Extended wear soft lenses can be worn for 24 hours or more. The FDA and most eye care practitioners recommend a maximum wearing period of 7 days. The lenses must then be removed overnight for cleaning and disinfection. The major advantage of extended wear lenses is convenience. Daily wear soft lenses provide the same level of comfort and vision as extended wear soft lenses. The popularity of extended wear soft lenses has decreased in the last few years due to the reported increased risk of infection.

Disposable Soft Lenses

Disposable soft lenses are designed to eliminate the complications of lens deposits by planned lens replacement. Lens deposits can interfere with vision, cause corneal irritation and contribute to ocular infection. In addition, disposable lenses offer the patient the convenience of reduced lens care.

Disposable lenses are approved for daily wear and extended wear. It is recommended that the lenses be discarded after 1, 2 or 4 weeks or 3 months of wear. The doctor will prescribe the replacement schedule for each patient. If a disposable lens is not discarded immediately after lens removal, it should be cleaned with a surfactant cleaner and stored in a disinfection solution.

CONTACT LENS CARE PRODUCTS

Products for use with contact lenses possess the same general characteristics of all ophthalmic products; they are sterile, isotonic and free of particulate matter. Additionally, product formulations contain various components to achieve specific goals of contact lens care.

Although all contact lenses serve similar functions in correcting visual defects, each distinct type of lens material requires a unique lens care program. In selecting appropriate lens care solutions, it is essential to correctly identify the type of lens the patient is using.

Hard and Rigid Gas Permeable Lenses

Similar lens care is used for the hard and RGP lenses. Products include wetting/soaking/disinfection solutions, cleaning agents, lubricants and rewetting solutions.

When a rigid contact lens is removed from the eye, it may be covered with lipids, proteins, eye makeup and other debris. After removal, the lens should immediately

be cleaned with a *surfactant cleaner*. Improper cleaning can contribute to a lens surface buildup, which can interfere with vision and potentially cause corneal irritation.

Rigid lenses should be soaked overnight in a *wetting/soaking/disinfecting solution*.
This solution has four major functions:

1. To enhance the lens surface wettability
2. To maintain the lens hydration similar to that achieved during daily contact
   lens wear
3. Lens disinfection
4. To act as a mechanical buffer between the lens and the cornea

It is not uncommon for a rigid lens patient to experience dryness after several hours
of wear. This is especially true with RGP lens patients because of the hydrophobic
nature of some lens material. *Rewetting drops* can provide temporary relief by rinsing debris off the lens surface and rewetting the eye and the lens.

Many clinicians routinely recommend the weekly use of an enzyme (papain) cleaner
with RGP lenses. This weekly cleaning process is very effective in removing protein
deposits from the lens surface. A protein film on an RGP lens can decrease vision
and cause giant papillary conjunctivitis.

Soft Contact Lenses

Soft contact lens care systems are designed to clean, disinfect and re-wet the
lenses. The first step is proper cleaning. Cleaning the lens gently in the palm of the
hand with a *daily surfactant cleaner* will remove fresh lipids, oils and other environmental debris. Soft lenses should be cleaned thoroughly with a surfactant cleaner
each time a patient removes a lens. After cleaning the lens, it should be thoroughly
rinsed with a soft lens *rinsing/storage solution.* All rinsing/storage solutions contain
0.9% saline. Some are available with no preservatives in unit-dose vials or aerosol
containers. Other saline solutions contain preservatives to decrease microorganism
growth. Use of saline made with salt tablets should be discouraged because of the
risk of contamination and infection (see Precautions).

Enzymatic cleaners are generally used on a weekly basis. They are more effective in
removing protein deposits than surfactant cleaners because they contain proteolytic
enzymes (papain, pancreatin or subtilisin). Most enzymes are dissolved directly in
saline, but the subtilisin enzyme tablet can be dissolved in a hydrogen peroxide disinfection solution.

Soft lens *disinfection* is the most important step in soft lens care. Disinfection is
achieved by using a thermal (heat) or chemical (cold) system.

Thermal disinfection was the first system approved for soft contact lenses. A heat
unit specially designed for soft lenses is used for 10 minutes at 80° C. This procedure will kill most microorganisms that are dangerous to the eye. Recently,
Acanthamoeba keratitis has become a concern of many clinicians. Heat disinfection
is the most effective procedure to successfully kill *Acanthamoeba*; however, heat
disinfection cannot be used with all soft lens materials. Also, the continued use of
heat can shorten the life of a soft lens.

RECOMMENDED DISINFECTION TIMES FOR SOFT LENSES			
System	Manufacturer	Disinfection Time (minimum)	Neutralization Time (minimum)
Allergan Hydrocare Cleaning and Disinfecting	Allergan	4 hours	none
Aosept	Ciba Vision	6 hours[1]	6 hours[1]
Disinfecting Solution	Bausch & Lomb	4 hours	none
Flex-Care	Alcon	4 hours	none
Lens Plus Oxysept System	Allergan	10 minutes	10 minutes
Lensept	Ciba Vision	55 minutes	5 minutes
MiraSept System	Wesley-Jessen	10 minutes	10 minutes
Opti-Free	Alcon	4 hours	none
Opti-Soft	Alcon	4 hours	none
ReNu Multi-Purpose	Bausch & Lomb	4 hours	none
Soft Mate	Sola/Barnes-Hind	4 hours	none
Soft Mate Consept	Sola/Barnes-Hind	10 minutes	10 minutes

[1] One-step method: Disinfection and neutralization occur together for a total of 6 hours.

The original chemical soft lens disinfection systems used thimerosal with either chlorhexidine or a quaternary ammonium compound. These systems had a high incidence of sensitivity reactions. Various hydrogen peroxide care systems are currently available in the US. Most systems require two steps to achieve disinfection and hydrogen peroxide neutralization; one system combines disinfection and neutralization in a single step. Hydrogen peroxide (3%) is a very effective disinfection agent and can be used with all soft lens polymers. However, hydrogen peroxide care systems can be complex and expensive. Generic peroxide solutions should not be substituted for solutions that have been formulated for contact lenses. They may be contaminated with heavy metals, have different concentrations of hydrogen peroxide or use stabilizers that may discolor soft lenses.

In the last few years, two new chemical soft lens care systems have been introduced into the US marketplace – *Opti-Free* by Alcon and *ReNu* by Bausch & Lomb. Polyquad (polyquaternium – 1) and Dymed (polyammopropylbiguamide) are the disinfection agents utilized in these care systems. Both are simple to use and may therefore increase patient compliance. These two chemical systems have become the care system of choice for the majority of soft lens patients.

DRUG INTERFERENCE WITH CONTACT LENS USE		
Drug	RGP[1]/Hard/Soft Lens	Action
Anticholinergics (eg, *Isopto Atropine*)	RGP, hard, soft	Tear volume decreased
Antihistamines, sympathomimetics	RGP, hard, soft	Tear volume decreased, blink rate decreased
Chlorthalidone (eg, *Hygroton*)	RGP, hard, soft	Causes lid or corneal edema
Clomiphene (eg, *Clomid*)	RGP, hard, soft	Causes lid or corneal edema
Diuretics, Thiazide (eg, *HydroDiuril*)	RGP, hard, soft	Tear volume decreased
Dopamine (eg, *Dopastat*)	soft	Discoloration of contact lenses
Epinephrine, topical (eg, *Epifrin*)	soft	Discoloration of contact lenses
Fluorescein, topical (eg, *Ful-Glo*)	soft	Lens absorbs the yellow dye
Hypnotics, sedatives, muscle relaxants (eg, *Amytal*)	RGP, hard, soft	Blink rate decreased
Nitrofurantoin (eg, *Furadantin*)	soft	Discoloration of contact lenses
Oral contraceptives (eg, *Ortho-Novum*)	RGP, hard, soft	Increased stickiness of mucus; corneal lid edema due to fluid retention properties of estrogens
Phenazopyridine (eg, *Pyridium*)	soft	Discoloration of contact lenses
Phenolphthalein (eg, *Modane*)	soft	Discoloration of contact lenses
Phenylephrine (eg, *Neo-Synephrine*)	soft	Discoloration of contact lenses
Iodine Groups (eg, *Phospholine Iodide*)	soft	Discoloration of contact lenses
Primidone (eg, *Mysoline*)	RGP, hard, soft	Causes lid or corneal edema
Rifampin (eg, *Rifadin*)	soft	Lens absorbs drug, causing orange discoloration
Sulfasalazine (eg, *Azulfidine*)	soft	Yellow staining
Tetracycline (eg, *Achromycin*)	soft	Discoloration of contact lenses
Tricyclic antidepressants (eg, *Elavil*)	RGP, hard, soft	Tear volume decreased

[1] Rigid gas permeable.

Soft lens rewetting solutions permit the lubrication of the soft lens while it is on the eye. Most patients find these rewetting drops minimally effective in reducing dryness. Maximum relief can be achieved by removing the lens, cleaning it with a daily surfactant cleaner and thoroughly rinsing it with a rinsing/storage saline solution.

PRECAUTIONS FOR CONTACT LENS USE

Acanthamoeba Keratitis

Soft contact lens wearers who use homemade saline solution are at risk of developing *Acanthamoeba* keratitis, a serious and painful corneal infection. This infection may cause blindness or impaired vision. Homemade saline solutions (nonsterile) may be used during the thermal disinfection phase but NOT after disinfection.

Drug Interference with Contact Lens Use

Systemic medications may affect the physiology of the cornea, lids and tear system. In addition, many drugs may discolor soft contact lenses. Pharmacists and eye-care practitioners should be aware of the interaction of systemic medications and contact lenses (see table p. 244).

Products listed on the following pages are grouped as follows:

CONTACT LENS SOLUTIONS	
Type of Lens	**Type of Solution**
Hard	Storage/Soaking Wetting Cleaning Cleaning/Soaking Wetting/Soaking Cleaning/Soaking/Wetting Re-wetting
Rigid Gas Permeable	Cleaning/Soaking Wetting/Soaking Cleaning
Soft	Rinsing/Storage Chemical Disinfection Surfactant Cleaning Enzymatic Cleaning Re-wetting

N. Rex Ghormley, OD, FAAO
Contact Lens Consultants, St. Louis

For More Information

Aquavella JV, Rao GN. Contact Lenses. Philadelphia, PA: J.B. Lippincott Co., 1987.

Barr JT, ed. Contact Lens Pocket Guide. Irvine, CA: Allergan Optical Corporation, 1987.

Bennett ES, Grone RM, eds. Rigid Gas-Permeable Contact Lenses. New York, NY: Professional Press Books, Fairchild Publications, 1986.

Chun MW, Weissmann BA. Compliance in contact lens care. *Am J Optom Physiol Opt* 1987; 64:274-76.

Collins MJ, Carney LG. Patient compliance and its influence on contact lens wearing problems. *Am J Optom Physiol Opt* 1986;63:952-56.

Duane TD, ed. Clinical Ophthalmology. Philadelphia, PA: J.B. Lippincott Co., 1988.

Lowther GE, et al. The Pharmacist's Guide to Contact Lenses and Lens Care. Atlanta, GA: CIBAVision Corporation, 1988.

Mondino BJ, et al. Corneal ulcers associated with daily wear and extended wear contact lenses. *Am J Ophthalmol* 1986;102:58-65.

Smith MB. Contact lens care systems. *Contact, The Eye Care Journal for Pharmacists* 1988;1:14-22.

HARD (PMMA) CONTACT LENS PRODUCTS

Conventional hard lenses are made of a rigid hydrophobic polymer, polymethyl-methacrylate (PMMA). For optimum comfort, these lenses require care with separate wetting, cleaning and soaking solutions.

STORAGE/SOAKING SOLUTIONS, Hard Lenses

Storage/soaking solutions maintain the lens in a state of hydration, prevent growth of microbial contamination and possibly remove debris from the lens surface through chelation or solvation. Discard used soaking solutions and replace with fresh solution daily.

				C.I.*
otc	Soakare (Allergan)	Solution: 0.01% benzalkonium chloride and 0.25% EDTA	In 120 ml.	190

WETTING SOLUTIONS, Hard Lenses

Wetting solutions contain surfactants to facilitate hydration of the hydrophobic hard lens surface. These solutions include methylcellulose and derivatives, polyvinyl alcohol, povidone, some newer polymers, preservatives and buffering agents. These agents increase solution viscosity and act as a physical cushioning agent between lens and cornea.

				C.I.*
otc	Adapt (Alcon)	Solution: Adsorbobase with 0.004% thime- rosol and 0.1% EDTA	In 15 ml.	46
otc	Liquifilm Wetting (Allergan)	Solution: Hydroxypropyl methylcellulose, NaCl, KCl, polyvinyl alcohol, 0.004% benzalkonium chloride and EDTA	In 60 ml.	12
otc	Sereine (Optikem)	Solution: Buffered solution with 0.1% EDTA and 0.01% benzalkonium chloride	In 60 and 120 ml.	6
otc	Stay-Wet (Sherman)	Solution: Polyvinyl alcohol, hydroxyethyl cellulose, povidone, NaCl, KCl, sodium carbonate, 0.01% benzalkonium chloride and 0.025% EDTA	In 30 ml.	12
otc	Wetting (Sola/Barnes-Hind)	Solution: Polyvinyl alcohol with 0.004% benzalkonium chloride and 0.02% EDTA	In 60 ml.	8

CLEANING, SOAKING AND WETTING SOLUTIONS, Hard Lenses   C.I.*

otc	Total (Allergan)	Solution: Buffered isotonic solution with polyvinyl alcohol, benzalkonium chloride and EDTA	In 60 and 120 ml.	335

* Cost Index based on cost per 30 ml storage/soaking solutions, cleaning, soaking and wetting solutions and 1 ml wetting solutions.

WETTING/SOAKING SOLUTIONS, Hard Lenses   C.I.*

otc	**Sereine** (Optikem)	**Solution:** Buffered isotonic solution with 0.1% EDTA and 0.01% benzalkonium chloride	In 120 ml.	90
otc	**Soaclens** (Alcon)	**Solution:** Wetting agents, 0.004% thimerosal, 0.1% EDTA and buffering agents	In 120 ml.	162
otc	**Wetting & Soaking** (Sola/Barnes-Hind)	**Solution:** Buffered isotonic solution with octylphenoxy (oxyethylene) ethanol, povidone, polyvinyl alcohol, propylene glycol, hydroxyethyl cellulose, 0.005% chlorhexidine gluconate, 0.02% EDTA and NaCl	Thimerosal free. In 120 ml.	132
otc	**Wet-N-Soak Plus** (Allergan)	**Solution:** Buffered isotonic solution with polyvinyl alcohol, EDTA and 0.003% benzalkonium chloride	In 120 and 180 ml.	152

REWETTING SOLUTIONS, Hard Lenses

Rewetting solutions are intended for use directly in the eye in conjunction with a contact lens. These products improve wearing time by rehydrating the lens, which may become dry and contaminated during wear. The principal components of these solutions are wetting agents.

C.I.*

otc	**Adapettes** (Alcon)	**Solution:** Buffered isotonic solution with povidone and other water-soluble polymers, sorbic acid and EDTA.	Thimerosal free. In 15 ml.	38
otc	**Adapt** (Alcon)	**Solution:** Povidone and other water soluble polymers with 0.004% thimerosal and 0.1% EDTA	In 15 ml.	46
otc	**Clerz 2** (Alcon)	**Solution:** Isotonic solution with hydroxyethyl cellulose, poloxamer 407, NaCl, KCl, sodium borate, boric acid, sorbic acid and EDTA	Thimerosal free. In 5 and 15 ml.	29
otc	**Lens Fresh** (Allergan)	**Solution:** Buffered isotonic solution with hydroxyethyl cellulose, NaCl, sodium borate, boric acid, 0.1% sorbic acid and 0.2% EDTA	Thimerosal free. In 15 ml.	29
otc	**Lens Lubricant** (Bausch & Lomb)	**Solution:** Buffered isotonic solution with povidone, polyoxyethylene, 0.004% thimerosal and 0.1% EDTA	In 15 ml.	28
otc	**Lens-Wet** (Allergan)	**Solution:** Buffered isotonic solution with polyvinyl alcohol, NaCl, 0.002% thimerosal and 0.01% EDTA	In 15 ml.	42
otc	**Opti-Tears** (Alcon)	**Solution:** Isotonic solution with dextran, NaCl, KCl, hydroxypropyl methylcellulose, 0.1% EDTA and 0.001% polyquaternium-1	Thimerosal free. In 15 ml.	36
otc	**Stay-Wet** (Sherman)	**Solution:** Polyvinyl alcohol, hydroxyethyl cellulose, povidone, NaCl, KCl, sodium carbonate, 0.01% benzalkonium chloride and 0.025% EDTA	In 30 ml.	12

* Cost Index based on cost per 30 ml wetting/soaking solution and 1 ml rewetting solution.

CLEANING SOLUTIONS, Hard Lenses

Cleaning solutions contain surfactant cleaners to facilitate removal of oleaginous, proteinaceous and other types of debris from lens surface. To adequately clean, physically rub the lens in the palm of the hand with solution and rinse with a sterile saline solution or water.

				C.I.*
otc	Clens (Alcon)	Solution: 0.02% benzalkonium chloride and 0.1% EDTA	In 60 ml.	16
otc	LC-65 (Allergan)	Solution: Buffered cleaning agent with 0.001% thimerosal and EDTA	In 15 and 60 ml.	31
otc	MiraFlow Extra Strength (Ciba Vision)	Solution: 20% isopropyl alcohol, poloxamer 407 and amphoteric 10	Preservative free. In 15 ml.	15
otc	Opti-Clean (Alcon)	Solution: Buffered isotonic solution with Tween 21, hydroxyethyl cellulose, polymeric cleaners, 0.004% thimerosal and 0.1% EDTA	In 12 and 20 ml.	37
otc	Opti-Clean II (Alcon)	Solution: Buffered isotonic solution with Tween 21, polymeric cleaners, 0.1% EDTA and 0.001% polyquaternium-1	Thimerosal free. In 12 and 20 ml.	37
otc	Opti-Zyme Enzymatic Cleaner (Alcon)	Tablets: Highly purified pork pancreatin	Preservative free. In 4s, 8s, 24s, 36s and 56s.	52
otc	Resolve/GP (Allergan)	Solution: Buffered solution with cocoamphocarboxyglycinate, sodium lauryl sulfate, hexylene glycol, alkyl ether sulfate and fatty acid amide surfactants	Preservative free. In 30 ml.	16
otc	Sereine (Optikem)	Solution: Surfactants and rewetting agents with 0.1% EDTA and 0.01% benzalkonium chloride	In 60 ml.	6
otc	Sila Clean 20/20 (Professional Supp.)	Solution: Benzalkonium chloride and EDTA	In 60 ml.	NA
otc	Titan (Sola/Barnes-Hind)	Solution: Polyoxyethylene, polyoxypropylene block polymer, tris (hydroxymethyl) amino methane, hydroxyethyl cellulose, 2% EDTA and 0.13% potassium sorbate	Thimerosal free. In 30 ml.	24

CLEANING AND SOAKING SOLUTIONS, Hard Lenses   C.I.*

otc	Clean-N-Soak (Allergan)	Solution: Surfactant cleaning agent with 0.004% phenylmercuric nitrate	In 120 ml.	178
otc	de•STAT (Sherman)	Solution: Lauryl sulfate salt of imidazoline, octylphenoxypolyethoxyethanol, 0.01% benzalkonium chloride and 0.25% EDTA	In 118 ml.	102

* Cost Index based on cost per 30 ml cleaning and soaking solution and 1 ml cleaning solution.

RIGID GAS PERMEABLE CONTACT LENS PRODUCTS

Silicone/acrylate and fluorocarbon polymers are used in rigid gas permeable (RGP) contact lenses. Lens care regimens include the use of a surfactant cleaner, enzyme cleaner and storage in a chemical disinfecting solution. Patients should be advised to follow the lens care protocol provided by the lens manufacturer or the instructions of their doctor.

DISINFECTING/WETTING/SOAKING SOLUTIONS, RGP Lenses   C.I.*

otc	**Boston Advance Conditioning Solution** (Polymer Tech)	**Solution:** Buffered hypertonic solution with hydrophilic polyelectrolytes and cellulose polymers, 0.0015% polyaminopropyl biguanide and 0.05% EDTA	In 120 ml.	5
otc	**Boston Conditioning Solution** (Polymer Tech)	**Solution:** Buffered hypertonic solution with hydrophilic polyelectrolytes and cellulose polymers, 0.05% EDTA and 0.006% chlorhexidine gluconate	In 120 ml.	5
otc	**Flex-Care Especially for Sensitive Eyes** (Alcon)	**Solution:** Buffered isotonic solution with NaCl, sodium borate, boric acid, 0.1% EDTA and 0.005% chlorhexidine gluconate	In 360 ml.	2
otc	**Stay-Wet 3** (Sherman)	**Solution:** NaCl, KCl, polyvinyl pyrrolidone, polyvinyl alcohol, hydroxyethyl cellulose, 0.02% sodium bisulfite, 0.1% benzyl alcohol, 0.05% sorbic acid and 0.1% EDTA	Thimerosal free. In 30 ml.	13
otc	**Wet-N-Soak Plus** (Allergan)	**Solution:** Buffered isotonic solution with polyvinyl alcohol, EDTA and 0.003% benzalkonium chloride	In 120 and 180 ml.	4
otc	**Wetting & Soaking** (Sola/Barnes-Hind)	**Solution:** Buffered isotonic solution with octylphenoxy (oxyethylene) ethanol, povidone, polyvinyl alcohol, propylene glycol, hydroxyethyl cellulose, 0.005% chlorhexidine gluconate, 0.02% EDTA and NaCl	Thimerosal free. In 120 ml.	4
otc	**Wetting and Soaking** (Bausch & Lomb)	**Solution:** Buffered hypertonic solution with a cationic cellulose derivative polymer, 0.006% chlorhexidine gluconate and 0.05% EDTA	Thimerosal free. In 118 ml.	4

CLEANING/DISINFECTING/SOAKING SOLUTIONS, RGP Lenses   C.I.*

otc	**de•STAT 3** (Sherman)	**Solution:** Lauryl sulfate salt of imidazoline, octylphenoxypolyethoxyethanol, 0.1% benzyl alcohol and 0.5% EDTA	Thimerosal free. In 118 ml.	4

SURFACTANT CLEANING SOLUTIONS, RGP Lenses   C.I.*

otc	**Boston Advance Cleaner** (Polymer Tech)	**Solution:** Surfactant solution with alkyl ether sulfate, ethoxylated alkyl phenol, triquarternary cocoa-based phospholipid and silica gel	In 30 ml.	5
otc	**The Boston Cleaner** (Polymer Tech)	**Solution:** Surfactant solution with alkyl ether sulfate and silica gel	Preservative free. In 30 ml.	5

* Cost Index based on cost per ml.

SURFACTANT CLEANING SOLUTIONS, RGP Lenses (Cont.)   C.I.*

otc	**Concentrated Cleaner** (Bausch & Lomb)	**Solution:** Surfactant solution with alkyl ether sulfate and silica gel	Preservative free. In 30 ml.	14
otc	**Gas Permeable Daily Cleaner** (Sola/Barnes-Hind)	**Solution:** Ethoxylated polyoxypropylene glycol, tris (hydroxymethyl) amino methane, hydroxyethyl cellulose, 0.13% potassium sorbate and 2% EDTA	Thimerosal free. In 30 ml.	16
otc	**LC-65** (Allergan)	**Solution:** Buffered cleaning agent with 0.001% thimerosal and EDTA	In 15 and 60 ml.	31
otc	**Opti-Clean** (Alcon)	**Solution:** Buffered isotonic solution with Tween 21, hydroxyethyl cellulose, polymeric cleaners, 0.004% thimerosal and 0.1% EDTA	In 12 and 20 ml.	37
otc	**Opti-Clean II** (Alcon)	**Solution:** Buffered isotonic solution with Tween 21, polymeric cleaners, 0.1% EDTA and 0.001% polyquaternium-1	Thimerosal free. In 12 and 20 ml.	37
otc	**Resolve/GP** (Allergan)	**Solution:** Buffered solution with cocoamphocarboxyglycinate, sodium lauryl sulfate, hexylene glycol, alkyl ether sulfate and fatty acid amide surfactants	Preservative free. In 30 ml.	16

ENZYMATIC CLEANERS, RGP Lenses   C.I.*

otc	**Enzymatic Cleaner For Extended Wear** (Alcon)	**Tablets:** Highly purified pork pancreatin	Preservative free. In 12s.	47
otc	**Opti-Zyme Enzymatic Cleaner** (Alcon)		Preservative free. In 4s, 8s, 24s, 36s and 56s.	52
otc	**ProFree/GP Weekly Enzymatic Cleaner** (Allergan)	**Tablets:** Papain, NaCl, sodium carbonate, sodium borate and EDTA	In 16s and 24s.	30

REWETTING SOLUTIONS, RGP Lenses   C.I.*

otc	**Wet-N-Soak** (Allergan)	**Solution:** Borate buffered solution with hydroxyethyl cellulose and 0.0060% WSLP	In 15 ml.	32

* Cost Index based on cost per ml or tablet.

SOFT (HYDROGEL) CONTACT LENS PRODUCTS

Soft (hydrogel) contact lenses are made of hydrophilic polymers. Hydrogel lenses must be maintained in a hydrated state in physiological saline to prevent them from becoming brittle. Hydrogel lenses will absorb many substances; therefore, use only solutions specifically formulated for hydrogel lenses. In addition, these lenses must be disinfected either by heating or by soaking in a chemical solution. *Heating a lens in solutions used for chemical disinfection may cause the lens to become opaque.*

Soft lens solutions are especially formulated to be compatible with, and to meet the particular needs of, soft contact lenses. Of particular importance to soft lens care is the need for thorough cleaning to remove deposits which coat and may discolor the lens, especially when subjected to asepticizing by heating.

> **Warning:**
>
> Do NOT use conventional (hard) lens solutions on soft contact lenses. Use caution in product selection. Not all products are intended for use in all types of soft lenses.

SURFACTANT CLEANING SOLUTIONS, Soft Lenses

Cleaning solutions are used for daily prophylactic cleaning to prevent the accumulation of proteinaceous (mucus) deposits and to remove other debris.

			C.I.*
otc	**Cleaner** (Ciba Vision)	**Solution:** Isotonic solution with cocoamphocarboxyglycinate, sodium lauryl sulfate, hexylene glycol, 0.2% EDTA and 0.1% sorbic acid	Thimerosal free. In 15 ml. — 28
otc	**Lens Clear** (Allergan)		Thimerosal free. In 15 ml. — 26
otc	**DURAcare** (Blairex)	**Solution:** Hypertonic solution with salt buffers, detergents, 0.004% thimerosal and 0.1% EDTA	In 30 ml. — 19
otc	**DURAcare II** (Blairex)	**Solution:** Buffered hypertonic solution with salt buffers, ethylene and propylene oxide, octylphenoxypolyethoxyethanol, lauryl sulfate salt of imidazoline, 0.1% sodium bisulfite, 0.1% sorbic acid and 0.25% EDTA	Thimerosal free. In 30 ml. — 20
otc	**LC-65** (Allergan)	**Solution:** Buffered cleaning agent with 0.001% thimerosal and EDTA	In 15 and 60 ml. — 25
otc	**Lens Plus Daily Cleaner** (Allergan)	**Solution:** Buffered surfactant solution with cocoamphocarboxyglycinate, sodium lauryl sulfate, hexylene glycol, NaCl and sodium phosphate	Preservative free. In 15 and 30 ml. — 21
otc	**MiraFlow Extra Strength** (Ciba Vision)	**Solution:** 20% isopropyl alcohol, poloxamer 407 and amphoteric 10	Preservative free. In 15 ml. — 20

* Cost Index based on cost per 1 ml.

SURFACTANT CLEANING SOLUTIONS, Soft Lenses (Cont.)   C.I.*

otc	**Opti-Clean** (Alcon)	**Solution:** Buffered isotonic solution with Tween 21, hydroxyethyl cellulose, polymeric cleaners, 0.004% thimerosal and 0.1% EDTA	In 12 and 20 ml. 37
otc	**Opti-Clean II** (Alcon)	**Solution:** Buffered isotonic solution with Tween 21, polymeric cleaners, 0.1% EDTA and 0.001% polyquaternium-1	Thimerosal free. In 12 and 20 ml. 37
otc	**Pliagel** (Alcon)	**Solution:** NaCl, KCl, poloxamer 407, 0.25% sorbic acid and 0.5% EDTA	Thimerosal free. In 25 ml. 17
otc	**Preflex Especially for Sensitive Eyes** (Alcon)	**Solution:** Buffered isotonic solution with NaCl, sodium phosphate, tyloxapol, hydroxyethyl cellulose, polyvinyl alcohol, sorbic acid and EDTA	In 30 ml. 18
otc	**Sensitive Eyes Daily Cleaner** (Bausch & Lomb)	**Solution:** Buffered isotonic solution with NaCl, hydroxypropyl methylcellulose, poloxamine, sodium borate, 0.25% sorbic acid and 0.5% EDTA	In 30 ml. 12
otc	**Sensitive Eyes Saline/Cleaning Solution** (Bausch & Lomb)	**Solution:** Buffered isotonic solution with boric acid, poloxamine, sodium borate, NaCl, 0.15% sorbic acid and 0.1% EDTA	In 237 ml. 9
otc	**Sof/Pro-Clean** (Sherman)	**Solution:** Buffered hypertonic salt solution with ethylene and propylene oxide, octylphenoxypolyethoxyethanol, lauryl sulfate salt of imidazoline, 0.004% thimerosal and 0.1% EDTA	In 30 ml. 12
otc	**Sof/Pro-Clean (s.a.)** (Sherman)	**Solution:** Buffered hypertonic salt solution with ethylene and propylene oxide, octylphenoxypolyethoxyethanol, lauryl sulfate salt of imidazoline, 0.1% sodium bisulfite, 0.1% sorbic acid and 0.25% EDTA	Thimerosal free. In 30 ml. 13
otc	**Soft Mate Protein Remover** (Sola/Barnes-Hind)	**Solution:** Alkyl carboxylic acid amine condensate, alkyl imidazoline dicarboxylate, polyoxyalkylene dimethylpolysiloxane, EDTA and borate buffers	Preservative free. In 8 ml bottles of 4s, 8s and 12s. 7
otc	**Soft Mate Daily Cleaning for Sensitive Eyes** (Sola/Barnes-Hind)	**Solution:** Isotonic solution with NaCl, octylphenoxy (oxyethylene) ethanol, hydroxyethyl cellulose, 0.13% potassium sorbate and 0.2% EDTA	In 30 ml. 18

* Cost Index based on cost per ml.

RINSING/STORAGE SOLUTIONS, Soft Lenses

Use these solutions for rinsing and storage of hydrogel lenses in conjunction with heat disinfection. Prepared saline solutions for soft lenses are alkaline, which helps minimize mucus accumulation; they may contain chelating agents (EDTA) which prevent calcium deposits from forming. Thimerosal-free preserved saline solutions may be used by patients sensitive to thimerosal or mercury-containing compounds. Preservative-free solutions are for patients intolerant to preservatives. Salt tablets are available to make saline solution; however, these solutions are nonsterile and contain no preservatives; use only with heat disinfection methods.

PRESERVED SALINE SOLUTIONS, Soft Lenses   C.I.*

otc	Alcon Saline (Alcon)	Solution: Buffered isotonic solution with NaCl, borate buffer, sorbic acid and EDTA	Thimerosal free. In 240 and 360 ml.	19
otc	Hydrocare Preserved Saline (Allergan)	Solution: Buffered isotonic solution with NaCl, sodium hexametaphosphate, boric acid, sodium borate, 0.01% EDTA and 0.001% thimerosal	In 240 and 360 ml.	50
otc	Opti-Soft (Alcon)	Solution: Buffered isotonic solution with NaCl, borate buffer, 0.1% EDTA and 0.001% polyquaternium-1. *For lenses with 45% or less water content*	Thimerosal free. In 240 and 360 ml.	76
otc	ReNu (Bausch & Lomb)	Solution: Buffered isotonic solution with NaCl, boric acid, 0.00003% polyamino-propyl biguanide and EDTA	In 240 and 360 ml.	28
otc	Saline Solution (Bausch & Lomb)	Solution: Buffered isotonic solution with boric acid, NaCl, 0.001% thimerosal and EDTA	In 355 ml.	20
otc	Sensitive Eyes (Bausch & Lomb)	Solution: Buffered isotonic solution with boric acid, NaCl, sodium borate, 0.1% sorbic acid and 0.025% EDTA	Thimerosal free. In 118, 237 and 355 ml.	33
otc	Soft Mate Saline (Sola/Barnes-Hind)	Solution: Isotonic solution with NaCl, 0.13% potassium sorbate and 0.025% EDTA	Thimerosal free. In 360 and 480 ml.	38
otc	Your Choice Sterile Preserved Saline Solution (Amcon)	Solution: Isotonic sterile aqueous solution with a borate buffer system, NaCl, 0.1% sorbic acid and EDTA	In 60 and 360 ml.	NA

* Cost Index based on cost per 30 ml.

PRESERVATIVE-FREE SALINE SOLUTIONS, Soft Lenses   C.I.*

otc	**Blairex Sterile Saline** (Blairex)	**Solution:** Buffered iso-tonic solution with NaCl, boric acid and sodium borate	In 90, 240 and 360 ml aerosol.	42
otc	**Unisol** (Alcon)		In 15 ml (25s).	82
otc	**Unisol 4** (Alcon)		In 120 ml.	43
otc	**Unisol Plus** (Alcon)		In 240 and 360 ml aerosol.	44
otc	**Your Choice Non-Preserved Saline Solution** (Amcon)		In 360 ml.	NA
otc	**Ciba Vision Saline** (Ciba Vision)	**Solution:** Buffered iso-tonic solution with NaCl and boric acid	In 90, 240 and 360 ml aerosol.	44
otc	**Lens Plus Sterile Saline** (Allergan)		In 90, 240, and 360 ml aerosol.	56

SALT TABLETS FOR NORMAL SALINE, Soft Lenses

Reconstitute tablets in container provided with Purified Water, USP. If pharma-ceutical grade water is not available, distilled water is preferred. These solutions are not sterile and are intended only for use in conjunction with heat disinfection regi-mens. Not for use in the eye. See Precautions on page 248.

                                                                 C.I.*

otc	**Marlin Salt System II** (Marlin)	**Tablets:** 250 mg	In 200s with 27.7 ml bottle.	1
otc	**Soft Rinse 250** (Soft Rinse Corp)		In 200s with 27.7 ml bottle.	1

* Cost Index based on cost per 30 ml or tablet.

ENZYMATIC CLEANERS, Soft Lenses

Enzymatic cleaning, by soaking in a solution prepared from enzyme tablets, is recommended once weekly. This is intended to remove protein and other lens deposits.

C.I.*

otc	**Enzymatic Cleaner for Extended Wear** (Alcon)	**Tablets:** Highly purified pork pancreatin *To make solution for soaking when diluted in preserved saline or sterile unpreserved saline solution.*	Preservative free. In 12s.	47
otc	**Opti-zyme Enzymatic Cleaner** (Alcon)		Preservative free. In 4s, 8s, 24s, 36s and 56s.	52
otc	**Vision Care Enzymatic Cleaner** (Alcon)		In 24s.	19
otc	**Allergan Enzymatic** (Allergan)	**Tablets:** Papain, NaCl, sodium carbonate, sodium borate and EDTA *To make solution for soaking when diluted in sterile saline.*	In 12s, 24s, 36s and 48s.	41
otc	**ReNu Effervescent Enzymatic Cleaner** (Bausch & Lomb)	**Tablets:** Subtilisin, polyethylene glycol, sodium carbonate, NaCl and tartaric acid *To make solution for soaking when diluted in preserved saline or sterile unpreserved saline solution.*	In 10s, 20s and 30s.	37
otc	**ReNu Thermal Enzymatic Cleaner** (Bausch & Lomb)	**Tablets:** Subtilisin, sodium carbonate, NaCl and boric acid *To make solution for heat disinfection directly in lens carrying case.*	In 8s and 16s.	46
otc	**Soft Mate Enzyme Plus Cleaner** (Sola/Barnes-Hind)	**Tablets:** Subtilisin, poloxamer 338, povidone, citric acid, potassium bicarbonate, sodium carbonate and sodium benzoate *To make solution for soaking when diluted in sterile saline.*	In 8s.	78
otc	**Ultrazyme Enzymatic Cleaner** (Allergan)	**Tablets:** Subtilisin A with effervescing, buffering and tableting agents *To make solution for soaking when diluted in 3% hydrogen peroxide disinfecting solution.*	In 5s, 10s and 20s.	87

* Cost Index based on cost per tablet or ml.

CHEMICAL DISINFECTION SYSTEMS, Soft Lenses

Chemical disinfection is an alternative to heat. Two-solution systems use separate disinfecting and rinsing solutions. One-solution systems use the same solution for rinsing and storage.

Warning: Lenses must not be disinfected by heating when using these solutions.

HYDROGEN PEROXIDE-CONTAINING SYSTEMS, Soft Lenses   C.I.*

otc	**Aosept** (Ciba Vision)	**Solution:** 3% hydrogen peroxide, 0.85% NaCl, sodium stannate, sodium nitrate and phosphate buffers	Thimerosal free. In 120, 240 and 360 ml.	53
otc	**Lensept** (Ciba Vision)	**Disinfecting Solution:** 3% hydrogen peroxide with sodium stannate, sodium nitrate and phosphate buffers	In 240 and 360 ml.	64
		Rinse and Neutralizer: Buffered isotonic solution with NaCl, sodium borate decahydrate, boric acid, bovine catalase, sorbic acid and EDTA	In 240 ml. Includes cup and holder.	64
otc	**MiraSept System** (Alcon)	**Disinfecting Solution:** 3% hydrogen peroxide with sodium stannate and sodium nitrate	Thimerosal free. In 30 and 120 ml.	38
		Rinse and Neutralizer: Isotonic solution with boric acid, sodium borate, NaCl, sodium pyruvate and EDTA	Thimerosal free. In 20 and 120 ml. Includes lens cup and holder.	83
otc	**Oxysept** (Allergan)	**Disinfecting Solution:** 3% hydrogen peroxide with sodium stannate, sodium nitrate and phosphate buffer	In 240 and 360 ml.	35
		Neutralizer Tablets: With catalase and buffering agents	In 12s and 36s. 12s include OxyTab cup.	17
otc	**Soft Mate Consept** (Sola/Barnes-Hind)	**Consept 1 Cleaning and Disinfecting Solution:** 3% hydrogen peroxide with polyoxyl 40 stearate, sodium stannate, sodium nitrate and phosphate buffer	Preservative free. In 120 and 240 ml.	69
		Consept 2 Neutralizing and Rinsing Spray: Isotonic solution with 0.5% sodium thiosulfate and borate buffers	Preservative free. In 240 ml.	54
otc	**Ultra Care** (Allergan)	**Disinfecting Solution:** 3% hydrogen peroxide with sodium stannate, sodium nitrate and phosphate buffer	In 360 ml.	NA
		Neutralizer Tablets: With catalase, hydroxypropyl methylcellulose and buffering and tableting agents	In 36s. Includes Allergan cup.	NA

* Cost Index based on cost per tablet or 30 ml.

NON-HYDROGEN PEROXIDE-CONTAINING, Soft Lenses C.I.*

otc	**Disinfecting Solution** (Bausch & Lomb)	**Solution:** Buffered isotonic solution with NaCl, sodium borate, boric acid, 0.001% thimerosal, 0.1% EDTA and 0.005% chlorhexidine	In 355 ml.	54
otc	**Flex-Care Especially for Sensitive Eyes** (Alcon)	**Solution:** Buffered isotonic solution with NaCl, sodium borate, boric acid, 0.1% EDTA and 0.005% chlorhexidine gluconate	In 360 ml.	69
otc	**Hydrocare Cleaning and Disinfecting** (Allergan)	**Solution:** Buffered isotonic solution with tris (2-hydroxyethyl) and bis (2-hydroxyethyl) tallow ammonium chloride, 0.002% thimerosal, sodium bicarbonate, sodium phosphates, HCl acid, propylene glycol, polysorbate 80 and polyhema	In 240 and 360 ml.	50
otc	**Opti-Free** (Alcon)	**Solution:** Buffered isotonic solution with citrate, NaCl, 0.05% EDTA and 0.001% polyquaternium-1	In 240 and 360 ml.	69
otc	**ReNu Multi-Purpose Solution** (Bausch & Lomb)	**Solution:** Isotonic solution with NaCl, sodium borate, boric acid, poloxamine, 0.00005% polyaminopropyl biguanide and 0.1% EDTA	In 240 and 360 ml.	55
otc	**Soft Mate** (Sola/Barnes-Hind)	**Solution:** Isotonic solution with NaCl, povidone, octylphenoxy (oxyethylene) ethanol, 0.005% chlorhexidine gluconate, 0.1% EDTA and borate buffer	Thimerosal free. In 240 and 360 ml.	74

REWETTING SOLUTIONS, Soft Lenses

May be used directly in the eye to rehydrate and improve comfort of hydrogel lenses.

C.I.*

otc	**Adapettes Especially for Sensitive Eyes** (Alcon)	**Solution:** Buffered isotonic solution with povidone and other water-soluble polymers, sorbic acid and EDTA	Thimerosal free. In 15 ml.	38
otc	**Clerz 2** (Alcon)	**Solution:** Isotonic solution with hydroxyethyl cellulose, poloxamer 407, NaCl, KCl, sodium borate, boric acid, sorbic acid and EDTA	Thimerosal free. In 5 and 15 ml.	29
otc	**Comfort Tears** (Sola/Barnes-Hind)	**Solution:** Isotonic solution with hydroxyethyl cellulose, 0.005% benzalkonium chloride and 0.02% EDTA	In 15 ml.	38
otc	**Lens Fresh** (Allergan)	**Solution:** Buffered isotonic solution with hydroxyethyl cellulose, NaCl, sodium borate, boric acid, 0.1% sorbic acid and 0.2% EDTA	Thimerosal free. In 15 ml.	29
otc	**Lens Lubricant** (Bausch & Lomb)	**Solution:** Buffered isotonic solution with povidone, polyoxyethylene, 0.004% thimerosal and 0.1% EDTA	In 15 ml.	28
otc	**Lens Lubricant** (Blairex)	**Solution:** Isotonic solution with borate buffer system, NaCl, hydroxypropyl methylcellulose, glycerin, 0.25% sorbic acid and 0.1% EDTA	Thimerosal free. In 15 ml.	23

* Cost Index based on cost per 30 ml non-hydrogen peroxide-containing systems and 1 ml rewetting solutions.

REWETTING SOLUTIONS, Soft Lenses (Cont.)   C.I.*

otc	**Lens Plus Rewetting Drops** (Allergan)	**Solution:** Buffered isotonic solution with NaCl and boric acid	Preservative free. In 0.3 ml (UD 30s).	34
otc	**Opti-Tears** (Alcon)	**Solution:** Isotonic solution with dextran, NaCl, KCl, hydroxypropyl methylcellulose, 0.1% EDTA and 0.001% polyquaternium-1	Thimerosal free. In 15 ml.	36
otc	**Sensitive Eyes Drops** (Bausch & Lomb)	**Solution:** Buffered solution with boric acid, sodium borate, NaCl, 0.1% sorbic acid and 0.025% EDTA	In 30 ml.	11
otc	**Soft Mate Comfort Drops For Sensitive Eyes** (Sola/Barnes-Hind)	**Solution:** Borate buffered solution with 0.13% potassium sorbate and 0.1% EDTA	Thimerosal free. In 15 ml.	36

* Cost Index based on cost per ml.

Systemic Drugs Affecting the Eye

The eye, due to its rich blood supply, multiple tissue types and relatively small size, is highly susceptible to toxic substances. Many systemically administered drugs have the potential to cause adverse ocular effects, and nearly all ocular structures are vulnerable. This section considers the most common drugs that are documented to cause ocular toxicity, summarizing the salient features of the ocular effects.

DRUGS AFFECTING THE CORNEA AND LENS

Antimalarial Drugs

Quinacrine, chloroquine and hydroxychloroquine can cause changes in the cornea. In the early stages, diffuse punctate deposits appear in the corneal epithelium, and later the deposits aggregate into curved lines that converge and coalesce just below the central cornea. These opacities take on a whorl-like configuration. Less than half of patients affected by corneal changes have visual symptoms consisting of halos around lights, glare and photophobia. Visual acuity usually remains unchanged. Once drug therapy is discontinued, both subjective symptoms and objective corneal signs disappear.

Chlorpromazine

Chlorpromazine is the only phenothiazine to cause changes in the cornea and lens. Lenticular pigmentation can vary from fine, dot-like opacities on the anterior lens surface to a central, lightly pigmented, pearl-like, opaque mass surrounded by smaller clumps of pigment. Corneal pigmentary changes occur almost invariably only in patients who have concomitant lens opacities. Corneal pigmentation occurs at the level of the endothelium and Descemet's membrane primarily in the interpalpebral fissure area. These ocular changes rarely reduce visual acuity, but patients may occasionally report glare, halos around lights or hazy vision. The pigmentary deposits are generally irreversible even when drug therapy is reduced or discontinued.

Indomethacin

The incidence of corneal toxicity associated with indomethacin therapy is 11% to 16%. The corneal lesions appear either as fine stromal, speckled opacities or have a

SYSTEMIC DRUGS AFFECTING THE EYE

Systemic Drug	Examples	Structure/Function Affected
Alcohol	alcohol	Extraocular muscles
Amiodarone	*Cordarone*	Cornea and lens
Antianxiety Agents	chlordiazepoxide (eg, *Librium)*	Extraocular muscles Causes cycloplegia
Anticholinergics	atropine scopolamine	Tear secretion Pupil (mydriasis) Causes cycloplegia
Antidepressants	amitriptyline (eg, *Elavil*)	Extraocular muscles Causes cycloplegia
Antihistamines	chlorpheniramine (eg, *Chlor-Trimeton*) diphenhydramine (eg, *Benadryl*)	Tear secretion Extraocular muscles Pupil (mydriasis) Causes cycloplegia
Antimalarials	chloroquine (eg, *Aralen Phosphate*) hydroxychloroquine (eg, *Plaquenil Sulfate*) quinacrine (eg, *Atabrine HCl*)	Cornea, lids, retina
Barbiturates	phenobarbital	Extraocular muscles
β-blockers	atenolol (eg, *Tenormin*)	Tear secretion Reduces intraocular pressure
Carbonic Anhydrase Inhibitors	acetazolamide (eg, *Diamox*)	Causes myopia
Central Nervous System Stimulants	amphetamines (eg, *Dexedrine*), cocaine, methylphenidate (eg, *Ritalin*)	Pupil (mydriasis) Lowers intraocular pressure
Chloramphenicol	eg, *Chloromycetin*	Optic nerve
Chlorpromazine	eg, *Thorazine*	Cornea and lens, lids Extraocular muscles
Corticosteroids	prednisone cortisol	Lens Elevates intraocular pressure
Digitalis Glycosides	digoxin (eg, *Lanoxin*)	Retina
Diuretics	hydrochlorothiazide (eg, *HydroDiuril*)	Causes myopia
Ethambutol	*Myambutol*	Optic nerve
Gold Salts	auranofin (*Ridaura*) gold sodium thiomalate (*Myochrysine*)	Cornea and lens Conjunctiva and lids Extraocular muscles
Indomethacin	eg, *Indocin*	Cornea, retina
Isotretinoin	*Accutane*	Conjunctiva and lids Tear secretion Retina
Opiates	morphine, codeine, heroin	Pupil (miosis)
Phenytoin	eg, *Dilantin*	Extraocular muscles
Psoralens	methoxsalen (*Oxsoralen*)	Cornea and lens
Quinine	eg, *Quinamm*	Retina
Salicylates	aspirin (eg, *Bayer*)	Extraocular muscles
Sulfonamides	sulfisoxazole (*Gantrisin*)	Causes myopia
Tamoxifen	*Nolvadex*	Retina
Tetracycline	eg, *Sumycin*	Conjunctiva and lens
Thioridazine	eg, *Mellaril*	Retina

whorl-like distribution resembling that of chloroquine keratopathy. These changes diminish or disappear within 6 months after discontinuing indomethacin. No definite relationship has been established between dosage of drug and corneal changes.

Photosensitizing Drugs

Photosensitizing drugs are compounds that absorb optical radiation and undergo a photochemical reaction, resulting in chemical modifications of tissue. The *psoralen* compounds are classic examples of photosensitizing drugs and are widely used by dermatologists to treat psoriasis and vitiligo. This treatment, commonly referred to as PUVA therapy, involves administering methoxsalen (*Oxsoralen*) or related compounds, followed by exposure to UV radiation. Cataract formation is well documented in patients undergoing PUVA therapy.

Gold Salts

Following prolonged administration, gold salts can be deposited in various tissues of the body, a condition known as chrysiasis. Ocular chrysiasis can involve the conjunctiva, cornea and lens. Corneal chrysiasis consists of numerous gold deposits that appear as yellowish-brown, violet or red particles distributed irregularly in the stroma. The deposition of gold usually spares the peripheral 1 to 3 mm and superior ¼ to ½ of the cornea, and the deposits tend to localize to the posterior stroma. Lenticular chrysiasis appears as fine dust-like, yellowish, glistening deposits in the anterior capsule or anterior subcapsular region.

Corticosteroids

Systemic steroids can produce posterior subcapsular (PSC) cataracts that are clinically indistinguishable from complicated cataracts and cataracts caused by exposure to ionizing radiation. They often cannot be distinguished from age-related PSC cataracts. Even if the steroid dosage is reduced or discontinued, the cataract usually remains unchanged. Visual impairment is rare in patients with steroid-induced PSC cataracts. Most patients retain visual acuity of 20/40 or better, but patients may report light sensitivity, frank photophobia, reading difficulty or glare.

Amiodarone

Amiodarone causes a distinctive keratopathy early in the course of treatment. The onset may be as early as 6 days following initiation of treatment, but it more commonly appears after 1 to 3 months of therapy. Virtually all patients will demonstrate corneal changes after 3 months of treatment. The corneal deposits are bilateral and are initially similar to the horizontal configuration of a Hudson-Stahli line, but eventually assume the configuration of a whorl-like opacity in the corneal epithelium. Once amiodarone therapy is discontinued, the keratopathy gradually resolves within 6 to 18 months. Lenticular opacities generally cause no visual symptoms, but moderate to severe keratopathy can lead to complaints of blurred vision, glare, halos around lights or light sensitivity. Visual acuity is usually normal.

DRUGS AFFECTING THE CONJUNCTIVA AND LIDS

Isotretinoin

Ocular complications of isotretinoin (*Accutane*) include blepharoconjunctivitis, dry eye symptoms, contact lens intolerance and subepithelial corneal opacities. There appears to be a dose-dependent relationship between isotretinoin therapy and blepharoconjunctivitis.

Chlorpromazine

Discoloration of the conjunctiva, sclera and exposed skin has been reported with phenothiazine therapy. The discoloration is usually slate blue. Melanin-like granules have been observed in the superficial dermis.

Tetracyclines

Conjunctival deposits similar to those seen in epinephrine-treated glaucoma patients have been reported in patients treated with oral tetracycline. These deposits appear as dark-brown to black granules in the palpebral conjunctiva. When observed under ultraviolet light, the brown pigment concentrations give a yellow fluorescence characteristic of tetracycline.

DRUGS THAT DECREASE AQUEOUS TEAR SECRETION

Anticholinergics

Dryness of mucous membranes is a common side effect of anticholinergic drugs since atropine and related agents inhibit glandular secretion in a dose-dependent manner.

Antihistamines

H_1 antihistamines have varying degrees of atropine-like actions including the ability to alter tear film integrity. Both aqueous and mucin production may decrease with use of systemic antihistamines.

Isotretinoin

Dry eye symptoms are commonly reported with use of systemic isotretinoin. The incidence has been estimated to be as high as 20%, and about 8% of patients experience contact lens intolerance.

Beta-Blockers

Reduced tear secretion is a reported side effect of oral β-blockers. Most of the reported cases have occurred with practolol (not available in the US), but other β-blockers have also been implicated in patients with dry eye syndrome.

DRUGS CAUSING MYDRIASIS

The iris is an excellent indicator of autonomic activity because of the delicate balance between adrenergic and cholinergic innervation to the iris dilator and sphincter muscles, respectively. Adrenergic and cholinergic agents can thus easily influence pupil size and activity.

Anticholinergics

Drugs with pronounced anticholinergic action, such as *atropine* or related compounds, can cause significant mydriasis. Systemic administration of at least 2 mg of atropine can cause pupillary dilation and cycloplegia. Both mydriasis and reduced pupillary light response can occur when transdermal scopolamine (*Transderm Scop*) is used for 3 or more days. This usually occurs through direct contamination of the eye by rubbing with fingers following application of the patch.

Central Nervous System Stimulants

Central nervous system stimulants, such as the *amphetamines, methylphenidate* and *cocaine*, can cause mydriasis. Likewise, central nervous system depressants, such as *phenobarbital* and the antianxiety agents, can dilate the pupil through their action on the adrenergic division of the autonomic nervous system.

DRUGS CAUSING MIOSIS

Opiates (eg, heroin, morphine and codeine) characteristically constrict the pupil. Systemically administered *anticholinesterase agents* can also cause miosis.

DRUGS AFFECTING EXTRAOCULAR MUSCLES

Drugs affecting the autonomic nervous system, central vestibular system, or causing extrapyramidal effects may cause nystagmus, diplopia, extraocular muscle palsy or oculogyric crisis. Nystagmus can be caused by intoxication with *salicylates, phenytoin, antihistamines, gold salts* and *barbiturates*. Diplopia has been associated with the *phenothiazines, antianxiety agents* and *antidepressants*. *Alcohol* can impair both smooth pursuits and saccades.

DRUGS CAUSING MYOPIA

Systemically administered *sulfonamides*, when given orally or as vaginal suppositories or creams, can induce transient myopia. The myopia is acute in onset and subsides within days or weeks following withdrawal of the medication. *Diuretics* and *carbonic anhydrase inhibitors* may also cause myopia.

DRUGS CAUSING CYCLOPLEGIA

Drugs with mild anticholinergic properties (eg, *antianxiety agents, antihistamines* and *tricyclic antidepressants)* and agents with strong anticholinergic effects (eg, *atropine* and *scopolamine*), can dilate the pupil and cause dry eye symptoms, but the cyloplegic effects are less commonly encountered in clinical practice. The most common drugs associated with clinical cycloplegia include *chloroquine* and the *phenothiazines*.

DRUGS AFFECTING INTRAOCULAR PRESSURE

Drugs known to be capable of dilating the pupil can cause acute or subacute angle-closure glaucoma if the anterior chamber angle is narrow. *Steroids* are widely known to elevate intraocular pressure in the presence of open angles. Other drugs, such as *β-blockers*, can reduce intraocular pressure.

DRUGS AFFECTING THE RETINA

Chloroquine and Hydroxychloroquine

Chloroquine maculopathy consists of a granular hyperpigmentation surrounded by a zone of depigmentation, which is surrounded by another ring of pigment. This clinical picture can vary in intensity, but is pathognomonic of chloroquine retinopathy and is referred to as a "bull's eye" lesion. Variations of pigmentary disturbances can occur, and some patients may show retinal changes resembling retinitis pigmentosa.

Thioridazine

Thioridazine can cause significant retinal toxicity, leading to reduced visual acuity, color vision changes and disturbances of dark adaptation. These symptoms usually occur 30 to 90 days after treatment is begun. The fundus appearance is often normal during the early stages, but within several weeks or months a pigmentary retinopathy develops, characterized by clumps of pigment developing first in the periphery and then progressing toward the posterior pole.

Quinine

Acute vision loss is common in *quinine* toxicity (eg, overdose due to attempted suicide) and frequently consists of a clinical presentation of no light perception along with dilated and nonreactive pupils. In the early stages, visual fields usually demonstrate concentric contraction, and improvement of the visual fields may require days or months, but the field loss can sometimes become permanent.

Talc

Tablets of medication intended for oral use contain inert filler materials, such as talc (magnesium silicate), cornstarch, cotton fibers and other substances. Chronic drug abusers may prepare a suspension of medication for injection by dissolving the crushed tablet of *cocaine, methylphenidate, codeine* or other narcotic in water. The solution is then boiled and filtered through a crude cigarette or cotton filter prior to injection. The talc particles eventually embolize to the retinal circulation and produce a characteristic form of retinopathy. Multiple, tiny, yellow-white, glistening particles are scattered throughout the posterior pole and are more numerous in the capillary bed and small arterioles of the perimacular area. Retinal neovascularization can also occur.

Cardiac Glycosides

Digitoxin and *digoxin* can cause changes in color vision and impairment of vision. Various visual phenomena often precede cardiac abnormalities as the earliest symptoms of digitoxin intoxication. A common symptom is snowy vision, wherein objects appear to be covered with frost or snow.

Indomethacin

Indomethacin can induce pigmentary changes of the macula and other areas of the retina. The lesions usually consist of discrete pigment scattering and fine areas of depigmentation around the macula.

Tamoxifen

Tamoxifen can cause white or yellow refractile opacities in the macular and paramacular area, with or without macular edema. The patient can experience reduced visual acuity associated with the macular lesions, and the visual fields can demonstrate abnormalities.

Isotretinoin

Isotretinoin therapy in dosages of 1 mg/kg body weight daily can impair dark adaptation with or without excessive glare sensitivity. Once therapy is discontinued, both the abnormal dark adaptation and abnormal electroretinogram (ERG) usually resolve within several months.

DRUGS AFFECTING THE OPTIC NERVE

Ethambutol

Ethambutol can cause ocular symptoms of reduced visual acuity, color vision changes and visual field loss. Signs of ocular toxicity can appear several weeks following initial therapy, but the onset of ocular complications usually occurs several months after treatment is begun. The primary ocular manifestation of ethambutol toxicity is retrobulbar neuritis.

Chloramphenicol

Chloramphenicol causes both optic neuritis and retrobulbar neuritis. There is severe bilateral reduction of visual acuity accompanied by dense central scotomas. The optic discs are usually edematous and hyperemic, the retinal veins are engorged and tortuous and hemorrhages are often seen. Optic atrophy is a late complication.

Jimmy D. Bartlett OD, DOS
University of Alabama at Birmingham

For More Information

Bartlett JD, Jaanus SD, eds. Clinical Ocular Pharmacology, ed. 2. Boston, MA: Butterworth, 1989.

Bartlett JD. Ophthalmic toxicity by systemic drugs. In: Chiou GCH, ed. Ophthalmic Toxicology. New York, NY: Raven Press, 1993;169-219.

Fraunfelder FT. Drug Induced Ocular Side Effects and Drug Interactions. Philadelphia, PA: Lea & Febiger, 1989.

Fraunfelder FT, Meyer SM. The national registry of drug-induced ocular side effects. *J Toxicol Cutaneous Ocul Toxicol* 1982;1:65-70.

Grant WM. Toxicology of the Eye, ed. 2. Springfield, IL: Charles C. Thomas, 1974.

Koneru PB, et al. Oculotoxicities of systemically administered drugs. *J Ocul Pharmacol* 1986;2:385-404.

Drugs With Unlabeled Ophthalmic Uses

For many years, the drug package insert was interpreted as a legal standard for drug use. However, the legal implications of the package insert have been challenged, and in some cases, various courts have recognized that drugs may be used for clinical indications other than those specified in the package insert. It is possible for prescribed dosage schedules to differ from those specified in the package insert if such a schedule is consistent with sound scientific rationale and medical practice. It has not, however, been clearly established whether an approved drug may be used for an unapproved (unlabeled) purpose without first obtaining an application for an Investigational New Drug (IND).

Since it has been recognized that the package insert may not contain the most recent information about a drug, it is now generally agreed that the clinician should be free to use a drug for an indication not in the package insert if two conditions have been met:

1. When such use is part of the rational practice of medicine intended for the benefit of the patient;

2. Documented evidence exists for use of a drug in the manner prescribed.

Under these circumstances an IND is not required; however, if the drug has not been demonstrated to be useful for an unlabeled purpose, then it is considered to be experimental, and an IND should be obtained.

When using an approved drug for an unlabeled purpose, the patient should be informed regarding the nature of the intended therapy, and the practitioner is advised to obtain the patient's written permission (informed consent) before beginning treatment. Since drug-related side effects are a significant cause of malpractice litigations, it is essential that patients understand the risks of potential side effects. In determining what constitutes sound medical practice in malpractice litigations, the package insert is admissible into evidence, but it does not establish conclusively the standards of acceptable practice or that departure from the directions contained in the package insert constitutes negligence. One of the best protections against un-favorable malpractice verdicts is to prescribe medications in the best interests of the patient according to rational standards of practice.

The drugs listed in the following table have been approved by the Food and Drug Administration (FDA), but not for the ophthalmic purposes listed. Each agent, how-ever, has been documented to be useful for the diagnosis or therapy of certain ocu-lar conditions.

DRUGS WITH UNLABELED OPHTHALMIC USES		
Generic *(Trade)*	Labeled Indication	Unlabeled Ophthalmic Use
Acetylcysteine *(Mucomyst)*	Mucolytic agent in broncho-pulmonary conditions	Topical mucolytic treatment of vernal, giant papillary conjunctivi-tis, filamentary keratitis
Acyclovir *(Zovirax)*	Treatment of genital herpes simplex	Treatment of epithelial HSV keratitis
Aminocaproic acid *(Amicar)*	Antifibrinolytic agent for the treat-ment of excessive bleeding	Oral treatment of traumatic hyphema
Aspirin (eg, *Bayer*)	Anti-inflammatory, analgesic, anti-pyretic agent	Oral treatment of vernal conjunctivitis
Fluorescein sodium (eg, *Fluorescite*)	Topical or IV diagnostic ophthalmic dye	Oral fluorography for diagnosis of retinal vascular diseases
Sodium hyaluronate *(Amvisc)* Chondroitin sulfate *(Viscoat)*	Viscoelastic agents in intraocular surgery	Topical treatment of severe dry eye disorders
Suprofen *(Profenal)*	Prevention of intraoperative miosis during cataract extraction	Topical treatment of contact lens-associated GPC

ACETYLCYSTEINE

Acetylcysteine *(Mucomyst)* has been approved for use as a mucolytic agent in acute and chronic bronchopulmonary conditions. The agent is administered by nebulization for its local effect on the bronchopulmonary tree. The product contains disodium edetate and sodium hydroxide and, thus, has a significant odor accompanying its clinical use. When used on the eye, acetylcysteine dissolves mucous threads and decreases tear viscosity. The drug is commonly prepared for topical ocular use by diluting the commercial preparation to 2% to 5% in artificial tears or physiologic saline.

ACYCLOVIR

Acyclovir *(Zovirax)* has been approved for treatment of genital herpes simplex (HSV). During initial episodes of the disease, oral acyclovir can decrease the duration of viral shedding and healing time of the genital lesions, decrease the severity of symp-toms and reduce the development of new lesions. Acyclovir ointment is also approved for treatment of initial genital herpes, and IV acyclovir seems to be effec-tive for severe initial episodes of the disease. Acyclovir is also the treatment of choice for biopsy-proven herpes simplex encephalitis. In the treatment of HSV kerati-tis, 3% acyclovir ointment may be useful to treat epithelial involvement. Although acyclovir is effective for treating HSV epithelial keratitis, there is no clear superiority of the drug when compared with other commercially available antiviral agents.

AMINOCAPROIC ACID

Aminocaproic acid (eg, *Amicar*) is an antifibrinolytic agent approved for treatment of excessive bleeding from systemic hyperfibrinolysis and urinary fibrinolysis. The drug may also be useful for the treatment of some patients with traumatic hyphema. Some studies have shown the drug to be effective in reducing the rate of rebleeding from about 30% to 3% or 4%. Dosage is 100 mg/kg body weight every 4 hours to a maximum dose of 30 g daily. It may be possible to administer one-half of this dosage to reduce side effects while maintaining efficacy. It has been established that the drug is ineffective in children.

ASPIRIN

The efficacy of salicylates in the treatment of ocular inflammation has been infrequently studied in human models, but several reports have suggested that aspirin may be valuable for intractable cases of vernal conjunctivitis. Patients who remain symptomatic following treatment with cromolyn sodium, steroids, or a combination of agents may demonstrate improvement in both symptoms and signs when aspirin is added to the therapeutic regimen.

FLUORESCEIN SODIUM

Fluorescein sodium (eg, *Fluorescite*) is approved for topical and IV use (Ophthalmic Dyes, p. 12). Oral fluorography was reintroduced in 1979, allowing fluorescein studies without the potential systemic effects attributable to IV fluorescein. Various studies using oral fluorography have established this technique as a viable alternative for the diagnosis of certain retinal vascular diseases. The procedure is especially useful for conditions in which late dye leakage is expected. Oral fluorography is performed using either bulk powder fluorescein sodium USP or the commercially available vials of 10% injectable fluorescein sodium. The dosage typically used is 1000 mg to 1500 mg of fluorescein sodium mixed with a citrus drink and allowed to cool in crushed ice.

VISCOELASTIC AGENTS

Sodium hyaluronate *(Amvisc)* and chondroitin sulfate *(Viscoat)*, are approved as vitreous replacement substances and for use during intraocular surgery to protect the corneal endothelium (p. 202). When prepared as a 0.1% topical solution in saline, sodium hyaluronate may be beneficial for patients with severe dry eye syndromes. The beneficial effects of sodium hyaluronate have been attributed to its viscoelastic properties, which lubricate and protect the ocular surface. Most patients achieve control of symptoms with topical instillation up to 4 times daily.

SUPROFEN

When used as a 1% solution, topically applied suprofen, a propionic acid derivative, has been shown to be superior to placebo in the treatment of contact lens-associated giant papillary conjunctivitis (GPC). In a randomized, double-masked comparison, suprofen provided a greater reduction of both signs and symptoms such as papillae and mucous strands.

Jimmy D. Bartlett OD, DOS
University of Alabama at Birmingham

For More Information

Absolon MJ, Brown S. Acetylcysteine in keratoconjunctivitis sicca. *Br J Ophthalmol* 1968;52:310-16.

Collum LMT, et al. Randomized double-blind trial of acyclovir and idoxuridine in dendritic corneal ulceration. *Br J Ophthalmol* 1980;64:766-69.

DeLuise VP, Peterson WS. The use of topical Healon tears in the management of refractory dry-eye syndrome. *Ann Ophthalmol* 1984;1:823-24.

Duane TD, ed. Clinical Ophthamalogy. Philadelphia, PA: J.B. Lippincott Company, 1988.

Hung SO, et al. Oral acyclovir in the management of dendritic herpetic corneal ulceration. *Br J Ophthalmol* 1984;68:398-400.

Irwin R. Practical aspects of oral fluorography. *J Ophthal Photog* 1981;4:16-18.

Jackson WB, et al. Treatment of herpes simplex keratitis: Comparison of acyclovir and vidarabine. *Can J Ophthalmol* 1984;19:107-111.

Kelley JS, Kincaid M. Retinal fluorography using oral fluorescein. *Arch Ophthalmol* 1979;97:2331-32.

Kraft SP, et al. Traumatic hyphema in children. Treatment with epsilon-aminocaproic acid. *Ophthalmology* 1987;94:1232-37.

Kutner B, et al. Aminocaproic acid reduces the risk of secondary hemorrhage in patients with traumatic hyphema. *Arch Ophthalmol* 1987;105:206-08.

Limberg MB, et al. Topical application of hyaluronic acid and chondroitin sulfate in treatment of dry eyes. *Am J Ophthalmol* 1987;103:194-97.

McGetrick JJ, et al. Aminocaproic acid decreases secondary hemorrhage after traumatic hyphema. *Arch Ophthalmol* 1983;101:1031-33.

Mengher LS, et al. Effect of sodium hyaluronate (0.1%) on break-up time (NIBUT) in patients with dry eyes. *Br J Ophthalmol* 1986;70:442-47.

Meyer E, et al. Efficacy of antiprostaglandin therapy in vernal conjunctivitis. *Br J Ophthalmol* 1987;71:497-99.

Mindel JS, Goldstein JI. Non-approved use of Food and Drug Administration approved drugs. *Am J Ophthalmol* 1979;88:626-28.

Noble MJ, Cheng H. Oral fluorescein and cystoid macular edema: Detection in aphakic and pseudophakic eyes. *Br J Ophthalmol* 1984;68:221-24.

Palmer DJ, et al. A comparison of two dose regimens of epsilon aminocaproic acid in the prevention and management of secondary traumatic hyphemas. *Ophthalmology* 1986;93:102-08.

Potter JW, et al. Oral fluorography. *J Am Optom Assoc* 1985;56:784-92.

Roth SH. Drug use, the package insert, and the practice of medicine. *Arch Intern Med* 1982;142:871-72.

Stuart JC, Linn JG. Dilute sodium hyaluronate (*Healon*) in the treatment of ocular surface disorders. *Ann Ophthalmol* 1985;17:190-92.

Wood TS, et al. Suprofen treatment of contact lens associated GPC. *Ophthalmology* 1988;96:822-26.

Orphan and Investigational Drugs

In addition to the Food and Drug Administration (FDA) approved drugs and the drugs with unlabeled ophthalmic uses (p. 271), two other groups of drugs are of interest to eye-care practitioners: Investigational New Drugs (INDs) and Orphan drugs. INDs are drugs currently under investigation by the FDA. Orphan drugs are drugs made available by manufacturers for rare diseases.

ORPHAN DRUGS

The term "orphan drug" first appeared in the medical literature in a 1968 editorial. It was used to disclaim nonapproved substances as drugs and included compounds such as lithium carbonate, d-xylose and sodium fluoride. These products were frequently labeled "for chemical purposes, not for drug use," "for research use only, not for clinical use," and "for manufacturing use only." Orphan drug has since been applied to drugs and devices used in the treatment or diagnosis of rare diseases.

The FDA established the Office of Orphan Products Development in 1982. These products consist of drugs, biologicals (eg, vaccines), medical devices and foods for the diagnosis, treatment or prevention of rare diseases.

GOVERNMENT INCENTIVES TO ASSIST IN ORPHAN DRUG DEVELOPMENT

♦ Developers of orphan drugs have 7 years of exclusive licensing, during which time the product may not be marketed by another company in the US without the sponsor's permission.

♦ Developers may claim up to 63% of the cost of clinical investigations as a tax credit.

♦ The FDA can grant up to $70,000 in support of a sponsor's orphan drug clinical research. The Orphan Drug Act authorizes $4,000,000 per year for these research grants.

♦ The FDA can assist sponsors of orphan drugs in the development of investigational guidelines and protocols.

♦ When appropriate, the FDA can modify approval requirements for specific orphan drugs (eg, modify the size of study populations).

♦ The FDA can assign to orphan drugs a high review priority. The review phase (time from a new drug application submission to approval) for nine orphan drugs receiving approval in 1985 and 1986 was 2.7 years.

Tatro, DS. Orphan drugs. *Drug Newsletter* 1988 Apr;7(4):26.

Ophthalmic drugs established by the FDA as Orphan Drugs are listed below. Orphan Drugs that have bibliographies in *Ophthalmic Drug Facts* are indicated by an asterisk (*) following the generic drug name.

ORPHAN DRUGS		
Drug Generic *(Trade)*	**Indication**	**Manufacturer/Sponsor**
Bromhexine *(Bisolvon)*	Treatment of mild to moderate kerato-conjunctivitis sicca in patients with Sjogren's Syndrome.	Boehringer Ingelheim 90 East Ridge P.O. Box 368 Ridgefield, CT 06877
Clostridium Botulinum Toxin Type A *(Dysport)*	Treatment of blepharospasm.	Porton Products, Ltd. 727 15th Street, NW Washington, DC 20005
Clostridium Botulinum Type F Neurotoxin	Treatment of spasmodic torticollis and essential blepharospasm.	Porton Products, Ltd. 727 15th Street, NW Washington, DC 20005
Cyclosporine *(Optimmune)*	Treatment of severe keratoconjunctivitis sicca associated with Sjogren's Syndrome.	University of Georgia College of Veterinary Medicine Athens, GA 30602
Cyclosporine 2% Ophthalmic Ointment *(Sandimmune)*	Treatment of high risk corneal transplant and keratoconjunctivitis sicca associated with Sjogren's Syndrome.	Sandoz Corporation 59 Route 10 East Hanover, NJ 07936
Dehydrex	Treatment of recurrent corneal erosion unresponsive to conventional therapy.	Holles Labs 30 Forest Notch Cohasset, MA 02025
Epidermal Growth Factor, Human	Acceleration of corneal epithelial re-generation and healing of stromal incisions from corneal transplant surgery and in non-healing corneal defects.	Chiron Corporation 4560 Horton Street Emeryville, CA 94608
Fibronectin	Treatment of non-healing corneal ulcers or epithelial defects that have been unresponsive to conventional therapy and whose underlying cause has been eliminated.	Chiron Ophthalmics with New York Blood Center 310 E. 67th Street New York, NY 10021
Filgrastim (granulocyte colony stimulating factor [G-CSF]); *(Neupogen)*	Treatment of AIDS patients with CMV treated with ganciclovir.	Amgen Inc. 1900 Oak Terrace Lane Thousand Oaks, CA 91320-1789
Gangliosides, Sodium Salts *(Cronassial)*	Treatment of retinitis pigmentosa.	Fidia Pharmaceutical Corp. 1775 K Street, NW Washington, DC 20006
GM-6001 *(Galardin)*	Treatment of corneal ulcers, topical formulation.	Glycomed, Inc.
Levocabastine 0.05%*	Treatment of vernal keratoconjunctivitis.	Iolab Pharmaceuticals 500 Iolab Drive Claremont, CA 91711
Lodoxamide tromethamine (Alomide)	Treatment of vernal conjunctivitis.	Alcon Labs
Pilocarpine HCl	Treatment of xerostomia induced by radiation therapy for head and neck cancer; xerostomia and keratoconjunctivitis sicca in Sjogren's syndrome.	MGI Pharma, Inc.

* Bibliography available in *Ophthalmic Drug Facts*.

ORPHAN DRUGS		
Drug Generic *(Trade)*	Indication	Manufacturer/Sponsor
Ofloxacin	Treatment of bacterial corneal ulcers.	Allergan, Inc. 2525 DuPont Dr. Irvine, CA 92713-1599
Propamidine 0.1% *(Brolene)*	Treatment of Acanthamoeba keratitis.	Bausch and Lomb, Inc. 1400 N. Goodman Street Rochester, NY 14692
Thymoxamine HCl* *(Thymoxid)*	Reversal of phenylephrine-induced mydriasis in patients who have narrow anterior angles and are at risk of developing an acute attack of angle-closure glaucoma following mydriasis.	Iolab Pharmaceuticals 500 Iolab Drive Claremont, CA 91711
Tretinoin	Squamous metaplasia of the ocular surface epithelia (conjunctiva and/or cornea) with mucous deficiency and keratinization.	Spectra Pharmaceuticals 155 Webster Street Hanover, MA 02339
Vision AID	Treatment of Retinitis pigmentosa.	Platon J. Collipp, MD

The Orphan Drug Act has provided an environment for the development of products for rare diseases and should continue to facilitate this process. In 1984, the Orphan Drug Act was amended to define a rare disease or condition as that which (a) affects fewer than 200,000 persons or (b) affects more than 200,000 persons and for which the manufacturing company has no reasonable prospect of recovering research and development costs from sales within the US. Occasionally, a drug which is already commercially available may achieve orphan status for an indication that does not involve a large patient population. The incentives provided by both the Orphan Drug Act and other federal initiatives make it possible for commercial manufacturers to produce drugs for FDA approval at minimal costs. Individuals with rare diseases can be assured that efforts will continue to be made to find a treatment.

Published information about orphan drugs is made available by various agencies. These sources can be contacted to obtain information about the acquisition or availability of an orphan drug product.

INFORMATION SOURCES FOR RARE DISEASES AND ORPHAN DRUG TREATMENT		
Organization	Information	Telephone
National Organization for Rare Disorders (NORD) 1182 Broadway, Suite 402 New York, NY 10001	Information on rare diseases and their treatment	(203) 746-6518
Federal Register: Dockets Management Branch (HFA-305) Food and Drug Administration Room 4-62 5600 Fishers Lane Rockville, MD 20857	List of orphan drugs and biologicals, designated uses, sponsor's name and address. Available under Docket #84N-0102	not available
National Information Center for Orphan Drugs and Rare Diseases (NICODARD) P.O. Box 1133, Department HP Washington, DC 20013-1133	General information on orphan drugs and rare diseases	(800) 456-3505 (301) 565-4167
Office of Orphan Products Development (HF-35) Food and Drug Administration 5600 Fishers Lane Rockville, MD 20857	Technical information on orphan drug product development, product availability, research grants, drug sponsorship	(301) 443-4718

Tatro, DS. Orphan Drugs. *Drug Newsletter* 1988 Apr;7(4):26.
* Bibliography available in *Ophthalmic Drug Facts.*

INVESTIGATIONAL NEW DRUGS

The FDA is responsible for determining if a new drug is safe and effective before it is approved for marketing. During the IND process, scientific and statistical information about the drug is gathered. The FDA cannot release information pertaining to formulas, manufacturing processes or identification of patients involved in clinical trials. However, the Freedom of Information Act does allow release of specially prepared information which does not contain trade or confidential information.

NEW DRUG DEVELOPMENT		
Stage	Description	Duration
Preclinical Trials	Research and development, initial drug synthesis and animal testing	1 to 3 years (average 18 months)
IND filing	Allows interstate transport and human testing	30 days
Clinical Trials		2 to 10 years (average 5 years)
Phase I:	Determine drug safety, tolerance, pharmacokinetics. In 20 to 100 normal adult males.	Several months
Phase II:	Given to 100 to 200 people with the disease to determine effectiveness and dose response.	Up to 2 years
Phase III:	Assessment of safety and efficacy in 800 to 1000 patients. Studies include drug interactions, use in the elderly and in liver and kidney disease.	1 to 4 years
NDA Review	NDA submitted to FDA for approval to market	2 months to 7 years (average 24 months)
Post-market surveillance	Adverse reaction reporting, survey/samples and inspections	Ongoing

A practitioner may obtain a Treatment IND allowing the use of IND drugs in a controlled situation. There are two ways to obtain a Treatment IND: 1) Contact the drug sponsor or 2) contact the FDA directly.

The sponsor usually provides a practitioner with technical information about the drug and a description of the approved treatment protocol. When the sponsor is unwilling to provide the treatment protocol, an individual may contact the FDA. The practitioner must meet all of the FDA's requirements for a Treatment IND. The FDA must respond to the request for a Treatment IND within 30 days of the application.

Selected ophthalmic drugs currently undergoing investigation by the FDA are listed on the following table. Investigational drugs which have bibliographies in *Ophthalmic Drug Facts* are indicated by an asterisk (*) following the drug name. Every effort has been made to ensure the information in the table is accurate. However, information on investigational drugs is often incomplete.

INVESTIGATIONAL DRUGS			
Drug Name Generic *(Trade)*	**Developmen- tal Stage**	**Class/Use**	**Manufacturer/ Sponsor**
Acarbose *(Glucobay)*	NDA pending	Treatment of diabetic retinopathy.	Miles Inc.
Anakinra *(Antril)*	Development	Treatment of ocular inflammation, primarily allergic conjunctivitis.	Insite Vision
Anakinra (interleukin-1 [IL-1] receptor antagonist) *(Antril)*	Development	Treatment for ocular inflammation, primarily allergic conjunctivitis.	Synergen, Inc.
Azelastine HCl	Development	Eyedrop formulation (ophthalmological indications; pediatric use).	Wallace Laboratories
Brimonidine	Phase III	Treatment for glaucoma.	Allergan, Inc.
	Phase III	Treatment of intraocular pressure spike post-laser surgery.	Allergan, Inc.
Bromhexine[1] *(Bisolvon)*	Clinicals	For treatment of mild to moderate keratoconjunctivitis sicca in patients with Sjogrens syndrome.	Boehringer Ingelheim
Carbomer gel	Phase II	Treatment of moderate to severe dry eye syndromes.	Alcon
CI-949	Phase 1/11	Treatment of allergic and inflammatory conditions, including conjunctivitis.	Parke-Davis Group (Warner-Lambert)
Colforsin	Phase II	For treatment of glaucoma.	Hoechst AG
Corneal Mortar	Preclinicals	Wound healing agent for use in radial keratotomy.	Chiron Corporation
Dexamethasone	Clinicals	Anti-inflammatory, using Molecusol delivery system.	Pharmatec, Inc.
Dorzolamide (Trusopt)	Phase III	Topical carbonic anhydrase inhibitor for glaucoma.	Merck
Ebastine (RP-64305)	Phase III	Treatment for seasonal or perennial allergic rhinitis with conjunctivitis.	Rhone-Poulenc Rorer, Inc.
Epidermal Growth Factor (EGF)	Clinicals	Healing agent for use in eye injuries, corneal ulcers, corneal transplants and radial keratotomy procedures.	Alcon with Creative Biomolecules
	Phase I/II trials inactive	For corneal ulcers and corneal transplants.	Amgen
	Phase II	For corneal defects and ophthalmic surgeries.	Chiron Ophthalmics
Ethacrynic Acid (EY-105)	Phase I/II	Drug incorporating ELY-105 to increase intraocular pressure following eye surgery.	Telor Ophthalmic
	Preclinicals	Drug incorporating EY-105 for long-term use in controlling intraocular pressure and glaucoma.	Telor Ophthalmic
Fibronectin[1]	Phase III	For treatment of corneal wounds and keratitis sicca. For unresponsive non-healing corneal ulcers or epithelial defects.	Chiron Ophthalmics and New York Blood Center

* Bibliography available in *Ophthalmic Drug Facts*.
[1] Orphan Drug.

INVESTIGATIONAL DRUGS (Cont.)			
Drug Name Generic *(Trade)*	Developmen- tal Stage	Class/Use	Manufacturer/ Sponsor
Fluorometholone *(MethaSite)*[1]	NDA Pending (Approvable March 1991)	For treatment of allergic conjunctivi- tis and reduction of post-operative eye inflammation.	Insite Vision
Fluorometholone *(MethaSite)*[1]	Approvable March 9, 1991	For treatment of allergic conjunctivi- tis and reduction of post-operative eye inflammation.	CIBA-GEIGY Corporation
Foscarnet Sodium (Trisodium phosphonoformate)		Combined with dideoxyinosine (ddl) *(Videx)*/treatment of CMV retinitis.	Astra Pharma- ceutical Pro- ducts, Inc. (AB Astra)
Ganciclovir (DHPG) (RS-21592-000)	Phase III	Combined with beta interferon (IFN)/ treatment of CMV retinitis, IV formulation.	Syntex Corporation
Ganciclovir-CDS	Development	Treatment of cytomegalovirus infec- tions of the brain and retina, using chemical delivery system (CDS).	Pharmatec, Inc.
Gangliosides, Highly Purified *(Cronassial)*[2]	Phase II	For treatment of retinitis pigmentosa.	Fidia Pharmaceutical
Human Superoxide Dismutase (hSOD)	Preclinicals	To block onset of cataracts.	Nova Pharma- ceutical with Duke University
Hyaluronic Acid (HA)*	NDA filed	For use in ophthalmic surgery.	Alcon Labs with Genzyme
Hyaluronic Acid (HA)	Clinicals	Artificial tears for treatment of dry eye syndrome and for ophthalmic surgery.	Bio-Technology General Corp.
(Hyall)	PMA filed	For use in ophthalmic surgery.	Fidia Pharma- ceutical/Spectra Pharmaceutical
(OP-DOO5)	Recommended for approval by FDA commit- tee	For use in ophthalmic surgery.	Walnut Pharma- ceuticals (Akorn) with Staar Surgical
Immunotoxin, monoclonal anti- body (MAb)-based	Research	Proliferative vitreoretinopathy.	Houston Biotech- nology, Inc.
Indomethacin *(Indocin Ophthalmic Solution)*	NDA pending	For prevention of aphakic cystoid macular edema.	Merck
Ketanserin	IND filing planned Feb. 1990	For treatment of post-surgical intraocular pressure control.	Iolab Pharmaceuticals
Ketorolac *(Toradol)**	NDA pending	For treatment of post-surgical eye inflammation and cystoid macular edema.	Syntex
Levobunolol[1] (BetaSite)	Phase I/II	Treatment of glaucoma.	Insite Vision
Levobunolol/ Dipivefrin HCl	Phase III	Treatment of glaucoma.	Allergan, Inc.

* Bibliography available in *Ophthalmic Drug Facts*.
[1] DuraSite extended release delivery system.
[2] Orphan Drug.

INVESTIGATIONAL DRUGS (Cont.)			
Drug Name Generic *(Trade)*	Developmen- tal Stage	Class/Use	Manufacturer/ Sponsor
Levocabastine*	NDA filed	For treatment of allergic conjunctivitis.	Iolab Pharma-ceuticals with Johnson & Johnson
	Phase III[1]	For treatment of vernal keratoconjunctivitis.	Iolab Pharma-ceuticals with KV Pharmaceutical
Lodoxamide*	NDA filed	Mast cell inhibitor for treatment of vernal conjunctivitis.	Alcon Labora-tories Inc.
Loteprednol	Phase III	For treatment of giant papillary con-junctivitis and seasonal allergic conjunctivitis.	Xenon Vision
Metipranolol Hydrochloride (0.1%) *(OptiPranolol Ophthalmic Solution)*	NDA pending	For use in lowering intraocular pres-sure in patients with ocular hyper-tension or chronic open angle glaucoma.	Bausch & Lomb Pharmaceuticals Division (Bausch & Lomb, Inc.)
Metipranolol Hydrochloride/ Pilocarpine	Phase I	Combination product for lowering intraocular pressure in patients with ocular hypertension or chronic open angle glaucoma.	Bausch & Lomb Pharmaceuticals Division (Bausch & Lomb, Inc.)
Molgramostim (granulocyte macro-phage colony stimu-lating factor [GM-CSF]); *(Leucomax)*	Phase III	Biosynthetic granulocyte macro-phage colony stimulating factor (GM-CSF) in combination with ganciclovir *(Cytovene)*/treatment of CMV retinitis.	Sandoz Corporation
	Clinicals	Biosynthetic GM-CSF in combination with ganciclovir (DHPG, *Cytovene*)/ treatment for CMV retinitis, inj. form.	Schering-Plough Corporation
MSI-239	Preclinicals	Combined with erythromycin/oph-thalmic anti-infective, treatment for gram positive and gram negative bacteria including staphylococcus epidermis and gentamicin-resistant pseudomonas, topical solution (eye drop) formulation.	Magainin Phar-maceuticals, Inc.
MSI-404	Preclinicals	Anti-infective active against Acan-thamoeba, topical solution (eye drop) formulation.	Magainin Phar-maceuticals, Inc.
MSI-420	Preclinicals	Treatment for wound healing, pro-motion of corneal epitheliazation, topical (eye drop) formulation.	Magainin Phar-maceuticals, Inc.
Naboctate	Phase I	Antiglaucoma agent, oral dosage form.	H.G. Pars Phar-maceuticals Laboratories
	Phase II	Antiglaucoma agent, topical dosage form.	H.G. Pars Phar-maceuticals Laboratories
	Phase II (oral) Phase II (topical)	For treatment of glaucoma.	H.G. Pars Phar-maceutical Labs
OcuNex	Phase II	Treatment of dry eye syndrome, using RGD matrix peptide technol-ogy and promotion of healing after eye injuries, infections or eye surgery.	Telios Pharmaceuticals

* Bibliography available in *Ophthalmic Drug Facts.*

INVESTIGATIONAL DRUGS (Cont.)			
Drug Name Generic *(Trade)*	**Developmen- tal Stage**	**Class/Use**	**Manufacturer/ Sponsor**
Ofloxacin *(Oflox)*	NDA pending	Quinolone antibiotic, eye-drop formulation.	Allergan, Inc.
Pentigetide *(Pentyde)**	NDA pending	Human IgE (B) pentapeptide for treatment of allergic conjunctivitis.	Bausch and Lomb from Immunetech
Peptides	Research	Treatment for autoimmune diseases affecting the eye and peripheral and central nervous system.	Houston Bio-technology, Inc.
Phospholipase A-2 inhibitors (PLA-2)	Preclinicals	Anti-inflammatory.	Biogen, Inc.
Pilocarpine	Phase III	For treatment of glaucoma.	CIBA-GEIGY Corporation (CIBA-GEIGY Limited)
Pilocarpine *(PilaSite)*[1]	Phase III	For treatment of glaucoma.	Insite Vision
	Development	For treatment of glaucoma. Sustained release.	Liposome licensed to Escalen Ophthalmics
Porfimer sodium *(Photofrin)*	Phase II/III	Periocular and orbital neoplasms.	Quadra Logic Technologies/ American Cyanamid
Procaterol Ophthalmic	Phase II	Treatment of allergic conjunctivitis, solution formulation.	Otsuka America, Inc. (Otsuka Pharmaceutical)
Propamidine Isethionate 0.1% *(Brolene)**[2]	Phase III (patient enroll-ment terminated)	For treatment of Acanthamoeba keratitis.	Bausch and Lomb
Prostaglandin Prodrug	Phase I	Treatment of glaucoma.	Allergan, Inc.
Protein Phase Separation Inhibitors *(Opacitrol)*	Preclinicals	New class of compounds for prevention and retardation of cataracts/topical, oral and parenteral forms.	Oculon Corporation
Sorbinil	Phase II/III	Aldose reductase inhibitor.	Pfizer Laboratories
Tepoxalin	Phase II	For inhibition of intra-operative miosis; ocular inflammation.	Iolab Pharmaceuticals
Thymoxamine HCl *(Thymoxid)**[2]	NDA withdrawn	To reverse phenylephrine-induced mydriasis in patients with narrow anterior angles and a risk of developing acute angle-closure glaucoma following mydriasis.	Iolab Pharmaceuticals
Timolol (Gelrite)	Phase II/III	For treatment of glaucoma.	Merck
Timolol Maleate/ Pilocarpine *(Timpilo)*	NDA pending	Combination product for treatment of glaucoma.	Merck
Tissue Inhibitor of Metalloproteinase (TIMP)	Research	Treatment of corneal ulceration.	Celltech Ltd.
Tretinoin *(Lacramore)*	Clinicals	Stevens-Johnson syndrome (dry eye)[2] in active ocular pemphigoid.	Spectra Pharmaceutical

* Bibliography available in *Ophthalmic Drug Facts.*
[1] DuraSite extended release delivery system.
[2] Orphan Drug.

For Information on Investigational New Drugs

Hyaluronic Acid

Ahn JC, Seiff SR. Locating cut medial canaliculi by direct injection of sodium hyaluronate into the lacrimal sac. *Ophthalmic Surg* 1989 Mar;20(3):176-78.

Alpar AJ, et al. Comparison of *Healon* and *Viscoat* in cataract extraction and intraocular lens implantation. *Ophthalmic Surg* 1988 Sep;19(9):636-42.

Alpar JJ. Endothelial cell loss in different non-automated extracapsular nuclear evacuation techniques and the role of sodium hyaluronate. *Ophthalmic Surg* 1986 Nov;17(11):719-23.

Alpar JJ. Sodium hyaluronate in glaucoma filtering procedures. *Ophthalmic Surg* 1986 Nov;17(11):724-30.

Alpar JJ. The use of *Healon* in corneal transplant surgery with and without intraocular lenses. *Ophthalmic Surg* 1984 Sep;15(9):757-60.

Baldwin LB, et al. The use of visoelastic substances in the drainage of postoperative suprachoroidal hemorrhage. *Ophthalmic Surg* 1989 Jul;20(7):504-07.

Berke S, et al. Comparison of the effects of two viscoelastic agents, *Healon* and *Viscoat,* on postoperative intraocular pressure after penetrating keratoplasty. *Ophthalmic Surg* 1990;21:821-26.

Boyd JE, Glasser DB. Protective effects of viscous solutions in phacoemulsification and traumatic lens implantation. *Arch Ophthalmol* 1989 Jul;107(7):1047-51.

Broocker G, Lazenby GW. The use of sodium hyaluronate in intracapsular cataract extraction with insertion of anterior chamber intraocular lenses. *Ophthalmic Surg* 1981 Sep;12(9):646-49.

Cohen BZ, et al. Use of sodium hyaluronate in reformation and reconstruction of the persistent flat anterior chamber in the presence of severe hypotony. *Ophthalmic Surg* 1982 Oct;13(10):819-21.

Donzis PB, et al. Sodium hyaluronate in the surgical repair of Descemet's membrane detachment. *Ophthalmic Surg* 1986 Nov;17(11):735-37.

Drews RC. Sodium hyaluronate in the repair of perforating injuries of the eye. *Ophthalmic Surg* 1986 Jan;17(1):23-29.

Edelhauser HF, McDermott ML. Drug binding of ophthalmic viscoelastic agents. *Arch Ophthalmol* 1989 Feb;107(2):261-63.

Folk JC, et al. Sodium hyaluronate in closed vitrectomy. *Ophthalmic Surg* 1986 May;17(5):299-306.

Gruber PF, et al. Use of *Healon* for corneal trephination in penetrating keratoplasty. *Ophthalmic Surg* 1984 Sep;15(9):773.

Hills JF, et al. Corneal epithelial healing after penetrating keratoplasty using topical *Healon* versus balanced salt solution. *Ophthalmic Surg* 1987 Jul;18(7):525-28.

Jahnke G, et al. Hyaluronate binding to intact corneas and cultured endothelial cells. *Invest Ophthalmol Vis Sci* 1989 Oct;30(10):2132-37.

Lane SS, et al. Prospective comparison of the effects of *Occucoat, Viscoat,* and *Healon* on intraocular pressure and endothelial cell loss. *J Cataract Refract Surg* 1991;17:21-26.

Liesegang TJ. Viscoelastic substances in ophthalmology. *Surv Ophthalmol* 1990 Jan-Feb;34(4):268-93 (Review).

Lloyd J, Wilson RP. The place of sodium hyaluronate in glaucoma surgery. *Ophthalmic Surg* 1986 Jan;17(1):30-33.

Macy JI, et al. Combined use of sodium hyaluronate and tissue adhesive in penetrating keratoplasty of corneal perforations. *Ophthalmic Surg* 1984 Jan;15(1):55-57.

Mortimer C, et al. Efficacy of polyacrylamide vs. sodium hyaluronate in cataract surgery. *Can J Ophthalmol* 1991;26:144-47.

Raitta C, Vesti E. The effect of sodium hyaluronate on the outcome of trabeculectomy. *Ophthalmic Surg* 1991;22:145-49.

Ruusuvaara P, et al. Effect of sodium hyaluronate on immediate postoperative intraocular pressure after extracapsular cataract extraction and IOL implantation. *Acta Ophthalmol* 1990;68:721-27.

Sand BB, et al. Sodium hyaluronate and methylcellulose in extracapsular cataract extraction. A controlled study of the intraocular inflammation following the preoperative use of sodium hyaluronate and methylcellulose. *Acta Ophthalmol* 1991;69:65-67.

Toczolowski JR. The use of sodium hyaluronate for the removal of severely subluxated lenses. *Ophthalmic Surg* 1987 Mar;18(3):214-16.

Indomethacin

Ahluwalia BK, et al. A comparative study of the effect of antiprostaglandins and steroids on aphakic cystoid macular edema. *Indian J Ophthalmol* 1988 Oct-Dec;36(4):176-78.

Bazan NG. Metabolism of arachidonic acid in the retina and retinal pigment epithelium: Biological effects of oxygenated metabolites of arachidonic acid. *Prog Clin Biol Res* 1989;312:15-37 (Review).

Green K, et al. Topical indomethacin and prostaglandins in normal and aphakic rabbit eyes. *Curr Eye Res* 1988 Nov;7(11):1105-11.

Jampol LM. Pharmacologic therapy of aphakic and pseudophakic cystoid macular edema. 1985 update. *Ophthalmology* 1985 Jun;92(6):807-10 (Review).

Kraff MC, et al. Factors affecting pseudophakic cystoid macular edema: Five randomized trials. *J Am Intraocul Implant Soc* 1985 Jul;11(4):380-85.

Kraff MC, et al. Prophylaxis of pseudophakic cystoid macular edema with topical indomethacin. *Ophthalmology* 1982 Aug;89(8):885-90.

Mishima H, et al. The putative role of prostaglandins in cystoid macular edema. *Prog Clin Biol Res* 1989;312:251-64 (Review).

Miyake K. Indomethacin in the treatment of postoperative cystoid macular edema. *Surv Ophthalmol* 1984 May;28 (Suppl):554-68 (Review).

Miyake K, et al. Incidence of cystoid macular edema after retinal detachment surgery and the use of topical indomethacin. *Am J Ophthalmol* 1983 Apr;95(4):451-56.

Miyake K, et al. Hypotheses on the role of prostaglandins in the pathogenesis of epinephrine maculopathy and aphakic cystoid macular edema. *Prog Clin Biol Res* 1989;312:265-76.

Yamaaki H, et al. Iris angiography after cataract extraction and the effect of indomethacin eye drops. *Ophthalmologica* 1984;188(2):82-86.

Ketorolac

Buckley MM, Brogden RN. Ketorolac. A review of its pharmacodynamic and pharmacokinetic properties and therapeutic potential. *Drugs* 1990 Jan;39(1):86-109 (Review).

Flach AJ, et al. Effectiveness of ketorolac tromethamine 0.5% ophthalmic solution for chronic aphakic and pseudophakic cystoid macular edema. *Am J Ophthalmol* 1987 Apr;103(4):479-86.

Flach AJ, et al. Quantitative assessment of postsurgical breakdown of the blood-aqueous barrier following administration of 0.5% ketorolac tromethamine solution. A double-masked, paired comparison with vehicle-placebo solution study. *Arch Ophthalmol* 1988 Mar;106(3):344-47.

Flach AJ, et al. The effect of ketorolac tromethamine in reducing postoperative inflammation: Double-mask parallel comparison with dexamethasone. *Ann Ophthalmol* 1989 Nov;21(11):407-11.

Flach AJ, et al. The quantitative effect of 0.5% ketorolac tromethamine solution and 0.1% dexamethasone sodium phosphate solution on postsurgical blood-aqueous barrier. *Arch Ophthalmol* 1988 Apr;106(4):480-83.

Flach AJ, et al. The effect of ketorolac tromethamine solution 0.5% in reducing postoperative inflammation after cataract extraction and intraocular lens implantation. *Ophthalmology* 1988 Sep;95(9):1279-84.

Flach AJ, et al. Prophylaxis of aphakic cystoid macular edema without corticosteroids. A paired comparison, placebo-controlled double-masked study. *Ophthalmology* 1990;97:1253-58.

Fraser-Smith EB, Matthews TR. Effect of ketorolac on candida albicans ocular infection in rabbits. *Arch Ophthalmol* 1987 Feb;105(2):264-67.

Fraser-Smith EB, Matthews TR. Effect of ketorolac on *Pseudomonas aeruginosa* ocular infection in rabbits. *J Ocul Pharmacol* 1988 Summer;4(2):101-09.

Ling TL, Combs DL. Ocular bioavailability and tissue distribution of ketorolac tromethamine in rabbits. *J Pharm Sci* 1987 Apr;76(4):289-94.

Levocabastine

Abelson MB, Smith LM. Levocabastine. Evaluation in the histamine and compound 48/80 models of ocular allergy in humans. *Ophthalmology* 1988 Nov;95(11):1494-97.

Arriaga F, Rombaut N. Absence of central effects with levocabastine eye drops. *Allergy* 1990;45:552-54.

Bende M, Pipkorn U. Topical levocabastine, a selective H_1 antagonist, in seasonal allergic rhinoconjunctivitis. *Allergy* 1987;42(7):512-15.

Ciprandi G, et al. Levocabastine versus cromolyn sodium in the treatment of pollen-induced conjunctivitis. *Ann Allergy* 1990;65:156-58.

Feinberg G, Stokes TC. Application of histamine-induced conjunctivitis to the assessment of a topical antihistamine, levocabastine. *Int Arch Allergy Appl Immunol* 1987;82(3-4):537-38.

Odelram H, et al. Topical levocabastine versus sodium cromoglycate in allergic conjunctivitis. *Allergy* 1989 Aug;44(6):432-36.

Pecoud A, et al. Effect of a new selective H_1 receptor antagonist (levocabastine) in a nasal and conjunctival provocation test. *Int Arch Allergy Appl Immunol* 1987;82(3-4):541-43.

Pipkorn U, et al. A double-blind evaluation of topical levocabastine, a new specific H_1 antagonist in patients with allergic conjunctivitis. *Allergy* 1985;40(7):491-96.

Rimas M, et al. Topical levocabastine protects better than sodium cromoglycate and placebo in conjunctival provocation tests. *Allergy* 1990 Jan;45(1):18-21.

Vanden-Bussche G. Levocabastine hydrochloride. *Drugs Future* 1986;11(10):841-43.

Zuber P, Pecoud A. Effect of levocabastine, a new H_1 antagonist in a conjunctival provocation test with allergens. *J Allergy Clin Immunol* 1988;82(4):590-94.

Lodoxamide

Davies RJ, Moodley I. Antiallergic compounds. *Pharmacol Ther* 1982;17(3):279-97.

DiBraccio M, et al. 1,2-condensed derivatives of pyrimidine IV synthesis and pharmacological properties of N, N-disubstituted 4-amino-2H-pyrido-(1,2a)-pyrimidin-2-ones ꞏ... ꞏ- .mino-4H-pyrido-(1,2a)-pyrimidin-4-ones. *Farmaco Ed Sci* 1988;43(9):705-23.

Donnelly JJ, et al. Effect of diethylcarbamazine citrate and anti-inflammatory drugs on experimental onchocercal punctate keratitis. *Ophthalmic Res* 1987;19(3):129-36.

Hiroi J, et al. Effects of FR50948, a new orally active antiallergic agent, in experimental allergic models. *Jpn J Pharmacol* 1988;46(4):337-48.

Jenne JW, Szefler SJ. Report of the AAAI task force on guidelines for clinical investigation of non-bronchodilator antiasthmatic drugs: Workshop 2: Special pharmacologic considerations. *J Allergy Clin Immunol* supplement 1986;78(3):498-506.

Ofloxacin

Fisch A, et al. Ofloxacin in aqueous humour and lens. *J Antimicrob Chemother* 1987;20(3): 453-54.

Fukuda M, Sasaki K. Studies on intraocular distribution of ofloxacin eye drops. *Folia Ophthalmol Jpn* 1986;37:823-28.

Fukuda M, et al. Measurement of cephaloridine and ofloxacin in cul-de-sac. *New Ophthalmol* 1985;2(10):1450-53.

Hatano H, et al. Experimental study on preventive and therapeutic effects of DE-055 (ofloxacin) eye drops on corneal ulcer caused by *Pseudomonas aeruginosa*. *Jpn Rev Clin Ophthalmol* 1985;79:73-77.

Inoue S, et al. Penetration of ofloxacin eye drops (DE-055) into aqueous humor. *Jpn Rev Clin Ophthalmol* 1986;80:1121-24.

Mitsui Y, et al. Therapeutic effects of ofloxacin eye drops (DE-055) on external infection of the eye: Multicentral double blind test. *Jpn Rev Clin Ophthalmol* 1986;80:1813-28.

Mitsui Y, et al. Effect on ofloxacin ophthalmic solution in the treatment of external bacterial infections of the eye: Well-controlled multicentral study. *Folia Ophthalmol Jpn* 1986;37:1115-40.

Osato MS, et al. The comparative in vitro activity of ofloxacin and selected ophthalmic antimicrobial agents against ocular bacterial isolates. *Am J Ophthalmol* 1989 Oct 15;108(4):380-86.

Tamura O, Abe M. Preoperative sterilization and prevention of postoperative infection by ofloxacin eye drops (DE-055). *Jpn Rev Clin Ophthalmol* 1986;80:1104-16.

Pentigetide

Floyd RA, et al. Double-blind comparison of HEPP (IgE pentapeptide) 0.5% ophthalmic solution, USP 4% in patients having allergic conjunctivitis (Abstract). *ARVO* 1988;104.

Frick OL, et al. Pentigetide (HEPP) inhibition of canine anti-ragweed passive cutaneous anaphylaxis (PCA) (Abstract). 13th Conference *ICACI,* 1988.

Hahn GS. Immunoglobulin-derived drugs. *Nature* 1986;324:283-84.

Hahn GS, et al. Double-blind, placebo-controlled trial of HEPP (IgE pentapeptide) for injection (Abstract). *AAAI,* 1988.

Kalpaxis JG. Clinical comparison of IgE pentapeptide (HEPP) and cromolyn (*Opticrom*) in allergic conjunctivitis (Abstract 52). *Ann Allergy* 1982;58:291.

Kalpaxis JG, Thayer TO. Double-blind trial of pentigetide ophthalmic solution, 0.5%, compared with cromolyn sodium, 4%, ophthalmic solution for allergic conjunctivitis. *Ann Allergy* 1991;66:393-98.

Plummer JM, et al. Pentigetide (IgE pentapeptide) inhibits A23187-induced histamine and beta-hexosaminidase release from rat peritoneal mast cells in vitro (Abstract). *Ann Allergy,* 1988.

Prenner BM, et al. Preliminary results from a multicenter study of the antiallergy pentapeptide "HEPP" (Abstract 82). *Ann Allergy* 1984;52:240.

Thayer TO, et al. Pilot trial of pentigetide in the treatment of allergic conjunctivitis induced by ocular antigen challenge (Abstract). *Amer Coll Clin Pharm,* 1988.

Propamidine Isethionate

Berger ST, et al. Successful medical management of Acanthamoeba keratitis. *Am J Ophthalmol* 1990;110:395-403.

Cohen EJ, et al. Medical and surgical treatment of Acanthamoeba keratitis. *Am J Ophthalmol* 1987;103(5):615-25.

Davis RM, et al. Acanthamoeba keratitis and infectious crystalline keratopathy. *Arch Ophthalmol* 1987;105(11):1524-27.

Ficker L, et al. Acanthamoeba keratitis – resistance to medical therapy. *Eye* 1990;4:835-38.

John T, et al. Acanthamoeba keratitis successfully treated with prolonged propamidine isethionate and neomycin-polymyxin-gramicidin. *Ann Ophthalmol* 1990 Jan;22(1):20-23.

Johns KJ, et al. Corneal toxicity of propamidine. *Arch Ophthalmol* 1988;106(1):68-69.

McClellan K, Coster DJ. Acanthamoebic keratitis diagnosed by paracentesis and biopsy and treated with propamidine. *Br J Ophthalmol* 1987;71(10):734-36.

Moore MB, McCulley JP. Acanthamoeba keratitis associated with contact lenses: Six consecutive cases of successful management. *Br J Ophthalmol* 1989 Apr;73(4):271-75.

Wiens JJ, Jackson WB. Acanthamoeba keratitis: An update. *Can J Ophthalmol* 1988;23(3): 107-10.

Wright P, et al. Acanthamoeba keratitis successfully treated medically. *Br J Ophthalmol* 1985;69(10):778-82.

Yeoh R, et al. Acanthamoeba keratitis. *Br J Ophthalmol* 1987;71(7):500-03.

Sorbinil

Biersdorf WR, et al. Cone electroretinograms and visual acuities of diabetic patients on sorbinil treatment. *Doc Ophthalmol* 1988;69(3):247-54.

Christensen JE, et al. The effect of an aldose reductase inhibitor (Sorbinil) on diabetic neuropathy and neural function of the retina: A double blind study. *Acta Neurol Scand* 1985;71(2): 164-67.

Cunha-Vaz JG, et al. Effect of sorbinil on blood retinal barrier in early diabetic retinopathy. *Diabetes* 1986;35(5):574-78.

Frank RN. Aldose reductase inhibition. The chemical key to the control of diabetic retinopathy? *Arch Ophthalmol* 1990;108:1229-31.

Harati Y. Review: Diabetic peripheral neuropathies. *Ann Intern Med* 1987;107(3):546-59.

Jacobson M, et al. Diabetic complications in lens and nerve and their prevention by sulindac or sorbinil: Two novel aldose reductase inhibitors. *Invest Ophthalmol Visual Sci* 1983;24(10):1426-29.

Pitts NE, et al. Aldose reductase inhibitors in clinical practice. Preliminary studies on diabetic neuropathy and retinopathy. *Drugs* 1986;32(Suppl 2):30-35.

Pitts NE, et al. Clinical experience with sorbinil – an aldose reductase inhibitor. *Metab Clin Exp* 1986;35(Suppl 4):96-100.

Raskin P, Rosestock J. Aldose reductase inhibitors and diabetic complications. *Am J Med* 1987;83:298-306.

Robison WG, et al. Early retinal microangiopathy: Prevention with aldose reductase inhibitors. *Diabetic Med* 1985;2(3):196-99.

Robison WG, et al. Retinal capillaries: Basement membrane thickening by galactosemia prevented with aldose reductase inhibitor. *Science* 1983;221(4616):1177-79.

Sima AA, et al. Original article: Regeneration and repair of myelinated fibers in sural-nerve biopsy specimens from patients with diabetic neuropathy treated with sorbinil. *N Engl J Med* 1988;319(9):548-55.

Sorbinil Retinopathy Trial Research Group. A randomized trial of sorbinil, an aldose reductase inhibitor, in diabetic retinopathy. *Arch Ophthalmol* 1990;108:1234-44.

Thymoxamine

Chitkara DK, Hudson JM. Blepharoptosis caused by systemic thymoxamine (letter). *Am J Ophthalmol* 1991;111:524-25.

Diehl DL, et al. The influence of iris pigmentation on the miotic effect of thymoxamine. *Am J Ophthalmol* 1991;111:351-55.

Grehn F, et al. Thymoxamine: A miotic for intraocular use. *Graefes Arch Clin Exp Ophthalmol* 1986;224(2):174-78.

Haynes WL, et al. Inhibition of exercise-induced pigment dispersion in a patient with the pigmentary dispersion syndrome. *Am J Ophthalmol* 1990;109:601-02.

Lee DA, et al. Effect of thymoxamine on the human pupil. *Exp Eye Res* 1983 May;36(5):655-62.

McKinna H, et al. Reversal of tropicamide-induced mydriasis by thymoxamine eye drops. *Current Med Res Opin* 1988;11(1):1-3.

Relf SJ, et al. Thymoxamine reverses phenylephrine-induced mydriasis. *Am J Ophthalmol* 1988 Sep 15;106(3):251-55.

Rosenfield M, et al. The influence of alpha-adrenergic agents on tonic accommodation. *Curr Eye Res* 1990;9:267-72.

Saheb NE, et al. Thymoxamine versus pilocarpine in the reversal of phenylephrine-induced mydriasis. *Can J Ophthalmol* 1982 Dec;17(6):266-67.

Shah B, et al. Influence of thymoxamine eye drops on the mydriatic effect of tropicamide and phenylephrine alone and in combination. *Ophthalmic Physiol Opt* 1989 Apr;9(2):153-55.

Thompson DA, Drasdo N. The effect of 0.5% thymoxamine on the pattern-onset electroretinogram. *Doc Ophthalmol* 1989;72:47-54.

Wood JM, et al. Factors affecting the normal perimetric profile derived by automated static threshold LED perimetry. I. Pupil Size. *Ophthalmic Physiol Opt* 1988;8(1):26-31.

Wright MM, et al. Time course of thymoxamine reversal of phenylephrine-induced mydriasis. *Arch Ophthalmol* 1990;108:1729-32.

Excipient Glossary

Acetoxyphenylmercury, see Phenyl-mercuric acetate.

Acetylcysteine: Mucolytic agent that reduces viscosity.

Alcohol (ethanol, ethyl alcohol): Solvent and preservative.

Alkyl ether sulfate, see Sodium lauryl sulfate.

Amphoteric surfactants: Wetting, solubilizing and emulsifying agents.

Anhydrous Lanolin: An ointment from the wool of the sheep, containing not more than 0.25% water.

Anhydrous Liquid Lanolin: Used in the preparation of an absorbent ointment base.

Antioxidants: Prevent or delay deterioration of products by oxygen.

Ascorbic acid (vitamin C): Antioxidant at concentrations of 0.01% to 0.1%.

Astringents: Precipitate protein and help to clear mucus from the outer surface of the eye.

Baking soda, see Sodium bicarbonate.

Benzalkonium chloride: A quaternary ammonium antimicrobial and preservative. Preserves ophthalmic products at 0.01% to 0.02%. Most effective at pH 8.

Benzene ethanol, see Phenylethyl alcohol.

Benzethonium chloride: Preservative. Maximum concentration for direct instillation into the eye is 1:10,000.

Benzyl alcohol: Antimicrobial preservative at concentrations $\leq$ 2%. Solvent at concentrations $\geq$ 5%. Also used as a local anesthetic and antiseptic.

Benzyl carbinol, see Phenylethyl alcohol.

Berberine: Preservative in extraocular irrigating solutions.

Boric acid: Antiseptic and buffering agent at 2%.

Buffering agents: Substances which stabilize the pH of solutions against changes produced by the introduction of acids or bases.

Carbomer 934P: Suspending agent and emulsifier in suspensions and gels.

Carboxymethylcellulose sodium (sodium cellulose glycolate, sodium CMC, CMC): Viscosity increasing agent.

Catalase (bovine catalase): Enzymes which promote reactions involving the decomposition of hydrogen peroxide to water and oxygen.

Cellulose methyl ether, see Methylcellulose.

Cetanol, see Cetyl alcohol.

Cetyl alcohol (palmityl alcohol, cetanol): Used in ointments as a stiffening and emulsifying agent.

Cetylpyridinium chloride: Disinfectant used in a variety of preparations to treat minor infections.

Chlorhexidine: Antibacterial and antiseptic. Chlorhexidine acetate and chlorhexidine gluconate 0.01% are preservatives of ophthalmic drops. Chlorhexidine gluconate 0.002% and 0.006% are used for disinfection of contact lenses.

Chlorobutanol: Antimicrobial and preservative in ophthalmic products at concentrations of < 0.15% to 0.5%. Chlorobutanol should be used in solutions less than pH 5.

Chlorobutanol anhydrase, see Chlorobutanol.

Cholesterol: Emulsifying and solubilizing agent in ointments.

CMC, see Carboxymethylcellulose sodium.

Dextrans: Demulcents or wetting agents.

Dextrose: Tonicity agent.

Disodium hydrogen phosphate, see Sodium phosphate (Dibasic).

EDTA (edetates, ethylenediaminetetraacetic acid, edetate disodium, edetic acid): Antioxidant and antibacterial synergists. Sequesters trace metal ions which catalyze autooxidation reactions in concentrations ranging from 0.005% to 0.1%. Exerts bacteriostatic activity and enhances antibacterial activity of many preservatives (eg, benzalkonium chloride) in concentration of 0.1%.

Emollients: To protect or soften tissues and to prevent drying and cracking.

Ethylcellulose: Tablet binder.

Gelatin: Viscosity increasing agent.

Glycerin: Tonicity agent, lubricant and preservative.

Glyceryl monostearate (glycerol stearate, glycerol monostearate): Emulsifying and solubilizing agent.

Glycols, see Propylene glycol.

Hydrochloric acid: Acidifying agent.

Hydrogen peroxide: Disinfectant. A 3% solution that cleans by oxidizing foreign matter and removing organic and inorganic materials.

Hydroxyethyl cellulose: Viscosity increasing agent.

Hydroxypropyl methylcellulose (methyl hydroxypropylcellulose, methylcellulose propylene glycol ether): Viscosity increasing agent in ophthalmic drops and in artificial tear solutions in concentrations of 0.45% to 1%.

Hypertonicity agents, see Tonicity agents.

Isopropyl alcohol (isopropanol): Solvent and disinfectant.

Lanolin: Ointment base.

Lanolin Alcohol: Paraffin-base substance that contains 6% alcohol and is used in the preparations of water-in-oil creams and ointments.

Liquid paraffin, see Mineral oil.

Liquid petrolatum, see Mineral oil.

Mannitol (mannite, manna sugar, manita): Tonicity agent.

Mercurial preservatives, see Thimerosal.

Mercurothiolate, see Thimerosal.

Merphenyl nitrate, see Phenylmercuric nitrate.

Methylcellulose (cellulose methyl ether): Viscosity increasing agent in ophthalmic drops (0.5% to 1%) and contact lens wetting and soaking agents. Methylcellulose 1% to 2% may also be used.

Methylcellulose propylene glycol ether, see Hydroxypropyl methylcellulose.

Methyl glycol, see Propylene glycol.

Methyl hydroxypropylcellulose, see Hydroxypropyl methylcellulose.

Methylparaben, see Parabens.

Mineral oil (liquid petrolatum, liquid paraffin): Used in ointments.

Nonoxynol: Nonionic surfactant used in wetting agents and emulsifiers.

Octylphenoxy polyethoxyethanol: Surfactant.

Palmityl alcohol, see Cetyl alcohol.

Parabens (methylparaben, propylparaben): Parahydroxybenzoic acid esters effective against molds and fungi. Generally not used as single agents.

PEG, see Polyethylene glycol.

Petrolatum (petroleum jelly): Emollient and ointment base.

Petroleum jelly, see Petrolatum.

Phenylethanol, see Phenylethyl alcohol.

Phenylethyl alcohol (phenethyl alcohol, benzyl carbinol, benzene ethanol, phenylethanol): Preservative at concentrations of 0.25% to 0.5%. Used in combination with other preservatives.

Phenylmercuric acetate (acetoxyphenylmercury): A mercurial antimicrobial and preservative in ophthalmic drops in a concentration of 0.001% to 0.002%.

Phenylmercuric nitrate (merphenyl nitrate): A mercurial antiseptic, antimicrobial and preservative in ophthalmic drops at a concentration of 0.002%.

Phosphoric acid: Solvent.

Poloxamer: Wetting and solubilizing agent.

Polyethylene glycol (PEG, polyoxyethylene glycol): Solvent, gelling agent and solubilizer.

Polyethylene oxide sorbitan esters, see Polyoxyethylene sorbitan fatty acid esters.

Polyoxyethylene glycol, see Polyethylene glycol.

Polyoxyethylene sorbitan fatty acid esters (polysorbates 20, 60, 80; polyethylene oxide sorbitan esters): Wetting and solubilizing agents.

Polyoxyl 40 stearate: Surfactant.

Polyquaternium-1 (*Polyquad* by Alcon): Disinfection agent used in contact lens care systems.

Polysorbates 20, 60, 80, see Polyoxyethylene sorbitan fatty acid esters.

Polyvinyl alcohol (PVA): Suspending and viscosity increasing agent in ophthalmic products (1.4%).

Polyvinylpyrrolidone, see Povidone.

Potassium acetate: Alkalinizing agent.

Potassium bicarbonate, see Potassium citrate.

Potassium carbonate, see Potassium citrate.

Potassium chloride: Electrolyte.

Potassium citrate: Buffering agent and sequestering agent at concentrations of 0.3% to 2%.

Potassium phosphates: Buffering agents.

Potassium sorbate (2,4–hexadienoic acid potassium salt): Antimicrobial and preservative. Only effective below pH 6.5.

Povidone (Polyvidone, polyvinylpyrrolidone, PVP): Suspending and viscosity increasing agent.

Preservatives: Destroy or inhibit reproduction of microorganisms.

Propylene glycol (1,2–propanediol, propane-1,2–diol, methyl glycol): Humectant, solvent.

Propylparaben, see Parabens.

PVA, see Polyvinyl alcohol.

PVP, see Povidone.

Silica gel: Stabilizing and suspending agent.

Sodium acetate: Buffering agent.

Sodium acid carbonate, see Sodium bicarbonate.

Sodium acid sulfite, see Sulfites.

Sodium benzoate (benzoate of soda): Antifungal, bacteriostatic and preservative at concentration of 0.1%.

Sodium bicarbonate (sodium hydrogen carbonate, sodium acid carbonate, baking soda): Alkalinizing and buffering agent.

Sodium biphosphate, see Sodium phosphate (Monobasic).

Sodium bisulfite, see Sulfites.

Sodium borate: Alkalinizing agent.

Sodium carbonate: Alkalinizing agent.

Sodium cellulose glycolate, see Carboxymethylcellulose sodium.

Sodium chloride: Tonicity agent. Aid in obtaining isotonicity in ophthalmic solutions.

Sodium citrate (trisodium citrate, citrosodine, citnatin): Alkalinizing agent. Buffer in concentrations of 0.3% to 2%.

Sodium CMC, see Carboxymethylcellulose sodium.

Sodium ethylmercurothiosalicylate, see Thimerosal.

Sodium hexametaphosphate, see Sodium polymetaphosphate.

Sodium hydrogen carbonate, see Sodium bicarbonate.

Sodium hydroxide: Alkalinizing agent.

Sodium lauryl sulfate: Emulsifying, solubilizing and wetting agent.

Sodium metabisulfite, see Sulfites.

Sodium phosphate (Dibasic) (disodium hydrogen phosphate): Buffering agent.

Sodium phosphate (Monobasic) (sodium biphosphate): Acidifying agent.

Sodium propionate: Antifungal.

Sodium pyrosulphite, see Sulfites.

Sodium Thiosulfate: An antifungal agent.

Sorbic acid (2,4–hexadienoic acid, 2-propenylacrylic acid): Antimicrobial and preservative at 0.05% to 0.2%. Often used with other antimicrobials. Most effective at pH 4.5.

Sorbitan esters: Wetting, solubilizing and emulsifying agent.

Sulfites (sodium bisulfite, sodium metabisulfite, sodium acid sulfite, sodium pyrosulphite): Antioxidant at concentrations of 0.01% to 1%.

Tartaric acid: Buffering agent.

Thimerosal (mercurial preservatives, mercurothiolate, thiomersalate, sodium ethylmercurothiosalicylate): A mercurial antiseptic, antimicrobial and preservative at a concentration of 0.01% to 0.02%.

Thiomersalate, see Thimerosal.

Tonicity agents: Help ophthalmic solutions to be isotonic with natural tears.

Trisodium citrate, see Sodium citrate.

Tyloxapol: Nonionic surfactant. Wetting, solubilizing and emulsifying agent.

Viscosity-increasing agents: Slow drainage of the product from the eye, thus increasing retention time of the active drug. Increased bioavailability may result.

Wetting agents: Reduce surface tension, allowing the drug solution to spread over the eye.

White petrolatum, see petrolatum.

Manufacturer Index

Abbott Laboratories
D-305, Bldg. AP30 4E
One Abbott Rd.
Abbott Park, IL 60064
708-937-6100

Akorn, Inc.
100 Akorn Dr.
Abita Springs, LA 70420
504-893-9300

Alcon Laboratories, Inc.
6201 South Freeway
Ft. Worth, TX 76134
817-293-0450

Allergan Pharmaceuticals
2525 DuPont Dr.
Irvine, CA 92713-1599
714-752-4500

Alza Corporation
950 Page Mill Rd.
Palo Alto, CA 94304
415-494-5000

Amcon Laboratories
40 N. Rock Hill Rd.
St. Louis, MO 63119
314-961-5758

American Regent Laborato-ries, Inc.
One Luitpold Dr.
Shirley, NY 11967
516-924-4000

Apothecon
Div. of Bristol-Myers Squibb
P.O. Box 4000
Princeton, NJ 08543-4000
609-987-6800

Astra Pharm. Prod., Inc.
50 Otis
Westborough, MA 01581
508-366-1100

Bausch and Lomb Pharm.
8500 Hidden River Pkwy.
Tampa, FL 33637
813-975-7700

Bausch and Lomb, Consumer
1400 N. Goodman St.
Rochester, NY 14692
716-338-6000

Baxter Healthcare Corporation
1425 Lake Cook Rd.
Deerfield, IL 60015
708-940-5000

Becton Dickinson
P.O. Box 243
Cockeysville, MD 21030
301-584-8966

Blairex Labs., Inc.
4810 Tecumseh Ln.
P.O. Box 15190
Evansville, IN 47716-0190
812-476-8077

Burroughs Wellcome Co.
3030 Cornwallis Rd.
Research Triangle Pk,
  NC 27709
919-248-3000

Century Pharmaceuticals, Inc.
10377 Hague Rd.
Indianapolis, IN 46256
317-849-4210

Ciba Vision Care
2910 Amwiler Ct.
Atlanta, GA 30360
404-448-1200

Clintec Nutrition
Three Parkway North, Ste.
  500
Deerfield, IL 60015
708-940-5000

Cook-Waite Laboratories, Inc.
90 Park Ave.
New York, NY 10016
212-907-2712

Cynacon/Ocusoft
P.O.Box 429
Richmond, TX 77469
800-233-5469

Dakryon Pharmaceuticals
301 Utica Ave.
Lubbock, TX 79416
806-797-9941

Del Pharmaceuticals
565 Broad Hollow Rd.
Farmingdale, NY 11735
516-293-7070

Dista Products Co.
Div. of Eli Lilly
Bldg. 11/3 Lilly Corp. Center
Indianapolis, IN 46285
317-276-4000

Eagle Vision, Inc.
6263 Poplar Ave., Ste. 650
Memphis, TN 38119
901-767-3937

Elkins-Sinn
555 E. Lancaster Pike
St. Davids, PA 19087
215-971-5539

Fisons Consumer Health
P.O. Box 1212
Rochester, NY 14603-1212
716-475-9000

Fisons Corp.
P.O. Box 1766
Rochester, NY 14623
716-475-9000

Forest Pharmaceutical, Inc.
Subs. of Forest Labs., Inc.
2510 Metro Blvd.
Maryland Heights,
    MO 63043-9979
314-569-3610

Fougera and Co.
60 Baylis Rd.
Melville, NY 11747
516-454-6996

Geneva Pharmaceuticals
Subs. of Ciba-Geigy
2599 W. Midway Blvd.
P.O. Box 469
Broomfield, CO 80038-0469
800-525-2492

Goldline Laboratories, Inc.
1900 W. Commercial Blvd.
Ft. Lauderdale, FL 33324
305-491-4002

W. E. Hauck, Inc.
P.O. Box 1065
Alpharetta, GA 30239-1065
404-475-4758

**Health Maintenance
    Programs**
7 Westchester Plaza
Elmsford, NY 10523

Holles Laboratories
30 Forest Notch
Cohasset, MA 02025-1198
617-383-0741

Iolab Pharmaceuticals
Iolab Corporation
500 Iolab Dr.
Claremont, CA 91711
714-624-2020

Keene Pharmaceuticals Inc.
P.O. Box 7
Keene, TX 76059-0007
817-645-8083

Lacrimedics, Inc.
9008 Newby St.
Rosemead, CA 91770
800-367-8327

La Haye
2205 152nd Ave. N.E.
Redmond, WA 98052

Lavoptik Co., Inc.
661 Western Ave. N.
St. Paul, MN 55103
612-489-1351

Lederle Laboratories
Div. of American Cyanamid
    Co.
North Middletown Rd.
Pearl River, NY 10965-1299
914-732-5000

Lilly and Co.
Bldg. 11/3 Lilly Corp. Center
Indianapolis, IN 46285
317-276-2000

Lyphomed
Parkway N. Center 3
Deerfield, IL 60015-22548
708-317-8800

Major Pharmaceutical, Inc.
Michigan Division
3720 Lapeer Rd.
Auburn Hills, MI 48321
313-370-0680

Marlin Industries
P.O. Box 560
Grover City, CA 93483-0560
213-393-3644

Mayrand, Inc.
P.O. Box 8869
Greensboro, NC 27419
919-292-5347

McGaw, Inc.
ASCZ P.O. Box 19791
Irvine, CA 92713-9791
714-660-2000

Medtech Laboratories, Inc.
3510 N. Lake Creek, POB
    1108
Jackson, WY 83001
307-733-1680

Merck Sharp and Dohme
Div. Merck & Co.
WP 38M-2
West Point, PA 19486
215-661-5000

**H.L. Moore Drug Exchange,
    Inc.**
389 John Downey Dr.
New Britain, CT 06050
203-826-3600

Optikem International, Inc.
2172 S. Jason St.
Denver, CO 80223
303-936-1137

Optopics Laboratories, Corp.
Main Street, P.O. Box 210
Fairton, NJ 08320-0210
800-223-0865

Otsuka America
1201 Third Ave. Ste. 5300
Seattle, WA 98101

Parke-Davis
Div. of Warner-Lambert Co.
201 Tabor Rd.
Morris Plains, NJ 07950
201-540-2000

Pasadena Research
P.O. Box 5136
San Clemente, CA 92672
714-492-4030

Pfizer Laboratories
Div. of Pfizer, Inc.
235 E. 42nd St.
New York, NY 10017-5755
212-573-2323

Pharmafair, Inc.
205C Kelsey Ln.
Tampa, FL 33619
813-972-7705

Pharmics
P.O. Box 27554
Salt Lake City, UT 84127
801-972-4138

**Polymer Technology
    Corporation**
100 Research Dr.
Wilmington, MA 01887
800-343-1445

Professional Supplies, Inc.
1153 Main St.
Stevens Point, WI 54481
715-345-0404

Raway Pharmacal, Inc.
Lower Granit Rd.
Accord, NY 12404
914-626-8133

Roche Laboratories
Div. of Hoffman-La Roche,
    Inc.
340 Kingsland St.
Nutley, NJ 07110-1199
800-526-6367

Roerig Division
235 E. 42nd St.
New York, NY 10017
212-573-2323

Ross Laboratories
625 Cleveland Ave.
Columbus, OH 43215
614-227-3333

Rugby Labs., Inc.
898 Orlando Ave.
West Hempstead, NY 11552
516-536-8565

Sanofi Winthrop
200 East Oakton St.
Des Plaines, IL 60018
212-907-2000

Schein Pharmaceutical, Inc.
26 Harbor Park Dr.
Port Washington, NY 11050
516-625-9000

Scherer Laboratories, Inc.
315 Gilmer Ferry Rd.
Ball Ground, GA 30107
800-858-9888

**Schering-Plough
  Corporation**
2000 Galloping Hill Rd.
Kenilworth, NJ 07033
908-298-4000

Schering-Plough HealthCare
110 Allen Rd.
Liberty Corner, NJ 07938
908-604-1995

Sherman Laboratories, Inc.
P.O. Box 368
Abita Springs, LA 70420
504-893-0007

**SmithKline Beecham
  Pharm.**
P.O. Box 7929
Philadelphia, PA 19103
215-751-4000

Soft Rinse Corp.
2411 Third St. South
Wisconsin Rapids, WI 54494

Sola/Barnes-Hind
810 Kifer Rd.
Sunnyvale, CA 94086-5200
619-277-9873

**Spectra Pharmaceutical
  Service**
155 Webster St.
Hanover, MA 02339
617-871-3991

Stellar
1900 N.W. 44th St.
Pompano Beach, FL 33064
305-972-6060

Steris Laboratories, Inc.
620 N. 51st Ave.
Phoenix, AZ 85043
602-278-1400

Storz Ophthalmics
Subsid. American Cyanamid
  Co.
3365 Tree Court Industrial
St. Louis, MO 63122-6694
314-225-5051

Syntex Inc.
3401 Hillview Ave.
P.O. Box 10850
Palo Alto, CA 94303
415-855-5050

The Upjohn Company
7000 Portage Rd.
Kalamazoo, MI 49001
616-323-4000

**United Research
  Laboratories**
3600 Meadow Ln.
Bensalem, PA 19020-8546
215-638-2626

Vision Pharmaceuticals, Inc.
P.O. Box 400
Mitchell, SD 57301-0400
605-996-3356

Wyeth-Ayerst Laboratories
P.O. Box 8299
Philadelphia, PA 19101
215-688-4400

INDEX

This **Index** lists all generic names, brand names (*italics*) and group names included in *Ophthalmic Drug Facts*. Additionally, many drug tables, synonyms, pharmacological actions and therapeutic uses for the agents listed are included.

Index entries may refer to more than one form of a product (eg, tablets, solutions, suspensions, ointments) when all forms are included on a single page. Separate index entries are included when multiple forms of a product appear on different pages or when products are listed in more than one therapeutic group.

NOTES

NOTES

NOTES

NOTES

NOTES

NOTES

NOTES

NOTES

<u>NOTES</u>

NOTES

NOTES

NOTES

NOTES

ISBN 0-932686-69-9